Preface

I am pleased to present this second book of my titles of books on medical Astrology. I have tried and taken every effort to over come the flaws or inadequacy of information that I have given in my earlier book.

As an astrologer many clients who have visited me for seeking remedial measures for their various problems in life being chemical engineer and having worked in pharma sector for over 27 years I could see the basic anamolies people face are either related to their physical or psychological diseases and as such I started collecting detailed data form ancient Indian and global literature, refrred many large books like Kalyan Verma's Sravli, Garga Hora, Parashara and even Hippocrates but the common thing I found was as route cause of suffering is Karma and the birth time at which specific planets are occupied in specific constellations which made human suffer. To exactly pin point the same was difficult task. So also the detailed knowledge that was required with respect to the exact kind of the disease was absent. This was overcome due to unbelievable help that I have received form my friends in medical fraternity to whom I have reffered the clients to seek the treatment and get help to diagnose the disease. I am actually very much obliged and compelled to express my sincere and cordial thanks to them but the list is much bigger and can not be included here and as such I am expressing my heartiest thanks to all of those Doctors who helped me in compiling the data and presenting this book before you.

Further I can not remain silence but to express deep regards to my late wife Sau. Vidya Kulkarni who constanly stand by my side and got this difficult task completed.

ASTROLOGY OF DISEASE

Medical Astrology

By
Vijay Kulkarn

[Type the abstract of the document here. The abstract is typically a short summary of the contents of the document. Type the abstract of the document here. The abstract is typically a short summary of the contents of the document.]

Contents

A Greek Doctor and Philosopher Dr. Hippocrates (Born B.C. 0460) proposed that Human character was the result of the balance of four humors viz Blood, Phlegm, Yellow bile and Black bile were loosely before the advent connected in Astrology . In fact of modern medical science, in ancient times the physicians were advocated compulsory knowledge of Astrology and its relevance to various diseases Apart from administering the medicines on different lunar days and on different stellar days.

In Ayurveda , the diseases are classified in Tridoshas (three humors) to help to diagnose the disease.

The tridoshas for the planets are;

 1- Sun –   Bilious
 2- Moon-   Airy and Phlegmatic
 3- Mars-   Bilious
 4- Mercury- Airy, Bilious, and Phlegmatic
 5- Jupiter -   Phlegmatic
 6- Venus-   Airy
 7- Saturn-   Airy

The diseases or defects in organs are the result of either way of life producing stress or the environment that affect; the disease those occur as prenatal effect is termed as karmic one. So also the diseases those are caused due to genetic transfer are also termed as karmic effect. Here important thing to note is that the birth in any family or continent is due to karmic effect only. As such the major elements we can consider to analyze are

1) Diseases that are effect of genetically transferred deformities, or prenatal ailments; that exists right from birth like Autism.
2) The ailments those are the effect of environment that leads to suffering of certain organ or modifies the behavioral pattern.
3) The diseases those are the outcome of faulty habits or life style leading to slow growth of defects or degenerative changes in body.

   All can be first understood to have caused the specific impact on one or many organs of body, in modern world of luxury and stiff competition everybody is running the way he can and tries to get his part of chunk while ignoring the body and thus drives to disease. The very life style is also responsible for occurrence of new and unknown diseases every day in life. So also if we observe the world data not ancient but recent since 1720 we will understand that how this world has invited diseases which were not present before.

   In 1720 world had seen pandemic of Plague which caused many lives leaving human helpless for short time.

   In 1820 the epidemic of cholera was occurred which also claimed many lives leaving behind the trauma.

   In 1920 again Spanish flue and Polio was occurred to claim further many lives and leaving behind shock to mankind. These are only few prominent examples we have seen apart from the entry of many new unknown diseases in life of human being. When we try to understand such episodes it is always better to refer to observe unaffected people and understand the reasons; we here get surprised to note simple reasons these people have safeguarded themselves. When we take tour of history we find this treasure of information that states the shocking truth behind. One and foremost being the neurological function of these winners was, astonishing due to the strong Mercury under aspect of benefic like Jupiter which yield them the very common sense other people were missing. To elaborate further we can take example of person stayed in Ahmedabad, once badly hit city due to Cholera had followed the simple rules of food habits and drinking habits that were totally different from others. He had forced his family members to only eat freshly collected vegetables that too after cleaning with hot sodabicarb mixed water and drink only boiled and cooled water available in his own well further he forcefully sleep for eight hours a day and follow some simple exercises every day. This is how he could save his entire family when most of other citizens were becoming pray to the disease Cholera. This family had reported no symptoms of even cholera. Another example I had noted was when one of rich family gathered in hospital and waiting for their family members wellbeing; the person was suffering from Tuberculosis was on ventilator and counting his last breaths. Suddenly Doctor enters the room of that ICU intervenes the other specialists suggested that the patient may be advised to drink water admixed with common salt drop by drop from mouth. The effect was astonishing, after few hours the ventilator was required to be removed and after one weeks time patient was discharged. This is not miracle but the fact is at appropriate time the doctor who had suggested saline water therapy was appeared over there. If we try to find out the scientific reason the salt water had increased Sodium radical metabolism in body and triggered the growth of Immunoglobulin M; that helped recover the patient. There are many instances we find the patient otherwise could have been recovered succumbs to death. One classic example of one of my native I could quote here that one day healthy lady of the age of 55 with no ailment in body had recently checked for routine insitu medical examination and doctor had declared everything normal and right; but the next day she complained of some flatulence and gases trouble while returning from morning walk and within one hour became unconscious. When admitted to hospital doctor found massive cardiac arrest for which as usual CPR was carried and after some time administered some anticlogging or thrombosis preventive drug and reported she will be recovered shortly. Unfortunately after only 15 minutes doctor came again and declared the patient died of massive cardiac arrest. Here question is that how the day before doctor could not trace out single symptom that they could otherwise have treated. But well this can be diagnosed with study of Natives natal chart. The natal chart shows, the sun placed in eighth cusp is afflicted with malefic Rahu. So also the ascendant falls in Cancer Lord of eighth cusp is placed in dual nature zodiac, i.e. in Gemini. This gives the indication of sudden death due to cardiac arrest.

Further we can notice that we can find out the probable period of death with reference to placement of lord of ascendant and lord of eighth house. If both are in movable zodiac then the native may have long life of more than sixty four years, if lord of ascendant is in movable sign and lord of eighth house is in fixed sign then the life span may have up to sixty three years. Thirdly if lord of ascendant occupies moving zodiac and lord of eighth cusp is placed in dual nature zodiac then the native will be short lived. Although this is as rule generally applied there are certain other parameters too which are required to be studied along with.

The general table that gives above mentioned indications for information is given as under,

Type	Longevity above 65 years	UP TO 65 years	Short lived up to 32 years
1	Ascendant in movable sign and lord of eighth cusp is in also movable sign.	Ascendant in movable sign and lord of eighth cusp in fixed zodiac.	Ascendant in movable sign and lord of eighth cusp in dual nature zodiac.
2	Ascendant in fixed zodiac and lord of eighth cusp in dual nature zodiac.	Ascendant in fixed zodiac and lord of eighth cusp in movable sign.	Ascendant in fixed zodiac and lord of eighth cusp is also in fixed sign.
3	Ascendant in dual nature zodiac and lord of eighth cusp in fixed zodiac.	Ascendant in dual nature zodiac and lord of eighth cusp is also in dual nature	Ascendant in dual nature zodiac and lord of eighth cusp is in movable sign

		zodiac.	

If above chart is referred and according to significator method of KP system we can find out the time and date of death of native can be predicted with near accuracy.

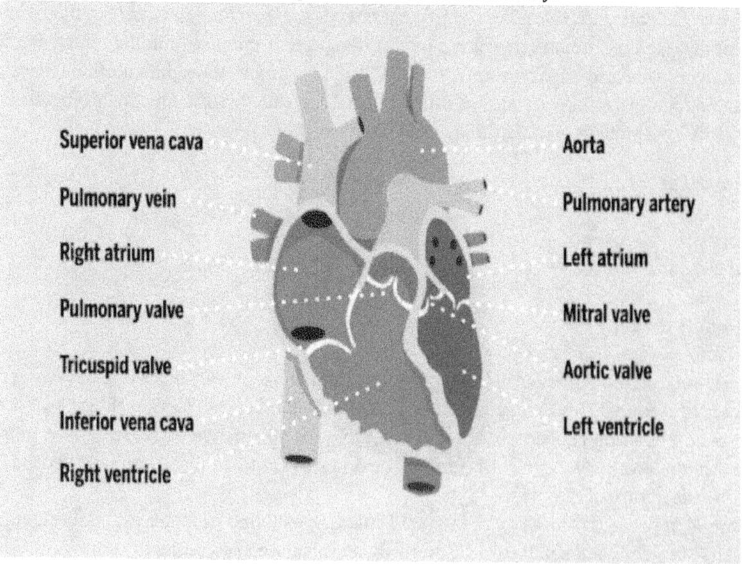

Chapter 2

Karmic effect and Disease

Every Human body and Psychology is prone to diseases of various natures. The types of diseases depend on **Ones Karma i.e. ones past deeds in the previous births.**

It is known fact that even in these days of advanced science and available tools for diagnosis many times it becomes difficult to find out the root cause of the disease and Doctor can't help Patients to the extent required. It is very well known that even in perfectly healthy body some complex chemical reaction takes place and we cannot get any early sign of the onset of the disease or ailments in the Body. It is still impossible for science to treat the victims of Cerebral Palsy or Cases of Autism.

Modern medical science has thrown a challenge to Astrologers by providing cure for many diseases and by developing menace to protect from epidemic diseases. Now here Astrologers to prove that

Astrology can go step further to than this and that can diagnose disease merely by looking at the Birth chart/Natal chart .If Doctor uses this clinical methods the Astrologer makes uses of his current transits of planets by proving the method of diagnosis equally better than doctor. It is common practice that doctor examines a person and finds out whether he is fit to carry out the tasks given and certify just by measuring chest, waist and weight of flesh. In due course of performance we have noticed many times that the person declared fit becomes invalid and doctor is unable to foresee the calamity or couldn't give word of advice.

An apparently healthy human dies suddenly of cardiac stroke even after declared fit or sometimes reverse that person declared as instate of advanced stage of some disease and doctor feel may have very short life slowly recover and then become fit to live long. What answer doctor have for these cases, they may say its fate and exactly here the Astrology helps us to know the exact cause. The date and time of birth are prefixed with reference to last birth karma so also the parents are pre fixed. This leads to the genetic disorders and diseases acquired due to life style of parents and relatives or that society. And as such the planetary disposition which we calculate with reference to birth data needs to be studied in detail to understand the cause and nature of disease.Traditional astrology is just the diagram or plans of building but where the details of information are incomplete and not accurate. AND FOR THIS Reason becomes difficult to interpret the hidden behavior of happenings in human body accurately. Late Prof. K.S. Krishnamurthy broke this barrier and made further detailed application of Astrology by giving due importance to

a) **Individual cusps**
b) **Planets**
c) **Stellar lords**
d) **Subs and sub lord**
e) **Significators.**
f) **Ruling planets theory**

Here we have co related the scientific way to get the clear concept in interpreting any event of life to the accuracy of seconds. This theory says that no planet is good or bad neither the cusp. It is the significance of the matter concerned that gives result in the affirmative or negative way. In modern medicine also the great psychiatrist Dr. Jung Carl made it a point to look into the Horoscope before determining the nature of the case.

In this method of predictive analysis the Rafael Table is considered accurate for understanding the cusps and its star lords and sub lords; this necessarily calculated according to the laws of Trigonometry. According to this Sion zero of cusp is calculated and KP ions subtracted to get Nirayan cusp. For diseases and severity sixth, eighth, and twelfth cusp and further sixth and eighth from theses cusps are considered. Planet, its occupancy, affliction, and aspect are taken into consideration; so also constellation, its lord and sub lords are studied to find out the probability of predictive analysis.

When any event takes place we can find out the the accurate timings by referring the Sun and Moon mahadasha, dasha lord, Antardasha and lord of antardasha with respect to their current transit is taken into consideration. If Jupiter and Ketu are the significator planets then we will have to find out their mahadasha and antardasha and when current transit of Jupiter in Sagittarius and in constellation of mula the event takes place. Prof. Krishnamurti estimated the yearly speed of ionansh 50.2388475 seconds which gives accuracy in finding sub lords of cusp and get the accurate predictive analysis.

In this padhati (system) western Yogas are accepted, 1) Law of conjoin 2) Ninety degrees 3) Square 5) Triangle 6) 240 degree 7) Half square i.e. 45 deg. And the effect depends on malefic or benefic planets and their cusps.

According to Indian system every planet has full aspect on seventh cusp from where the planet is placed and its own zodiac. Rahu and Ketu are shadow planets but are considered very important even though they don't own any zodiac, but their aspect or conjoin is of great important in deciding the exact cause and effect. No planet is considered good or bad but their occupancy or aspect or with which they are conjoined gives the effect. The retrograde or placed in malefic zodiac like consepts are not considered in this book. Important rules are---

1) Any planet is more important than the star lord for example any planet in Vishakha constellation is more important than Jupiter.
2) When any planet is placed in own constellation then its sub lord becomes its star lord.

3) Dasha lord is significator of one important and one supportive planet; and one one one cusp chain of dasha takes place and the predicted event happens.
4) All three dasha lord and their sub lord is also indicator of one important and one supportive cusp and the event takes place in this period.
5) In ruling planets also make chain of three and according to transit of Sun makes chain and exactly on that day the event happens.
6) Rahu and Ketu never becomes representative of each other and as such ther sub lord becomes their star lord.

In this Book the scientific method used to support any hypothesis is tested analyzed and statistical data already generated is used.

Chapter 3

Importance of Zodiacal Signs

Every person is afflicted by the Sun, The Moon, and the 12 signs of zodiac. This planet earth is part of the complete solar system and everything on earth is part of the complete solar system. So also everything on earth is inter-related to all the other spheres.

Each part of the body is ruled by a particular sign of zodiac. And the association of the sign of zodiac with various parts of the human body and the power they were believed to confer on them. How a specific part of the body or the organ placed under the governance of certain zodiacal sign is still a mystery un explained. Its origin is most probably due to Greeks or the Egyptians. Hippocrates father of

Medicine all under the power of heavenly bodies over human body and certain Egyptians apportioned certain parts of the body to signs and treated diseases by evolving the zodiacal regent of the part affected. Disease of the more important body organs were diagnosed according to the influence of the signs of the zodiac at the time and remedies were administered which were either acted by suggestion were in operative. Entire Universe is divided into 12 zodiac signs each being 30 Degrees named as Aries, Taurus, Gemini, Cancer, Virgo, Libra , Scorpio, Sagittarius, Capricorn, Aquarius,   and Pisces and the names of the planets are Sun, Moon, Mars , Mercury , Jupiter, Venus, Saturn , Kethu, Uranus, Neptune, and Pluto.

The twelve signs of the zodiac commencing from Aries in general and from the ascendant in particular governs the twelve important organs of the Human body and in addition to this planets of one sign will affect organs governed by that sign of the same element or constitution.

This is brief of the list.

1. Aries Governs Head, Face, Brain, Bones of Head, and Facial Bones.
2. Taurus governs Neck, Throat, Larynx, Cerebellum, Right eye, Bones of the Neck and cheeks.
3. Gemini governs Shoulder, Hands, Lungs, Blood, Breath, Shoulder blades, Bones of Arms.
4. Cancer governs breast, chest, stomach, digestive organs, bones of chest, and ribs.
5. Leo governs Heart, spinal cord, Nerves, and fiber, bones of the back.
6. Virgo governs Abdominal and umbilical region, Bowels, Intestines, Liver, Nervous system.
7. Libra governs Lumbar region, skin, kidneys, bones of Lumbar, Uterus, Bladder.
8. Scorpio governs Genital organs, Anus, Bladder, bones of pelvic area.
9. Sagittarius governs Hips, Thighs, Veins, Arteries, Buttock Bones and Thigh bones.

10. Capricorn governs Knees, Hands, Bones of Kneecap, joints, skin.
11. Aquarius governs Ankles, Feet, Circulatory system, Bones of ankles and shanks.
12. Pisces governs Feet, Toes, Lymphatic System, Left eye, bones of the feet.

Aries Leo and Sagittarius are fiery signs, and control the vitality of person. Taurus, Virgo, and Capricorn are earthy signs and controls bones, Flesh. Gemini, Libra, and Aquarius are airy signs and First House controls the breath. Cancer Scorpio and Pisces are watery signs and control the Human blood and Circulation.

So also the types of diseases depend upon ones karma or past deeds in previous births. Hindus believe that the Law of karma is responsible to attribute diseases, from time immemorial depending upon whether the karmic effect is Sanchita or Prarabdha. The cumulative effects of good or bad deeds in past births are felt in this birth in the form of good or bad health. Which is essential for a man's enjoying and suffering of life? This may be revealed in Karmic chart or Vidhi chart. Therefore Astrology is multidimensional science depicting the branches of knowledge from matrimonial, Mundane, electional, Horary, Medical etc.

Astrologically the Sun and Moon are the rulers of of our eyes, Saturn and Mars are directional lords and hence rulers of our ears. The Universe (Kalpurusha) And Parts of Human Body ,

The zodiac is divided into twelve Houses reckoning from Ascendant and each house commonly as Cusp is assigned to a specific part of the body.

These can be listed as below,

House (Cusp)	Parts of the body or nature
First House	Head, Face, Brain, Mind. (Personality)
Second House	Right eye, Nose, Tongue, Teeth, Ears, Fingers, Nails, Bones, Flesh.
Third House	Neck, Throat, Collar bones, Hands, Breathing, AND GROWTH.
Fourth House	Heart, Lungs, Chest, Blood.
Fifth House	Upper abdomen, Liver, Gall Bladder, Spleen, Intestine, mesentery.
Sixth House	Lower abdomen, Navel, Bones, Flesh, Anus, Kidneys.
Seventh House	Groins Semen, Female genitals and organs, Pineal gland, Uterus.
Eighth House	Reproductive organs, Urethra, Seminal Vesicles.
Ninth House	Thighs, Limbs, Femoral Arteries.
Tenth House	Knees, Ankles, Metatarsal bones, heels.
Eleventh House	Shanks, Breathing, Left ear.
Twelfth House	Feet, Blood, Left Eye.

Then comes Constellations, there are 27 constellations and each Zodiac occupies two and quarter parts of constellations. Each Constellation further divided into four Parts that is Charana Thus each Zodiac occupies Nine Parts .All this can be summarized as bellow.

Ashvini -- Controls Head, Cerebral Hemisphere, Frontal Lobes.

Bharani – Controls Cerebrum, Diencephalon, Cerebellum, Brain stem, Lateral Sulks (Fissure)

Krattika-- Controls Forehead, Eyes, Precentral Gyrus, Superior Frontal Gyrus, Motor Speech Area.

Krattika 3rd and 4th padas- Neck, Thyroid, Wind pipe, Larynx, Tonsils, Lower Jaws.

Rohini- Face, Mouth, Tongue, Palate, Atlas, Cervical Vertebrae.

Mrugshirsha 1st Pada – Face, Upper jaw, Cheeks, Arteries, Jugular artery, Veins, Occipital.

Mrugshirsha 2nd pada – Pre Occipital Lobe, Medulla Oblongata, Parietal lobe.

Mrugashirsha 3rd pada- Sensory Speech Area, Temporal Lobes, Vocal cords, Thymus gland.

Mrugashirsha 4th pada- Arms, Ears, Upper ribs, Food pipe.

Ardra – Throat, Shoulders, Collar bones, Shoulder blades.

Punarvasu 1 and 2nd padas – Ear internal delicate bones and diaphragm.

Punarvasu 3rd and 4th padas- Lungs, Respiratory system, Chest, Stomach, Pancreas, Liver.

Pushya - Lungs, Epigastric Region, Ribs.

Ashlesha- Lungs posterior part, Lower gastric area, Esophagus, Gall bladder, Lower part of Liver.

Magha - Heart, Spinal cord, Spleen, Aorata.

Purva phalguni – Cardiac region, Major Arteries, Valves in Heart.

Uttara phalguni 1st and 2nd Padas - Spinal cord C15 to C25 Vertebrae, Lower ribs.

Uttara phalguni – 3RD AND 4TH PADAS – Small Intestine, Appendix, Duodenum, Diaphragm.

Hasta – Large intestine, Bowels, Colon, Enzyme secreting Glands.

Chitra 1st pada – Belly, Pelvis, Bones in this region.

Chitra 2nd padas – Kidneys, Hernia, Lumbar region, Vasomotor system.

Chitra 3rd and 4th padas – Kidneys Glomerules, Blood Filtration System.

Swati -- Skin, Urethra, Urinary Bladder.

Vishakha 1st, and 2nd padas – Urine drain system, Pancreas.

Vishakha 3rd and 4th padas – Genital organs, Rectum, Prostate, Descending Colon.

Anuradha -- Bladder lower port, Bones near Genital organs, Lumbar 4th, 5th and 6th Vertebrae.

Jyeshtha - Anus, Cervix, Uterus, Ovary, Fallopian tubes.

Moola - Hips, Thighs, Ilium, Sciatica Nerve.

Purvashadha – Thighs, Femoral bones, Sacral region, Lumen, Veins.

Uttarashadha 1st and 2nd padas - Thighs, Femur arteries.,

Uttarashadha 3rd 4th padas – Skin, Knees, Tibia and Fibula.

Sravan –Lymphatic vessels, Skin, Supra renals.

Dhanishtha – 1st 2nd padas –knee cap, Tendons, Ligaments, Ankles, Veins.

Dhanishtha 3rd, 4th padas- Limbs, Portion between knees and Ankles.

Shatatarka- Calf, Ligaments, muscles, Tendons.

Purvabhadrapada- Back portion of Ankles, Heels, Ligaments, Lower portion of feet, Fingers of feet.

Uttarabhadrapada- Metatarsal bones, Skin of Feet.

Revati – Joints of Feet bones.

Chapter 5

Constellations and Body Organs (ii)

An Indian system of ASTROLOGICAL predictive analysis called as Krishnamurthi Paddhati is first method of predictive diagnosis and proved since years most accurate. In this system of Diagnosis the 360 degrees of Zodiac is divided into 249 subs and these subs and sub lords are playing major role in predictive analysis of the diseased part of Body. Further to it Sub lord is Key factor for particular incidence in life and to determine the nature of the effect that may undergo.

In Astrology sixth House is considered as the House of defects or Diseases and the Lord of this cusp defines the affected part of the Body and with intensity or severity of the disease.

We have to further study the relation between Parts of Body and each sub lord, and to understand this we may have to first tabulate the following chart which is self explanatory.

Each Zodiac with Lord of zodiac, Lord of the Constellation and sub lord of the Constellation denoting the specific Body part can be tabled as given under. .

Sub No	Zodiac	Planetary Combination for Constellation	Body Parts or organs affected
01	Aries	Mars / Ketu /Ketu	Nostril , middle bone of the nostril
02		Mars / Ketu / Venus	Eye ball, Retina, Ocular Hydro pressure,

No	Sign	Planets	Body Part
			Optic Nerve, Lenses tissues
03		Mars/ Ketu / Sun	Frontal Occipital Lobe, Ophthalmic Ganglion
04		Mars / Ketu / Moon	
05		Mars / Ketu / Mars	Parietal lobes, Diencephalon , Ear drum,
06		Mars / Ketu / Rahu	
07		Mars / Ketu / Jupiter	Parietal occipital Gyrus, Parietal Occcipital Sulcus , Cornea, Blood supply capillaries of eye
08		Mars / Ketu / Saturn	Optic Disc, Optic nerve, Retina .
09		Mars/Ketu/ mercury	Cochlea, Ear drum, Eustachian tube
10		Mars / Venus / Venus	Ophthalmic nerve , ear external lobe, Medulla oblongata.
11		Mars / Venus /Sun	Upper lid and Lowe lid of eye, veins of eye.
12		Mars / Venus /Moon	Lachrymal sack watering of eyes, color of eye.
13		Mars / Venus /Mars	Great cerebral vein, Arachnoids granulation , Superior saggital sinus.
14		Mars/Venus/Rahu	Medulla oblongata
15		Mars /Venus / Jupiter	Confluence of sinuses, Median aperture .
16		Mars/ Venus / Saturn	Maxillofacial tissues, Lower and upper Jaws,
17		Mars / Venus / Mercury	Otorhino nerves, lateral aperture of Luscha, Strait sinus , Central canal.
18		Mars / Venus / ketu	Sub arachnoids space, Choroid plexus, Lingual gyrus.
19		Mars / Sun / Sun	Optic chiasm, Mammillary Body, Calcarine fissure.
20		Mars / Sun / Moon	Anterior commisure, Cuneum, Splenium corpus collasum, choroid plexus.
21		Mars / Sun / Mars	Hypothalamic sulcus, Lamina terminalis, Genu of corpus collasum.
22		Mars / sun / Rahu	Singulate gyrus, Septum pellucidium, Fornix, Masa intermedia.
23	Taurus	Venus / Sun / Rahu	Anterior chamber of aqueous body, Vitreous body, Optic disc.
24	Taurus	Venus /Sun /Jupiter	Frontal Lobe , Temporal Lobe.
25		Venus / Sun /Saturn	Maxillofacial Skeleton and Flesh, Pallet, Facial muscles, Facial skin.
26		Venus / Sun / Mercury	Teeth, Lips , Gums , Chin.
27		Venus / Sun /Ketu	Mandibular notch , Ramaus mandible, Trapezious Muscles, Jugulodigastric node.
28		Venus /Sun / Venus	Zygomatic Arch, Angular Optic Arteries , and Vein, Superficial Parotid Nodes.
29		Venus / Moon / Moon	Iris, Cilliary Body Structure, Fovea, The centre of macula, Choroid Layer.
30		Venus/Moon/ Mars	Carotid, Auditary tube, Eustachian tube
31		Venus / Moon /Rahu	Sternocleidomastoid, Trapezium, Masseter.
32		Venus / Moon/ Jupiter	Orbicularis ,Zygomatic Major,TemporalisMasseter.
33	Taurus	Venus / Moon /Saturn	Cricoid cartilage, Median cricothyroid ligament Thyroid cartilage, Mucosa of posterior Tracheal wall.
34		Venus / Moon /Mercury	Dorsum of tongue, Volstpapilae, Polstopharyngeal arch, Soft palate, Orifice of submandibular duct, Sublingual papillae.
35		Venus / Moon /Ketu	Ursula, Adenoids, Tonsils, Epiglottis, Upper Oesophagus, Subglottic Space, Vocal cords.
36		Venus / Moon /Venus	Buccal mucosa, Hard palate, Trigon, Alveolar Ridges, Ovula, Gum, Teeth, Soft tissue Under tongue.
37		Venus / Moon / Sun	Olfactory (CN1),Ophthalmic (CNV1),Maxillary (CNV2)Cranial nerves, Incus, Stapes,Maleus.
38		Venus/Mars/Mars	Optic(CNII), Oculomotor(CNIII), Trochlear(CNIV)

			Trigeminal(CNV),Occipital bor,PalatineBone, Lacrimal bone, Paranasal Sinuses.
39		Venus/ Mars/ Rahu	Cervical Fascias, Hyoid Bone, Thyroid gland, Parathyroid gland, Facial Arteries, Cervical Plexus.
40		Venus/ Mars / Jupiter	Gingiva, Incisors ,Canines, Premolars, Molar teeth, Maxillary (CNV2) , Mandibular (CNV3).
41		Venus/ Mars/ Saturn	Abduces Nerve, Vestibulocochlear nerve, Accesary nerve, Vagus nerve, Glossopharyngeal nerve, Hypoglossal Nerve.
42	Gemini	Mercury / Mars /Mercury	Supraspinatus Muscles, Infra spinatus muscles, Acromin , Greater tubercle of humerus, teres minor muscles, deltoid muscles, Posterior cutaneous nerve.
43		Mercury / Mars / Ketu	Tendons of triceps , Branchi muscles, Medial intermescular septum, Ulnar nerve, anconeus muscles, Flexor carpi, Branchiioradialis muscles.
44		Mercury / Mars / Venus	Exterior carpi ulnaris, Median nerve, Musculocutaneus nerve, Palmer digital nerve, Radial nerve, Accessorycephalic vein, Axillary artey Bascilic vein, Deep palmer artery.
45		Mercury / Mars /Sun	Mediastinum, Plural cavities, Intercostal muscles, Intercostal neurovascular bundles.
46		Mercury / Mars / Moon	Pectoralis Major, Serratius anterior, Lattisimus dorsi.
47		Mercury / Rahu / Rahu	Longhead of triceps, Teremajor muscles, Subclavious.
48		Mercury / Rahu /Jupiter	Biceps brachii, Coracobrachialis, Bicipital Aponeurosis, Brachialis.
49		Mercury /Rahu / Saturn	Humerus, Greater tubercle, Lesser tubercle, Bicipital groove, Shaft of Humerus, Subclavian Artery, Deltoid tuberosity, Medial epicondyl.
50		Mercury / Rahu / Mercury	Cephalic vein, Branchial plexus, Musculo cutaneous Nerve, Axillary median and radial .
51		Mercury /Rahu /Ketu	Extensor digitorum, Palmaris Pollicis, Extensor pollicis brevis, Flexor digitorum profoundus, Pronator teres.
52		Mercury/ Rahu/ Venus	Pisiform traquetrum, Lunate scaphoid, Hamate, Capitate, Trapezoid, Trapezium, 8TH AND 9TH Ribs, Metacarpels, Phalanges and joints.
53		Mercury/ Rahu / Sun	Palmaris longus, Sternum, Elbow Joint, Pisiform Triquetrum, Lunate, scaphoid Hamate, 8th and 9th ribs., Metacarpels, Phalanges.
54		Mercury /Moon / Rahu	10th,11th Rib, Proximal and inter pharyngeal joints, Avascular necrosis, extrinsic ligaments, intrinsic ligaments, Radial artery palmer branch, h.
55	Gemini	Mercury / Rahu/ Mars	Flexor digitorum , Radiocarpel joints, Distal Radio ulnar Joint, Proximal carpel joints, distal carpel. 12th rib, Longus scapula.
56		Mercury/ Jupiter/ Jupiter	Deltoid tuberosity, Posterior circumflex HumeralArtery.
57		Mercury/ Jupiter/Saturn	Pulmonary artery, Primary branchi, Secondary Branchi, Tertiary branchi, Branchioles, Cardiac alveolar artery, Alveolar duct, Pulmonary vein.
58		Mercury/ Jupiter/ Mercury	Convex surface of diaphragm, caria hilum, Broncho pulmonary lymph nodes, Pulmonary Plurae, Azygos, Ascending lumbar vein.
59		Mercury/Jupiter/ Ketu	Biceps branchi, Coraco oranchits, BicipitalAponeurosis, Branchialis.
60		Mercury/ Jupiter/ Venus	Carpel Flexor Retinaculum, Carpel Tunel, Carpel Muscle tendons, Carpel Nerve.
61		Mercury/ Jupiter/Sun	Posterior part of carpel, Dorsal intrasseous.
62		Mercury/ Jupiter/ Moon	Fleshy part of Carpel, Carpel Nerve.
63	Cancer	Moon/ Jupiter/ Moon	Sternoclavicular joint, Suprasternal joint, Sternal manubrium, Verebral canal, Pericardial cavity.
64		Moon/ Jupiter/Mars	Intercostals muscles, Brachial plexus, Trachea, Esophagus, Posterior Inter costal veins, Main Bronchus, Pericardiophrenic veins.
65		Moon/ Jupiter/ Rahu	Tracheal Tube, Clavicle vertebrae, Thoracic vertebrae, Acromial facet, Bones of dorsal trunk.
66		Moon/ Saturn/ Saturn	Esophagus, Thoracic aorta , Sympathetic trunk, Pericardium, Branchocephalic Trunk, Pulmonary Apex.
67		Moon/ Saturn/ Mercury	Superior Vena cava, Bronchopulmonay segment, Right pulmonary artery, Left

Sub NO.	Zodiac	Planetary combination for constellation	Body parts or organ affected
			branch of cephalic vein, Cervical part of parietal pleura.
68		Moon/Saturn/Ketu	Hepatic artery, Cystic artery, Common hepatic duct, Cyclic duct , Gall bladder , Supramesocolic part of peritoneal cavity, Inguinal ligament Apo neurosis of the mobliques muscles .
69		Moon/ Saturn / Venus	Thoracic lateralis, Thoracoepigastrica, Linea alba, Paraumbilicales.
70		Moon/ Saturn/ Sun	Transversal fasica, Abdominus externas, Thoracic cord of connective tissue, Sternum, Symphysis linea.
71		Moon/ Saturn/Moon	6th and 7th Ribs, Renal cortex, Nephron, Renal Medula, Renal papilla of Pyramid, Supra renals.
72		Moon/Saturn/Mars	Falciform ligament of liver, Left triangular ligament, Caudate lobe, Coronary ligament, Hepatic veins, Quadrate lobe, Common bile duct.
73		Moon/ Saturn/ Rahu	Caudate process, Fissure for teres ligament. Proximal port of Common bile duct.
74		Moon/ Saturn / Jupiter	9th Rib, Supraspinatus, Teres minor, Acromin, carecoid subscapuaris, Humerus, Scapula , Capsular ligament.
75		Moon/Mercury/Mercury	Principal pancreatic duct, Accessory pancreatic duct, Pancreatic neck, Spleen, Splenic artery.
76		Moon/ Mercury / ketu	Gall bladder, Cystic duct, Hepatic duct, Fundus, Hepatopancreatic ampulla of vater.
77		Moon/Mercury/ Venus	Ileum, Large intestine, Cecum, Ileocecal sphincter, Superior Mesenteric Artery.
78		Moon/ Mercury/ Sun	Pulmonary alveoli, Right and Left Pulmonary artery, Pulmonary veins, Custodia recess.

Sub NO.	Zodiac	Planetary combination for constellation	Body parts or organ affected
79	Cancer	Moon/ Mercury/Moon	Lungs, Alveoli, Bronchioles, trachea.
80		Moon/Mercury/Mars	Diaphragm, Gray's anatomy plates, Floating ribs, Ensiform cartilage
81		Moon/Mercury/ Rahu	Right colic flexure, Left colic flexure, Epiploacae, Hausta, ileum
82		Moon/Mercury/Jupiter	Pancreas, Hepato pancreatic am pula, Hepatopancreatic sphincter
83		Moon/Mercury/ Saturn	Jejunun, Spleen, Lieberkunh glands,Alveoli,
84	Leo	Sun/Ketu/Ketu	Fossa, Ovalis, Pulmonary alveoli, Veins, Right atrium, left coronary artery
85		Sun/Ketu/ Venus	Trcuspid valve, Right ventricle, Left atrium Ascending aorta
86		Sun/Ketu/ Sun	Rt. Coronary artery, Aortic valve, Lt ventricle, Mitral valve
87		Sun/Ketu/ Moon	Epicardium, Myocardium, Pulmonary vein.
88		Sun/Ketu/ Mars	Descending aorta, Aortic arch, Inferior venacava, pulmonary trunk
89		Sun/Ketu/ Rahu	Pulmonary vein, Semilunar valve, Atrio ventricular valve., c. sinus
90		Sun/Ketu/ Jupiter	Atrio ventricular valve, Coronary sinus.
91		Sun/Ketu /Saturn	Right atrium, Rt. Ventricle, Ascending aorta, Aortic valves.
92		Sun/Ketu/Mercury	Pericardium, Heart muscles.
93		Sun/Venus/Venus	Function of mitral valve, Tricuspid valve, Aortic valve.
94		Sun/Venus/Sun	Function of coronary artery, Function of pulmonary artery.
95		Sun/Venus/Moon	Function of right atrium and right ventricle.
96		Sun/Venus/Mars	Function of coronary sinus, function of pulmonary artery.
97		Sun/Venus/Rahu	Function of superior venacava, and ascending aorta.
98		Sun/Venus/ Jupiter	Function of sub clavian artery, Descending venacava.
99		Sun/Venus /Saturn	Function of semilunar valves, Branchio cephalic trunk.
100		Sun/Venus/Mercury	Function of aortic arch, pulmonary vein.
101		Sun/Venus/Ketu	Fossa ovallis, Atria, Pumonary artery.
102		Sun/Sun/Sun	Function of cephalic vein, cervical port of parietal pleura.
103		Sun/Sun/Moon	Function of ventricles, Right pulmonary artery.
104		Sun/ Sun/Mars	Aortic valves, tricuspid valve.

No.	Sign	Dasha/Antardasha/Pratyantardasha	Body Part
105		Sun/Sun/Rahu	Function of left coronary artery, coronary sinus.
106	Virgo	Mercury/Sun/Rahu	Retroperitoneum, Visceral peritoneum,Supra pubic region.
107		Mercury/Sun/Jupiter	Perietal peritoneum, peripheral nerves of pelvic girdle.
108		Mercury/Sun/Saturn	Nerves system of hips and legs, caudal eminence.
109		Mercury/Sun/Mercury	Endometrium, Cervix, clitoris, ovaries.
110		Mercury/ Sun/ Ketu	Coccygeal vertebrae, Anococcygeal raphe, Glutious maximus.
111		Mercury/Sun/Venus	Coccydynia, sacro coccygeal teratoma, Intraarticular ligaments.
112		Mercury/Moon/Moon	Jevatur ani muscles, Femoral head,Femoral neck.
113		Mercury/Moon/ Mars	Function of diaphragm, Upper cartilage of nasal chambers.
114		Mercury/Moon/Rahu	Lower cartilage of nostrils, Skin septum, Nasal cavity.
115		Mercury/ Moon/Jupiter	Pancreas, Pancreatic body, Pancreatic tail.
116		Mercury/Moon/Saturn	Paraumbilicals, Circumphlex illium, Ileohypogastrium.
117		Mercury/Moon/Mercury	Recto uterine tubes, vesico uterine pouch, Ileocecal valve.
118		Mercury/Moon/Ketu	Vermiform appendix, Transverse colon,Ascending colon.
119		Mercury/Moon/Venus	Sigmoid colon, Rectal valves, Anal sphincters, Prepuce vault.
120		Mercury/Moon/Sun	Articular processes, Lumbar region.
121	Virgo	Mercury /Mars/ Mars	Duodenum, Jejunum, Common bile duct, esophageal sphincters.
122		Mercury/Mars/Rahu	Anorectal sphincters, Pyloric sphincters, Zollinger Ellison syndrome
123		Mercury/ Mars/Jupiter	Lumborum illiacum, crest of illium, Tensor foscica, Lateralis
124		Mercury/ Mars/Saturn	Coccyx, Mamillary processes, Detruser muscles, Bartholine glans.
125	Libra	Venus/Mars/ Mercury	Floating ribs, Pubic ramus, Sinus processes, Anterior/posterior ligaments
126		Venus/Mars/Ketu	Ilio lumbar ligament, bundle of lumbar,sacral,and coccygeal nerves.
127		Venus/Mars/Venus	Para umbilicals, Uterine tubes, Vesico uterus, uterine pouch,Vas defefrence
128		Venus/Mars/ Sun	Prostate Epididymis,Seminiferus tubules, intervertebral formina
129		Venus/ Mars/Moon	Supra renals, ureter, Purified blood vessels, Nephrons,Renal cortex.
130		Venus/ Rahu/Rahu	Renal vein,Renal nerve,Renal artery,Fllopian tubes,Cervix.
131		Venus/Rahu/Jupiter	Sciatic notch, Wings of illium, Iliac crest, Ischial spine,sacrum.
132		Venus/Rahu/Saturn	Rectouterine pouch,Coopers glands, Transversal fascica,.
133		Venus/Rahu/Mercury	Apex of bladder, Trigone, Meso nephric ducts, Detruser muscles,.
134		Venus/Rahu/ketu	Medial circumflex femoral artery, lateral femoralcircumflex, nrves.
135		Venus/Rahu/Venus	FoveaCapits, necktrochanters, Interochanteric crest.
136		Venus/Rahu/Sun	Renal fat pad, urethra, medular renal column, Renal papillae.
137		Venus/Rahu/Moon	Clycs,cortical blood vessels, Acruate bllod vessels, Renal capsule.
138		Venus/Rahu/Mars	Interlobular blood vessels, Renal nerve, Rena helium.
139		Venus/Jupiter/Jupiter	Mesonephric ducts, Ureteric lamina propia,Gluteus maximus.
140		Venus/Jupiter /Saturn	Spongiosum glans, Levatermuscles,pectineus psoasmajor.
141		Venus/Jupiter/Mercury	Flavum interspinus legaments, Supra spinus ligaments, Ovaries.
142		Venus/Jupiter/Ketu	Anterior and posterior longitudinal muscles, Uterine nerves.
143		Venus/Jupiter/Venus	Inferior mesonephric nerves, Inferior mesenteric vein.
144		Veins/Jupiter/Sun	Cecum, colon, Rectum,ileocecal valves, bulky ovaries,colitis.
145		Venus/Jupiter/Moon	Acetabulum labrum, Abturator artery, Puboformal ligament.
146	Scorpio	Mars/Jupiter/Moon	Urinary bladder, Somatic nervous system of pelvic girdle.
147		Mars/Jupiter/Mars	Intra artecular ligament, Sacrococcygeal ligament,Goblet cells.
148		Mars/Jupiter/Rahu	Intestinal glands,Brunners glands, secretion of gastroileal reflex.
149		Mars/Jupiter/Saturn	Epididymis, Vas deference, Seminal vesicles,erectile tissue,duct.
150		Mars/Saturn/Mercury	Splenic artery, Apedix, Mucosa associated lymphoid tissue.
151		Mars/Saturn/Ketu	Anorectal muscles, Rectal sphincters, Fascica external sphincter.
152		Maras/Saturn/Venus	Corpus spongiosum, Glans penis,Foreskin.
153		Mars/Saturn/Sun	Prrineal space, Urteric muscles, Lamina propia.
154		Mars/Saturn/Moon	Sphincters in Bladder, Detruser muscles.
155		Mars/Saturn/Mars	Vasa deference, Treitz, Fallopian tubes, Testicles.
156		Mars/Saturn/Rahu	Hepatic artey, Cystic artery, Cyclic duct, Falsiform ligament.

No.	Sign	Lord/Sub/Sub-sub	Body Parts
157		Mars/Saturn/ Jupiter	Caudate lobe,Fundus, Hepatopacreatic ampula, Superior mesenteric artery
158		Mars/ Mercury/Mercury	Sigmoid colon, tenae, ileum rectum.
159		Mars/Mercury/Ketu	Anal sphincter, epiplocae, haustra.
160		Mars/Mercury/Venus	Testosterone, Testicles , function of testosterone.
161		Mars/Mercury/Sun	Ileocecal sphincters, superior mesenteric artery.
162		Mars/Mercury/Moon	Cervix, Uterus, function of ovaries, Function of supra renala.
163		Mars/Mercury/Mars	Endometrium, Cavity in Uterus.
164		Mars/Mercury/Rahu	Function of endocrine gland related to Ovaries, Testicles.
165	Scorpio	Mars/Mercury/Jupiter	Renal pyramid, Renal papillae, glans penis cavernosum.
166		Mars/Mercury/Saturn	Seminiferous tubules, transversal fascica, Vesico uterine pouch
167	Sagittarius	Jupiter/Ketu/Ketu	Sacrum, Lumbar Lamina,Sacropulmotorygreates.
168		Jupiter/Ketu/Venus	Pubic symphysis, Illium ,Pubis, Ischium,Acetabulum.
169		Jupiter/Ketu/Sun	Posterior Rami,Spinal nerve,Illioguineal nerve, Sacral plexus.
170		Jupiter/Ketu/Moon	Genito femoral nerve,Lateral cutaneous nerve.
171		Jupiter/Ketu /Mars	Illeohypogastric nerve, Obturator nerve.
172		Jupiter/Ketu/Rahu	Femoral artery, Iguinal ligament, Profunda femoris artery.
173		Jupiter/Ketu/ Jupiter	Lateral femoral artery, Circumflex artery, Medial femoral artery.
174		Jupiter/Ketu/Saturn	Abductor canal, Politeal artery, Abductor hiatus.
175		Jupiter/Ketu/ Mercury	Gluteal artery, Greater sciatic artery.
176		Jupiter/Venus/Venus	Sciatic foramen, Piriformis.
177		Jupiter/Venus/Sun	Anteriar tibial artery, Posterior tibial artery, Fibular artery.
178		Jupiter/Venus/Moon	Deep fibular nerve, Tibioperoneal trunk.
179		Jupiter/Venus/Mars	Great sapheneous vein, Smal sapheneoua vein.
180		Jupiter/Venus/Rahu	Anterior tibial vein, Posterior tibial vein, femoral vein.
181		Jupiter/Venus/Jupiter	Superficial fascica, Deep fascica,visceral fascica.
182		Jupiter/Venus/Saturn	Superficial abductor, Extensor abductor, Internal iliac.
183		Jupiter/Venus/Mercury	Deep lateral rotator.
184		Jupiter/Venus/Ketu	Gluteal maximus, Gluteal artery,Gluteal minimus.
185		Jupiter/Sun/Sun	Vestibular glands, Somatic efferent fibers, Pudendal nerves.
186		Jupiter/Sun/Moon	Bulbocavernosus, Ischeocavernousus.
187		Jupiter/Sun/ Mars	Somatic efferent neurons, Sympathetic preganglionic nervs.
188		Jupiter/ Sun/ Rahu	Neural crest cells,Chromafin cells,Epinephrine,Chromogranins.
189	Capricorn	Saturn /Sun/Rahu	Interochanteric crest, Gluteal tuberosity, Linia aspera.
190		Saturn/Sun/Jupiter	Pectineal line,Popliteal fossa.
191		Saturn/Sun/Saturn	Lateral supracondylarline, Abductor tubercle.
192		Saturn/Sun/Mercury	Medial and lateral condylas, Epicondyle, intercondyle fossa.
193		Saturn/Sun/Ketu	Quadriceps femoris,Hamstrings,Sartorius.
194		Saturn/Sun/Venus	Rectus femoris,Vastus medialis,Gastrocenimus.
195		Saturn/Moon/Moon	Tibialis anterior, Soleus.
196		Saturn/Moon/Mars	Tibia,Fibula,ankle,Anterior and posterior arteries.
197		Saturn/Moon/Rahu	Sciatic and femoral nerve, Tibial arteries, Saphenous,Ankle joints.
198		Saturn/Moon/Jupiter	Tibial and fibular vein, Hinjed joints.
199		Saturn/Moon/Saturn	Temoral condyle, Plantar flexion.
200		Saturn/Moon/Mercury	Dorsiflexon, Calcanus , Talus.
201		Saturn/Moon/Ketu	Navicular,cuboid, Cunieform bones.
202		Saturn/Moon/Venus	Metatarsals and phalages.
203		Saturn/Moon/Sun	Lumbar vertebrae, Dorsal muscles, Central planter muscles.
204		Saturn/Mars/Mars	Medial and planter artery of foot, Deep Planter arch.
205		Saturn/Mars/Rahu	Superficial dorsal vein, Planter venousnetwork.
206		Saturn/Mars/Jupiter	Dorsal venous arch, marginal and digital vein.
207		Saturn/Mars/Saturn	Metatarsal veins, Medial nerves,Planter nerves, Digital nerves.
208	Aquarius	Saturn/Mars/Mercury	Posterior malleolus, medial malleolus,Tallus.

No.	Sign	Dasha	Description
209	Aquarius	Saturn/Mars/Ketu	Artereis and blood vessels of intestine, Chromogranin.
210		Saturn/Mars/Venus	Norepinephrine, Enkephaline, and nuero peptide in blood.
211		Saturn/Mars/Sun	Beta adrenoreceptors, Hypoglycemia, Epinephrine.
212		Saturn/Mars/Moon	Beta hydroxybutyric acid, and acetoacetic acid in lever.
213		Saturn/Rahu/Rahu	Subaracnoid space, coroid plexus, Aqueduct sylvious , Cisterna magna,
214		Saturn/Rahu/Jupiter	Sphenoid area, Zygoma,Mxilla mandible.
215		Saturn/Rahu/Saturn	Periodorsal artery, Middle cerebral artery,Central canal.
216		Saturn/Rahu/Mercury	Posterior cerebral artery, internal carotid artery.
217		Saturn/Rahu/Jupiter	Supraspinatus, Infra spinatus, teres minor, Acromin.
218		Saturn/Rahu/Venus	Subscapularis, Humerous scapularis,Capsular ligament.
219		Saturn/Rahu/Sun	Malleolus, Proturbance, ankles.
220		Saturn/Rahu/Moon	Main bronchus, Lobar bronchus, Segmental bronchus.
221		Saturn/Rahu/Mars	Cervical part of parietal pleura, Middle lobe of lungs.
222		Saturn/Jupiter/ Jupiter	Hepatic artery, Cystic artery, Cyclic duct.
223		Saturn/Jupiter/Saturn	Supra mesocolic part of peritoneal cavity,Inguinal ligMENT.
224		Saturn/Jupiter/Mercury	Thorasica lateralis, Para umbilicals,Thorasic cord of connective tissue.
225		Saturn/Jupiter/Ketu	Muscle obliqusabdominus, Tranversal fascica.
226		Saturn/Jupiter/Venus	Falsiform ligament, left triangular ligament.
227		Saturn/Jupiter/Sun	Interstitial fluid, Lymphatic system, Lymph cap.illaries.
228		Saturn/Jupiter/Moon	Lymphoid tissue, Endothelial lymphatic trunk,Tributaries.
229	Pisces	Jupiter/Jupiter/Moon	Lymph nodes, Tonsils, Spleen, Thymus inguinal
230		Jupiter/Jupiter/Mars	Peripheral nervous system, Ganglions, Glial cells.
231		Jupiter/Jupiter/Rahu	Enteric nervous system, Sensory strip, Motor strip.
232		Jupiter/Saturn/Saturn	Reward circuit, Ventral tegmental area, Neuclear accumbens.
233		Jupiter/Saturn/Mercury	Primary motor cortex, Cornea, Aqueous humour, Pupil.
234		Jupiter/Saturn/Ketu	Rentinas ganglious cell, Lateral geniculate nucleus.
235		Jupiter/Saturn/Venus	Secretion of endorphins and serotonins.
236		Jupiter/Saturn/Sun	Goal directed movements, Vetrious humour, Retina.
237		Jupiter/Saturn/Moon	Deccusation, conscious visual perception.
238		Jupiter/Saturn/Mars	Posterior communicating basilar, External carotid artery.
239		Jupiter/Saturn/Rahu	Pona hippocampus,Aygdala, Cingulate gyrus.
240		Jupiter/Saturn/Jupiter	Neuro transmitter synapse, Pleasure centres.
241		Jupiter/Saturn/Mercury	Dendrites, Nodes of ranvier, Axon terminals,Lymph capillaries.
242		Jupiter/Saturn/Ketu	Absorption of fat soluble vitamins, Villis in intestine.
243		Jupiter/Mercury/Venus	Cranum cortex,Cerebellum dura, Brain stem.
244		Jupiter/Mercury/Sun	Temporal lobes, Occipital lobes.
245		Jupiter/Mercury/Moon	Meninges, Corpus callosum, Frontal lobes.
246		Jupiter/Mercury/Mars	Broca area, Vernicle area.
247		Jupiter/Mercury/Rahu	Optic chaisma, Thalamus, Optic Tract.
248		Jupiter/Mercury/Jupiter	Mid brain, Optic nerve, Grey matter, White matter.
249		Jupiter/Mercury/Saturn	Centric nervous system, Functional M.R. imaging.

Chapter 6

Types of ailments and relation with Zodiac

As we look forward human being suffers from six major types of disease as

1. Physical ailment due to degenerative changes in body.
2. Physical ailments due to prenatal causes.
3. Physical ailments due to external factors as infection/sun stroke
4. Physical ailments cause of stress hormone cortisol.
5. Physical ailments due to accidental reasons.
6. Physical ailments due to psychosomatic factors.

1) All these can be perfectly predicted or diagnosed and appropriately treated in time with much lesser input of funds and efforts if we try to understand the very relation between different parts of body with respect to planetary aspect at that time or in birth chart. To understand it in si to we have to start understanding the age old predictive analysis method popularly called as Krishnamurthi Method or known as KP System or KP Method. We here try to understand that how Diagnosis Aries- This is of hot constitution and may give rise to Head related ailments including Neuralgia, Cerebral hemorrhage pains etc.
2) Taurus- Gives diseases related to tonsils, thyroid, Para thyroid, Cervical Syndrome , Venereal diseases, uterus related problems.
3) Gemini- This produces Pulmonary ailments , tuberculosis, Eoseonaphilia, pericardits.
4) Cancer- Gastric problems, jaundice, gallstones.
5) Leo - Anorexia, fainting, spinal ailments, Atherosclerosis, Anemia.
6) Virgo- Intestinal ailments, Chyle urea, Appendix related problem.
7) Libra – Urethra , kidney related diseases, Rheumatic syndrome, uterus ailments.
8) Scorpio – Bladder related problems, reproductive organ related problems.
9) Sagittarius- Pelvic region related ailments, Lumbar region pain.
10) Capricorn- Knee related diseases, dermatological problems, vitiligo.
11) Aquarius- Ankles, lower limb problems, varicose veins, eye related ailments.
12) Pisces- Feet, toes, drug addiction, deformities in feet.

Apart from these each planet also produce its impact on various organs of the body as briefed bellow.

1. Sun- Eye related issues, Hyperacidity, skin diseases, fracture, baldness, Head related problems.
2. Moon- Heart, lungs related ailments, ovaries related issues, nervous disorders, poisoning.
3. Mars- Ligaments tear, Blood related ailments, fevers, burns, tumors, Hypertension Rheumatism.
4. Mercury- Nerve disorders, Skin disorders, Psychological ailments, Paralysis.
5. Jupiter- Liver, Stomach, Colon ailments, Ear problems, Obesity, Enlargement of organs.
6. Venus- Reproductive organ related diseases, Pancreas related ailments, Bile stones.
7. Saturn- Rheumatic Arthritis, Spinal cord related issues, Loss of limbs, blindness.
8. Rahu- Respiratory disease, Leprosy, Splenomegaly, Cataract, Endocrine glands.
9. Ketu- Ano rectal problems, Speech disorder, Non diagnosable disease.

Apart from these some distant planets also yield much severe effect on our body as Uranus gives rise to accidents and head injury, Hysteria, premature birth , Abnormal growth. Neptune produces coma, epilepsy, narcotic poisoning, and allergy.

So also pathogenic effects of constellations are also worth noting,

1) Ashwini—Head injury, Cerebral hemorrhage, Cerebral tumors, insomnia, meningitis.
2) Bharani----Forehead pains, ailments, Eyes, Syphilis.
3) Krittika ----Fever, Malaria, Non healing wounds, Wounds due to explosion, Throat troubles.
4) Rohini -----Pulmonary and cough related problems, pain in lower limbs, edema.
5) Mrigshirsha- Injuries, Colorectal problems, piles, P.C.O.D., Fracture of elbow, Collarbones.
6) Ardra ----   Asthma, Ear problems, mumps, Eosinophillia.
7) Punarvasu-Pneumonia, Enlargement of heart, Iodine deficiency disorder, Anorexia, Liver.
8) Pushya   Tuberculosis, Gall bladder stones, Phthisis, Eczema, Pyorrhea.
9) Ashlesha - Nephritis, Hysteria, Hypochondria, Digestive system related complaints.
10) Magha --- Cardiac ailments, Painful back, Tachycardia, Palpitation.
11) Purvaphalguni- Vasculatis, Painful leg, Swelling of ankles, Tricuspid and pulmonary vaves.
12) Uttaraphalguni- German missiles, Hypertension, Migraine , Tumors in intestine, Colon.
13) Hastha----- Fatigue, Flatulence, Irritable bowel syndrome, Shortness of breath, Typhoid.
14) Chitra -----Ulcers, Amoebic dysentery, Leg pain, Cramps in legs, Itching, Insect bites.
15) Swati -----Poly urea, Chyle urea, Urethral diseases, Skin diseases, Psoriasis.
16) Vishakha—Diseases related to Endocrine glands, Abscissa, Diabetes, Vertigo, Prostate cancer.
17) Anuradha- Amenorrhea, Infertility, Constipation, Fracture of hip bones.
18) Jyeshtha—Leucorrhea, Bleeding piles, Fistula, Painful arms and Shoulders,.
19) Moola ----Loco motor Ataxia, Rheumatism, Lumbar diseases, and Respiratory diseases.
20) Purvashadha- Sciatica, Lung cancer, Hip gout, Swelling above knee, Rheumatoid Arthritis.
21) Uttarashadha- Paralysis of limbs, Eye infections, Gastric Ulcers, Thrombosis.
22) Sravana, -- Pleurisy, Anorexia, Auto immune diseases.
23) Dhanishtha-   Leg injury, Dry cough, Lameness, Eosinophillia, Varicose veins, Blood poisoning.
24) Shatataraka-   Guinea worms, Hypertension, Eczema, Fracture of Upper limbs.
25) Purvabhadrapada- Ventricular tachycardia, Swollen ankles, Hypotension, Dilated heart.
26) Uttara bhadrapada- Rheumatic Arthritis, Hernia, Colorectal Diseases.
27) Revaty-   Deformities of feet, Flatulence, Deafness, Nephritis, Ear Wounds.

Diseases and sub lords some notes....

In the K.P. system there are notable diseases or bodily ailments related to specific Sub lords with respect to indicator house in birth chart which are just charted here with are of great interest to our readers.

1. The Sixth house is house of ailments as we know all and Eighth house is house of defeat or danger so also Twelfth house refers to the Hospitalization.
2. The sub lord of Sixth house or cusp is the main deciding factor to indicate the onset of ailment along with other indicators about the diseases.
3. The probability for the onset of diseases normally depends up on both the Lord of Maha dasha Bhukti lord and Lord of Antar / prati anter dasha period. Planets related with the Sixth cusp and lord of First house produces the diseases in their conjoined periods.
4. In case sub lord of the sixth cusp is in twelfth house and is strong indicator of sixth cusp and ascendant first house or cusp then the native certainly suffers from an incurable diseases or ailments.

Astrological diagnosis of the disease or ailment as per K.P. Theory can be explained as given under,

1. The sub lord of sixth cusp is considered ,
2. Then constellation or star in which sub lord of sixth house is placed, is noted.
3. There after the zodiac in which the sub lord of sixth cusp is placed is noted,
4. Then the Zodiac sign in which the star lord of sixth cusp is placed is noted.

5. Then we have to refer the nature of the planet as in above and combine together
   With zodiac sign will give the clue about the nature of ailment.

Estimate the period of ailments

In case significator of sixth cusp is also the significator of Ascendant i.e. first house the disease will be caused,

1. Note down the significator of sixth and first house.
2. Then take common planets of 1st and sixth house .
3. Whenever the conjoined period of the significator will operate the native will have ailment.
4. As we know the sixth house of ascendant chart is the house of sickness, the significator of this house and First house i.e. ascendant indicates the ailment to native and the nature of disease can be found out from sub lord of the sixth cusp. So whenever Sub lord of any house which denotes a part of the Body will have some relation with first and sixth house, then only it can be said the native will suffer from the disease in that part of the body. The significator planet will signify the disease and the cuspal portion will indicate the affecting organ of the body.
5. The fatal disease is indicated by eighth house and its significators. The planet is considered malefic for health or part of life only when they have some connection with the house sixth, eighth and twelfth we can find out the disease and body part affected.

In case the sub lord of sixth house is in the constellation of Saturn then the disease is chronic one and if sub lord is also Saturn then it is of lingering nature may last for long time. If sub lord of sixth house is in connected to Mercury then complication will occur. In case the sub lord of sixth cusp is connected to mars then the disease will be acute and sudden, Planets in movable sign causes diseases of short duration and if common sign then the ailment will be of short duration but recurring nature. Normally planets in As such here are the types of signs, Aries Cancer, Libra and Capricorn are movable signs, Taurus, Leo, Scorpio Aquarius are fixed signs; and Gemini, Sagittarius , Pisces are common signs.

In diagnosing diseases we can certainly take this into account and can find out curable measures at an early stage so also we can develop disease fighting capacity of native's body.

As such most of the major accidents and fractures can be noted at an early stage and can easily be avoided by developing positive attitude and alertness.

6. Fixed sign causes ailments of prolonged nature and chronic with difficulty in recovery.
7. The psychology of disease and measures to take
8. The ever baffling of human problem has been the very sub conscious or the mind, the sub conscious is an elusive entity and as such we don't know where exactly it is located or what it is. Some show the head and others the heart as its location but in all the cases the breeding ground for some of the most destructive forces in the world is subconscious.

Mental disease is essentially one of the brain diseases and the Karak is Moon. The Moon governs the Brain and very nervous system called Central nervous system. It also governs the intellect and entire Peripheral nervous system. In case Moon is afflicted or adversely placed in the Horoscope, the native will suffer from general mood swing or anxiety, depression. Still this cannot be applied to all the cases of mental afflictions. Mind plays very important role in this case. The brain cells may or may not be affected. But brain is capable of producing any disease. And as such we can consider the brain is capable of producing disease as well as wonderfully can cure the disease. Thus Moon is the psychopaths and analysts can find the relation between fears, joy, grief, anger with that of disease. Here the fact is all natives experiencing these do not turn mad and Astrology only can explain this. The Horoscope of the native can speak for the disease and mindset. As such

Moon is planet of emotions and Mercury is planet of intelligence. And considering these we can find out beneficial combination of these two planets, Moon and Mercury in one house makes native intelligent. The Moon governs the mind and subconscious structures while Mercury controls the entire Nervous system and has a domain over the brain nerves. These two planets are responsible for maintaining mental stability and derive the response level to the drugs administered. Here Saturn being cause for melancholy and loneliness. In case Saturn and Rahu afflicts the Moon or Mercury in any house, the natives response level to drugs administered diminishes along with developing depression.

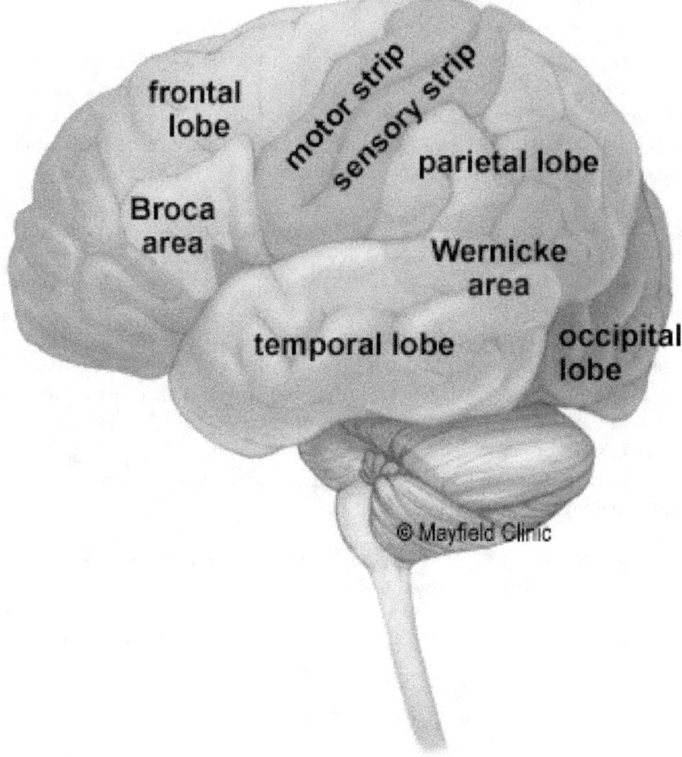

The Planetary combination described bellow may lead to mental illness or diseases.

1. The fifth house from Lagna rules over the capacity to think positively and wisdom to understand the way to mentally prepare to overcome the illness. Any affliction to this house by malefic may cause mental disease or depression.
2. The Jupiter is karak of fifth house and if afflicted in third house by malefic may cause mental complications.
9. Aries and Moon are responsible for all abnormal mental activities and astrology can illustrate the cause.
10. The Moon and Rahu in Lagna and malefic in fifth or ninth house may give rise to mental disorders.
11. The Moon and Mercury, if afflicted by Saturn or Rahu in Saturn's sign cause Hysteria and nervous disorders.
12. The Moon, Mars, Saturn, if conjoined in the eighth house give mental disorders.

13. Combination of Moon and Rahu, or Mercury and Saturn in Gemini or Virgo may also give rise to Psychological disorders.
14. If Jupiter and Saturn in twelfth house are afflicted by Mercury the native certainly suffers from Anxiety, Depression, and Fear and insecurity complex.
15. Sun in first house and Mars or Saturn in seventh house severe anxiety is noticed.
16. Saturn in lagna and Mars in fifth, seventh or ninth house severe depression is observed.
17. Jupiter in first house while Mars or Saturn in seventh house creates self destructive attitude and may cause even suicidal tendency.
18. Conjunction of Moon, Mars, and Saturn in eighth house is noticed to produce Hysteria.

Chapter 07

Psychological disorders

With reference to western Astrology based on Sion sign/Sun sign if neither the Moon, nor Mercury be in good aspect with ascendant or nor with each other then also psychological problems may occur; brain being unable to comprehend the situation. Gem reasoning and cancer is the sign of emotions, several afflictions to these signs by Moon or Mercury or other planets by using aspects cause psychological disorders.

As per K.P. the sixth house shows disease; eighth house threat and twelfth house hospitalization or surgery. The sub lord of sixth cusp is in the last and deciding factor about disease. Tendency to the disease also depends up on both the dasha lord bhuktilord and antardasha lord. Planets connected with the sixth house and lagna will produce disease in their conjoined periods. If the sub lord of sixth house is in twelfth house and becomes a strong significator of sixth house then the native will certainly suffer from an incurable disease. If the sub lord of sixth house is in seventh cusp and is connected to the cusps third fifth and ninth then Psycho-somatic aberrations is caused. Third house and the other cusps related to the brain are first, fifth and ninth. The better compatibility with adverse situations is denoted by ninth house and some lesser extent by third house. The sign Aries and the first cusp in zodiac governs the head and brain; and as such if Aries is afflicted the native naturally suffers from disease related to brain, so also if Sun is afflicted adversely or disposed adversely native gets ailments related to brain and head. If the sub lord of the sixth cusp is afflicted to Aries by cusps sixth, eighth and twelfth the native certainly will have to suffer severe depression and anxiety or may even produce Obsessive Compulsive Disorder. In case sub lord of sixth house is either Moon or Mercury/Sun is afflicted in the sign of Aries will give rise to dementia and often Alzheimer's syndrome. So also in case the sub lord of Sixth cusp is afflicted in sign Virgo which signifies entire nervous system, memory and thought producing will also cause nervous disorder.

As such we can sum up the inference that psychological; Nerve system related disorders are caused by Aries, Lord of ascendant, Mars, Moon, Mercury, Fifth and Sixth house. So also consciousness is signified by Fifth house, Lord of Fifth house and Mercury is significator of consciousness and mental disorders. Unconsciousness appears when these are afflicted seriously. This can be established by study of few Horoscopes mentioned bellow.

Case No. 001   Female born on 07th March 2007 Wednesday at 070500 hrs in Pune Maharashtra, The Ascendant or first House is Aquarius the Lord is Saturn placed in sixth house and is also a lord of twelfth house. Saturn is in the star of Mercury and sub lord is Rahu in sixth house. Also Mercury Lord of fifth house indicating mental status is seriously afflicted by Rahu and Ketu, as well Moon the characteristic of

Psych is placed in eighth house in Virgo having star lord Mars and Rahu is also seriously afflicted so also under aspect of Saturn from six Planet Position in Birth chart

Sr.No	Planet	Nirayan Deg /Min/ Sec.		Zodiac Lord	Star Lord	Sub Lord
01	Sun	Aquarius	022-08-16	Saturn	Jupiter	Saturn
02	Moon	Virgo	210-03-25	Mercury	Mars	Rahu
03	Mars	Capricorn	342-52-20	Saturn	Moon	Rahu
04	Mercury	Aquarius	001-31-29	Saturn	Mars	Mercury
05	Jupiter	Scorpio	294-27-14	Mars	Mercury	Rahu
06	Venus	Pisces	052-51-55	Jupiter	Mercury	Mars
07	Saturn	Cancer	175-48-41	Moon	Mercury	Rahu
08	Rahu	Aquarius	022-15-46	Saturn	Jupiter	Saturn
09	Ketu	Leo	202-15-46	Sun	Venus	Saturn
10	Uranus	Aquarius	020-48-24	Saturn	Jupiter	Jupiter
11	Neptune	Capricorn	356-31-09	Saturn	Mars	Jupiter
12	Pluto	Sagittarius	304-50-20	Jupiter	Ketu	Mars

Fifth house indicating severe mental retardation and irrecoverable mental disorder example

Cusp Position as per KP Chart

Cusp No.	Name	Nirayan Degree / Minute /Sec.		Zodiac Lord	Star Lord	Sub Lord
01	I	Aquarius	025-54-22	Saturn	Jupiter	Ketu
02	ii	Aries	037-21-35	Mars	Ketu	Venus
03	Iii	Taurus	039-38-49	Venus	Sun	Jupiter
04	Iv	Taurus	068-22-41	Venus	Mars	Saturn
05	V	Gemini	092-21-54	Mercury	Jupiter	Mercury
06	Vi	Cancer	114-18-23	Moon	Mercury	Sun
07	Vii	Leo	140-12-45	Sun	Venus	Ketu
08	Viii	Libra	174-34-20	Venus	Mars	Ketu
09	Ix	Scorpio	176-13-09	Mars	Jupiter	Rahu
10	X	Scorpio	204-58-04	Mars	Mercury	Saturn
11	Xi	Sagittarius	228-57-17	Jupiter	Venus	Saturn
12	Xii	Capricorn	250-53-46	Saturn	Moon	Venus

How to determine the House and the nature of the ailments

The sixth house is considered as the main house deciding the disease and the Lord of sixth house in this case is Moon and the star lord of sixth house is Mercury; the sub lord is Sun. The lord of sixth house causing ailments is placed in eighth house making it further severe. Here the star lord of sixth house is in Eighth house where the lord of eighth house is Mercury and placed in first house in conjunction with Rahu and Uranus becoming more vulnerable. The lord of first house is Saturn and placed in sixth house furthering the complication in diseases.   Important planet star lord of sixth house is Mercury and is main planet signifying the entire nervous system caused the current vulnerable status of the native. The native is not only suffering from Autism but also other complicated nervous disorders like hyper activity and sever insomnia with totally disturbed body clock. So also star lord of sixth house is Mars representing Aries; the significator of Head and brain. This is self explanatory that how the native suffers the disease denoted by sixth house and its relation with eighth house worsening the case further. Presently the native is under treatment with total focus on the Herbal drugs.   The fifth house is hose of mental diseases and the sub lord of is Mercury which is placed in First house having conjoined with Rahu and Uranus clearly indicates the complications in integrative nerves motor nerves, sensory receptors i.e. stimuli making conversion of sensory input into electrical signals or nerve impulses which are transmitted to brain cells. In brain cells which produce thought as the Moon is afflicted in eighth house and sixth house is under aspect of Saturn placed in sixth house. All these clarifies that the very thought producing centre in brain and the centre from where directions based on the integrated nervous signals are sent to different body organs is diseased. Moon in eighth house having no planets clearly implies that the disease is of chronic type and of lingering nature due to Moon under aspect of Saturn.

The sign Virgo is also tenanted by the malefic Saturn whose situation there results in severe insomnia. Rahu is also there in first house in conjunction with Mercury causing multiple psychic disorders. The sub lord of the sixth house is Sun which is afflicted by Rahu and Uranus making certain and lifelong irrecoverable damage to central nervous system and peripheral nervous system; and as the planets causing the disease are placed in invisible portion the zodiac. The native suffered from this mental ailment since December 2012 when Moon in Mars mahadasha when she was running Moons period and Rahu bhukti dasha. Moon own sixth house is in eighth house.

She suffered from this nervous disorder, living with her parents in a continuous semi-unconscious state leaving Doctors confused about exact diagnosis. Sign lord Saturn is in ninth house referred as house affecting the very intelligence and is afflicted with presence of Rahu and Saturn. The star lord of ninth house is Rahu and in ninth house with Saturn signifies the cusp clearly. The sub lord of First house is Mercury which is significator of entire nervous system and lord of fifth house is placed in fifth house with star lord Mars is placed in first house indicating first house, Fifth house and Mercury all are afflicted giving severe depression and totally deterred MMP1 chart indicating serious psychological disorders further aggravated by Saturn from 135degrees with evil aspect on Mars which is significator of third and tenth house.

The fifth house rules the intelligent ability and cognitive behavior; the sub lord of this cusp is Venus is also in fifth house negating the effect of fifth house seriously affecting the very consciousness of the native. Here we can assess the important house i.e. cusp no six or house of diseases is occupied by sign of cancer so also house of emotion is owned by Moon i.e significator of mental health with star lord Saturn and Sub lord being Mars. This sign lord is Moon is chief governor of the mental disease placed in Taurus a fixed sign in the star of Sun in fifth house complicating the very nature of disease making diagnosis difficult further. Moon is also under aspect from Rahu creating disease serious. The star lord of 6th house is Saturn and as lord of first house and twelfth house is in ninth house in his own star and sub so also Moon is also in the sub of Rahu in ninth cusp. The sub lord of sixth cusp is Mars and also a lord of third cusp i.e. Aries which controls the neuro -motor transmission system giving cognitive thought pattern i.e. stability. Mars in first house with the star of Jupiter in sixth cusp a fixed sign denoting chronic level of ailment to the native; and Mars being with sub lord Saturn, in first and twelfth house owner placed in ninth cusp signifies the ninth house along with Rahu indicates serious and long duration mental ailments. The sixth house cusp sub lord Mars is also aspecting to Leo in seventh house from first house; this is indicator of diseases related to brain and affliction therein. The sixth house sub lord Mars in First cusp which is invisible sign with Star Lord Jupiter in Seventh house another invisible sign creating diagnosis impossible. The ninth cusp house of higher intelligence is also afflicted by Saturn and Rahu so also the lord of sixth cusp is placed in forth house afflicted by Ketu and under aspect by Saturn and Rahu. As such the complications resulted in death of native on 14th October 1978 in Rahu mahadasha Rahu Anter dasha and Mercury prati anterdasha. Rahu dasha lord is in Ninth cusp with star lord Saturn also in same cusp and in his own sub representing Mars as discussed occupied first house in Aquarius a fixed sign and Rahu is in Scorpio which is also a fixed sign. Again further ninth house is inauspicious for Aquarius ascendant leading the death of the boy in Rahu Maha dasha Rahu Anter dasha that to in Mercury Prati antardasha cause Mercury is owner of eighth house referred as malefic house for longevity. The very nature of the death can be determined by the eighth cusp and its significators. Sub lord of eighth cusp is ketu a node conjoined with Moon and under aspect by Mars that too when Ketu is with the sub lord of Rahu. Here Scorpio

defines that death occurs through the attack by some body and sudden clarifies that the boy was beaten to death by some body.

Sr. No	Planet	Nirayan DEG-Min-Sec.	Zodiac lord	Star lord	Sub lord
01	Sun	079—29—04	Mercury	Rah	Mars
02	Moon	031—01—33	Venus	Sun	Rahu
03	Mars	322—14—38	Saturn	Jup	Saturn
04	Mercury	063—00—33	Mercury	Mar	Venus
05	Jupiter	126—18—10	Sun	Ket	Rahu
06	Venus	061—01—07	Mercury	Mar	Merc.
07	Saturn	213—32—43	Mars	Sat	Saturn
08	Rahu	223—06—31	Mars	Sat	Rahu
09	Ketu	043—06—31	Venus	Moo	Rahu
10	Uranus	098—12—39	Moon	Sat	Venus
11	Neptune	184—30—05	Venus	Mar	Venus
12	Pluto	336—51—05	Jupiter	Sat	Mercu.

Chapter 8

Epilepsy and horoscope

Epileptic episodes are the result of malfunctioning in brain; this is characterized by sudden interruption in Brain function resulting in temporary unconsciousness or fainting. The intensity of attack ranges from minor to major body reaction. The most known symptom is frequently occurring violent convulsions and in rare cases genetic transfer of the disease into child even then it is not hereditary. The major cause of this disease are either brain injury in natal phase or in central nervous system, emotional reasons or alcoholic/drugs influence.

According to Astrological views the Epilepsy is the disease produced by afflicted or weak Mars, Mercury, and or weak Moon placed in malefic house. Mercury being the major planet affecting the entire nervous system and functioning of neuro motor transmission system, Mars governs the cranial nerves and Blood supply to brain cells and the Moon that governs the very levels of Serotonins, and Endorphins in body giving cause for mood swing when any of or all of these get affected or under aspect of planets like Neptune or Uranus give rise to sudden temporary disruption in brain functioning. Affliction of these planets in Aries may produce Epileptic attacks; or Ketu in evil aspect to Moon, and/ or Mercury in Aries give mysterious diseases. The very intensity of attack and effect over other systems in body may be judged in accordance with the specific star lord or sub lord of the relevant zodiac in which above planets are placed and be treated accordingly. Here notable observation reveals that in many cases psychological treatment like Rational Emotive Therapy, C.B.T. along with routine medicines works wonders in controlling and often eliminating disease totally. The sign Aries and the ascendant i.e. first cusp represent the head, brain; and the diseases like Encephalitis, Epilepsy, and frequent loss of consciousness, suicidal tendency when afflicted severely or with Afflicted Moon and Mercury in these cusps.

Sun represents heart, skin, head, and constitution of native. Moon represents Lungs along with mood swing, sleep disorders; Mars indicates energy levels, cranial blood supply, Mercury being cause for entire nervous system functioning, sudden mood swing. So also following sub in zodiac sign Aries indicate Epileptic attacks and onset of disease;

Aries Mars/Ketu/Ketu 0 deg. 00 min. and 00 seconds to 0 deg. 46 min. 40 seconds
Mars/Ketu/Mars   4 deg 46min 40 seconds to 5 deg 33 min. 20 seconds
Mars/Ketu/Mercury   11 deg. 26 min 40 seconds to 13 deg. 20 min. 00 seconds produces the Epileptic attacks when along with these Moon and mercury are severely afflicted in horoscope.   The sixth house represents the disease and eighth cusp represents the threat of death along with twelfth cusp denotes hospitalization. The sub lord of sixth cusp is the only indicator about disease and onset depends on both the dasha lord, Bhukti/Antar dasha lord and Prati antardasha lord period. Planets connected with sixth cusp and ascendant will produce the disease in there conjoined periods. In case sub lord of the sixth cusp is in twelfth cusp gives the 5 Diagnostic indicators of the disease are as given under,

a) Note the sub lord of sixth cusp,
b) Find out star in which the sub lord of the sixth cusp is placed,
c) Note the zodiac sign in which sub lord of sixth cusp is placed,
d) Also note the zodiac in which the star lord of sub lord of the sixth cusp is placed.
e) Then study the nature of the planet as in above and combine with zodiac sign
   This will give the clue about intensity and nature of the disease; so also disease will be occurred during the conjoined periods of the significators of Ascendant and sixth cusp.

Case 003 woman born on 02 May 1971 at 04: 39 am in Tirunamanallur with Lat. 011:46N and Long. 079:25 E

In this Horoscope Ascendant falls in20:47:00 in Pisces ruled by Jupiter as sign lord and Mercury as Star lord with Venus Sub lord. The ascendant lord Jupiter is placed in ninth house ; the house of higher intelligence and as there are no planets in Jupiter's star the Jupiter signifies clearly of Ascendant house and therefore gives mental worries and instability of thought so also Jupiter is in the star of Saturn which is lord of twelfth house, and Jupiter is under aspect of Saturn from third house being known as malefic house as it falls eighth from eighth cusp; so also Jupiter is further afflicted by Neptune in ninth house as Neptune is planet of mystery. Lord of sixth cusp strong signification of the onset of disease; and the native suffers from irrecoverable disease. The star lord of ascendant is Mercury which is significator of the disease Epileptic attacks; also rules the brain function including nerve motor transmission is in its own star in ascendant cusp, afflicted by Venus which is lord of eighth cusp so also Mercury is in the sub of Saturn the lord of twelfth cusp said to be malefic house.

The ascendant sub lord Venus which is also lord of eighth cusp again a malefic house and as such affects the function of brain. Venus also in the star of twelfth cusp and in the sub of Jupiter in ninth house afflicted by Saturn from third cusp which is malefic and thus being lord of ascendant giving all the significators of first cusp are well connected with ascendant, eighth cusp and twelfth house making recovery impossible. So also the Ascendant is in aspect of Uranus from seventh cusp creating the disease further aggravated. The sign lord and sub lord of sixth cusp i.e. Sun which rules the head and cranial blood supply is placed in sign of Aries in second house which represents the again brain and head is the primarily indicator of onset of disease Epilepsy ; in addition Aries is under aspect of sign lord Mars a planet associated with disease Epilepsy and Apoplexy or insanity making Epileptic episodes accounted for.

Venus own the constellation of sixth cusp; the house of diseases, and Mercury the planet which influences the episodes of Epilepsy is in its own star in Ascendant making house afflicted so also being the lord of eighth house. The onset of disease starts in Mahadasha of Mercury and antar dasha of Venus which are placed in ascendant and

indicate the connection of disease with that of head and brain. In this case Sub lord of eighth cusp shows the disease that takes away life i.e. life is threatened; also Saturn owns the sub lord of the cusp eighth is in star with Sun which is lord of un tenanted sixth cusp showing some ailments at the close of life. Saturn is in third house should perhaps be considered the death –inflicting disease in preference to its constellation lord Sun in Aries in second cusp. Saturn's sign lord Venus is rising in ascendant is said to be denoting the proneness to the onset of Epilepsy as disorder of genetic type also. Saturn is also aspect the sign in ninth cusp relating to the uterus and ovaries. This indicates that the native may have afflicted by some disorder in reproductive system possibly related to uterus and cervix. Now one may well conclude that the present ailment of epileptic attacka of native is curable one. And as it is true to say that when in Mercury mahadasha and Moon antardasha up to October 15th 1982 the native got fully recovered. This can be better summarized that Epilepsy attacks can be diagnosed by the bellow given planetary combination in terms of KP theory.

The sixth cusp sub lord must either be Mercury , Mars or Sun and should have connection with Ascendant cusp, Sixth cusp, and eighth house; also it should be noted that Sign Aries with presence of Sun being afflicted by planets Sun, Mars , Mercury then we can simply predict that the native is suffering from Epilepsy attacks.

Sr. No.	Name of Planet Deg. Min. Sec.		Lord of zodiac	Star Lord	Sub Lord
01	Sun	017—33--56	Mars	Venus	Mars
02	Moon	103—37--36	Moon	Saturn	Rahu
03	Mars	275—38--54	Saturn	Sun	Mercury
04	Mercury	359—53--20	Jupiter	Mercury	Saturn
05	Jupiter	220—47--05	Mars	Saturn	Sun
06	Venus	346—39--24	Jupiter	Saturn	Jupiter
07	Saturn	030—34--45	Venus	Sun	Rahu
08	Rahu	296—12--07	Saturn	Mars	Jupiter
09	Ketu	116—12--07	Moon	Mercury	Jupiter
10	Uranus	166—58--05	Mercury	Moon	Saturn
11	Neptune	218—55--05	Mars	Saturn	Venus
12	Pluto	336—39--00	Jupiter	Saturn	Mercur

Chapter 9

Heart and Horoscope

Cardiac called as Heart is the foremost important organ of the body without which life is absent; as such it is also most complicated organ of the body after brain. As we know everybody is afraid of the problems related to heart and also it has now started occurring as common over vast range of age, cast, creed, race and gender. The main function of heart is to pump blood at pre specified rate efficiently to all parts of body and when any obstruction or defect appears in the pumping of blood results in cardiac problems may sometimes lead to cardiac failure or attack due to coronary thrombosis even after slightest exercises or sometimes breathlessness, vertigo, severe fatigue, etc. Astrologically Heart diseases may be classified into following categories.

1.   Sudden onset of cardiac arrest.

2. Slowly developed disease due to problems in valves of the system
3. Developed over prolonged period due to deposition of fat over arteries.
4. Psychologically associated cardiac problems.

First of all we shall have to understand the very function of heart; the heart is comprised of four chambers; Right Atrium, Right Ventricle, Left atrium and Left Ventricle. Deoxygenated Blood from all over the body is brought through superior and inferior vena cava into first right atrium from where it is transported to Right Ventricle and then into Lungs for exchange of gases through pulmonary artery and then oxygenated blood is transported Left Atrium thru pulmonary vein and finally into left Ventricle. This oxygenated blood then pumped into arteries for cellular respiration. In all these flow channels there are valves located in heart called as tricuspid, ventricular orifice or pulmonary valve which prevent back flow of blood. During prolonged disease these valves or blood vessels gets affected due to either fat deposition (called stenosis)or some other defects which causes poor blood supply to heart muscles. On the other hand if valves affected or pre natal defects failing to operate normal may intermix the deoxygenated and oxygenated blood leading to short of breathing or severe fatigue after even normal body movements. Here importance of correlating the science of Astrology with that of Human physiology; also accord helping early diagnosis the onset of problem and period when likely to occur. And as such timely medical aid can be provided to arrest or prevent the very onset of disease. In case in birth chart planetary position reveal the symptoms of infliction with appropriate defects the native may immediately be taken up with medical fraternity for treatment.

Internal View of the Heart

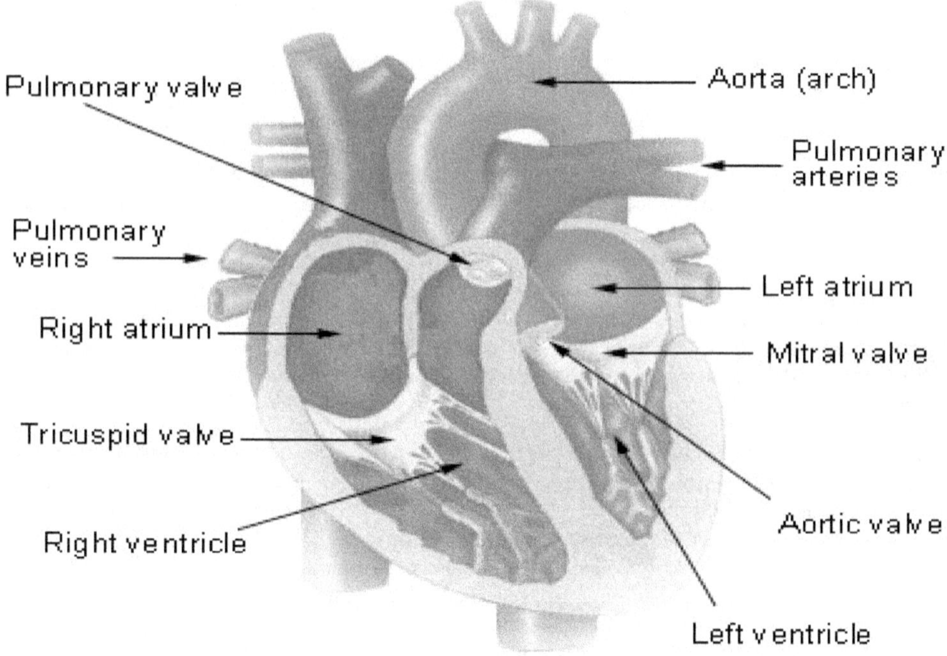

According to Horoscope fourth cusp from ascendant rules over the cardiac function including exchange of gases in lungs and the fifth sign of zodiac that is Leo governs the Heart in general so also Moon rules over Heart, along with Jupiter which rules the lungs. Mercury controls the very nerve supply to heart including electric signal supply to heart. Mars governs the brain and Sun in cancer may create problems; Aquarius or Pisces during their periods or at the time of birth; causes major problems related to heart. Moon in Gemini or Leo or during transit or even at the time of birth also gives the weakened heart. Malefic in Leo or Aquarius during their transit or at the time of birth also creates problems related to functioning of heart or even problems related to vessels and valves. When ascendant is in watery sign and the lord of ascendant in malefic house i.e. sixth, eighth, or twelfth are likely to develop problems specifically related to pumping of blood into Arteries. When the sign Leo or Aquarius and the fourth cusp are afflicted by Mars, Rahu, or Saturn the native shows symptoms of severe cardiac problems. When Saturn which governs the very breathing and exchange of gases in lungs afflicts the sign creates weakened heart.   The zodiac sign Cancer is major zodiac related to heart besides the sign Leo also represents the heart; The Moon and Sun signifies the heart where Sun rules the diseases of heart. When lord of fourth cusp placed in an inimical sign and weak, fourth house is occupied by Saturn or Rahu or Mars and Saturn, or Rahu and Mars or even retrograde Jupiter; which is under aspect from Mars indicates the pumping problems of the hearts in case not guarded by benefic planets. When Sun and Saturn conjoined in fourth cusp causes sinus as well as often ventricular tachycardia or in case under aspect from Mars and Rahu denotes the malfunctioning of heart valves. In case Mars and Ketu or afflicted Moon with two malefic in fourth cusp gives rise to either narrowing of vessels due to blockages or even abnormal heart rate causing severe problems. Coronary thrombosis or atherosclerosis i.e. sudden collapse of artery causes heart to cease the functioning; these results due to malefic influence of Mars in fourth house as Mars controls the blood circulation and exchange of gases in lungs. When in horoscope of any person if Mars is placed in fourth cusp produces Sinus tachycardia irrespective of zodiac sign and worsening it in case under aspect of malefic. Thus strength of fourth house importance and in any case either by association or by aspect with eighth cusp or lord of eighth cusp from any house indicates the heart disease; also significator for longevity i.e. Saturn may inflict the death of native due to cardiac malfunctioning; the key factors for cardiac diseases are Sun, Jupiter, Saturn, Moon, and zodiac sign Leo and specifically constellation Uttaraphalguni. The cardiac malfunctions are generally linked with the irregularities of blood pressure and operation of valves. The much dreaded planet Saturn is solitarily responsible for chronic or prolonged diseases; narrowing of vessels defects in vessel wall called vasculatis leading to poor blood supply to cardiac muscles. Where Heart the organ diseased or defected is indicated by presence of Saturn in fourth house or first house also indicates the natal defects or defects caused by particular other associated disease. As Sun is and or sign Leo is afflicted shows more proneness to the cardiac diseases, so also affliction of fourth house represents the indication of heart disease.   And along with these points if zodiac sign Cancer is afflicted anywhere in birth chart denotes the probability of cardiac defects.

Thus in short following conditions are necessary to be observed.   1) The ascendant, sixth house and significator of sixth house with significator of first house considered to diagnose the onset of cardiac problem.   2) Ascendant, Sun, Moon, and sixth cusp require to be assessed for fortified by status conjunction and aspect.

3) Strong and uninflected Sun and Moon are assets of health in birth chart. It ensures not only good health strong body and mind, and well defined cognitive functions. As we know heart receives deoxygenated blood from tissue of various body parts and oxygenated blood from lungs and then oxygenated blood is pumped to different tissues of body for cellular respiration and deoxygenated blood is pumped to lungs for exchange of

gases. And such acts as pumping organ. The following sub division of sensitive degrees in the sign Leo which governs the function of heart.

Degrees from and to having malefic affect	Zodiac lord	Star lord	Sub lord
00—00—00 to 00—46—40	Sun	Ketu	Ketu
03—40—00 to 04—46—40	Sun	Ketu	Moon
04—46—40 to 05—33—20	Sun	Ketu	Mars
09—20—00 to 11—26—40	Sun	Ketu	Saturn
11—26—40 to 13—20--00	Sun	Venus	Sun
29---13---20 to 30—00—00	Sun	Sun	Rahu

The lord of fourth cusp in natural zodiac, Moon governs entire thoracic region and nerve conduction and significator for heart. Moon is also said to govern mind which means Moon if afflicted results in anxiety and depression which in its turn increases stress hormone Cortisol that affects the digestive system and pulmonary function. Also Mars the lord of ascendant and eighth cup in natural horoscope afflicts Sun causes internal hemorrhage or thrombosis. Therefore effects of Planets Sun, Moon, Mars with zodiac Cancer and Leo including sixth, eighth and twelfth cusp certainly will indicate the onset of cardiac malfunction or other ailments.

Case no 004

A female born on 19 April 1967 at 03:50:00 am in Khopoli city of Maharashtra

This chart which shows Aquarius as ascendant, Venus lord of fourth house placed in own zodiac in fourth house, Sun in Aries in third house afflicted by Rahu also present in third house, The Moon in sixth house with Jupiter in Cancer and Uranus placed in seventh house in Leo aspecting Ascendant. Mars placed in Ninth house with ketu in Libra, and finally Neptune in Scorpio in tenth cusp aspecting fourth house. With reference to the primary observation it is clear that the First cusp is afflicted as under aspect of Uranus from Seventh cusp with Zodiac lord Saturn and Star lord Rahu afflicting the ascendant; Saturn placed in second house with Zodiac lord Jupiter, Star lord Saturn, and sub lord Mars which creates possibility of cardiac ailments. Sun placed in Aries and afflicted by Rahu in same Zodiac; so also the Seventh house Leo is afflicted with presence of Uranus. This indicates that the native will suffer from heart related problems. Fourth house as we see is under aspect from Neptune from Tenth house and zodiac lord of Neptune is Jupiter which aggravates the problem; the Moon in this chart which is creator of instability in mind and thereby aggravating stress is placed in sixth house, a malefic house known as cause of disease in own zodiac with star lord Mercury which its turn placed in second house and afflicted by Saturn with star lord also Saturn and sub lord Rahu indicating the abnormal heart function and gradual increase in Blood pressure with no known cause; Mercury also owner of eighth house indicating threat of disease with high intensity. Here as we see the Mercury is also owner of Fifth cusp which is house indicative of diseases associated with uterus leading to prolonged and persistent hormonal imbalance and further magnifying the nature of disease leading to onset of cardiac disease with constant hypertension from the period 19th February 2013 when Mahadasha of Sun was due in antardasha of Saturn and pratiantardasha of Mercury; a period when menopause occurred and hormonal imbalance got aggravated leading to sudden rise in hypertension. Also notable is that this is period when blockages in artery developed but not noticed in angiography which resulted in hypertension due to unknown cause. She suffered a lot since then till Sept 2019 when in Mahadasha of Moon with antardasha of Saturn and Prati antardasha of Rahu occurred. And this was period when she was advised to undergo Bypass surgery due to 99 % blockages in major artery supplying blood to Heart and was operated on 4th September 2019 when in Moon mahadasha with Saturn antardasha and Rahu prati antardasha. This surgery was successful as there was life threatening at that time.   Also it is worth noting that Ascendant Aquarius with star lord Rahu and under aspect fro Uranus was better placed during this period due to presence of Jupiter in

Sagittarius during period of surgery. Planetary position in birth chart is tabled below. So also it is worth noting that the metabolism in the body affected severely during this period causing skin problems, constant folic acid deficiency, gain in weight for no known reason, severe fatigue with loss of interest in living, and loss of control over management of emotions, leading to constant negative thought

Planetary position in birth chart as detailed bellow:-

Sr no	Planet	Zodiac	Degree: Minutes: Second	Zodiac Lord	Star Lord	Sub Lord
01	Sun	Aries	064:47:19	Mars	Ketu	Mars
02	Moon	Cancer	168:12:13	Moon	Mercury	Mercury
03	Mars	Libra	240:05:59	Venus	Mars	Mercury
04	Mercury	Pisces	043:16:35	Jupiter	Saturn	Rahu
05	Jupiter	Cancer	152:17:00	Moon	Jupiter	Rahu
06	Venus	Taurus	101:56:11	Venus	Moon	Rahu
07	Saturn	Pisces	042:16:00	Jupiter	Saturn	Mars
08	Rahu	Aries	074:12:35	Mars	Venus	Venus
09	Ketu	Libra	254:12:35	Venus	Rahu	Mercury
10	Uranus					

| 11 | Neptune | Scorpio | 270:15:15 | Mars | Jupiter | Moon |
| 12 | Pluto | Leo | 204:59:17 | Sun | Venus | Mercury |

Case 005

A male native born on 01st December 1989at 23:30: 00 in Pune city waked

The Horoscope of this person indicates the very afflicted Jupiter in eleventh cusp under aspect from Saturn, Uranus and Neptune and as lord of eighth house indicates short life. The ascendant Sun is placed in fourth cusp in Scorpio with lord of zodiac Mars star lord Saturn giving weak stature and there by affecting the function of heart, so also presence of Mars in third cusp indicate sudden and unwarranted onset of the disease. The fifth house is afflicted severely with presence of Satur, Neptune and Uranus under aspect of owner of malefic eighth house from eleventh cusp clearly denotes the sudden cardiac trouble. As it is evident from the chart that Moon with sub lord Rahu is also severely afflicted and further being conjoined with Saturn, Uranus and Neptune makes the native vulnerable to the disease related to cardiac. The ascendant Leo is also afflicted due to Star lord Ketu giving rise to unexpected sudden occurrence of cardiac failure. There was no sign of any symptoms showing any cardiac troublesuddenly develops the severe hyper acidity on 20th April 2019 requiring hospitalization due to breathlessness; presence of Ketu in twelfth house during Mahadasha of Rahu which is occupying Sixth house and Antardasha of the same planet Rahu. Here noticeable fact is that Mars from third house with star lord Venus occupying sixth house and afflicted due to Rahu leaves no chance of recovery or further treatment causing sudden infarction in cardiac muscles leading to death before even proper diagnosis is made. It is also note worthy that the person even when was advised adequate rest and overcome or get treated for insomnia ignored it as the significator Moon was also totally afflicted due to Saturn, Uranus and Neptune in Fifth house with sub lord also Saturn. Due to all these factors sudden death occurred on 20th April 2019. In this case it was worth noting that Sun was totally weak and was under aspect from Ketu placed in twelfth house leaving no time to take any measures for attending even emergency measures. When hospitalized the native was conscious complaining short breathing/breathlessness and the moment was taken on ventilator becomes unconscious leading to death within an hour's time.

Table showing planetary position is as given bellow.

Sr. No	Planet	Zodiac	Degrees: Minutes: Second	Lord of Zodiac	Star lord	Sub lord
01	Sun	Scorpio	105: 48:42	Mars	Saturn	Jupiter
02	Moon	Sagittarius	143: 44:45	Jupiter	Venus	Saturn
03	Mars	Libra	084: 55:18	Venus	Jupiter	Mercury
04	Mercury	Scorpio	117: 22:17	Mars	Mercury	Jupiter
05	Jupiter(R)	Gemini	315: 19:09	Mercury	Jupiter	Venus
06	Venus	Capricorn	150: 25:09	Saturn	Sun	Rahu
07	Saturn	Sagittarius	138: 26:45	Jupiter	Venus	Rahu
08	Rahu	Capricorn	176: 20:23	Saturn	Mars	Jupiter
09	Ketu	Ketu	356: 20:23	Moon	Mercury	Jupiter
10	Uranus	Sagittarius	130: 15:06	Jupiter	Ketu	Saturn
11	Neptune	Sagittarius	137: 12:11	Jupiter	Venus	Moon
12	Pluto	Libra	082: 21:08	Venus	Jupiter	Saturn

Case No 006

This is a case of male native; birth date is 11th May 1986 time 02:10:00 in Mumbai/Parel   this person born in Mumbai had healthy body till onset of the disease. The Horoscope shows Ascendant Aquarius is first afflicted by star lord Rahu of the cusp and under aspect of Saturn from tenth house creating serious ailments which are life threatening so also the Jupiter which gives longevity also is under aspect of Saturn and afflicted with Mars as star lord Mars which is placed in Sagittarius afflicted by Neptune creating ailments of myocardium. Sun placed in Aries with Mars as lord of zodiac with sub lord Saturn is afflicted and further weakened in conjunction with Rahu in same house having Ketu as sub lord. This weak Sun produces unexpected growth of tumor in body and also as Moon is also afflicted with sub lord Saturn and under aspect from Saturn and Uranus from tenth cusp making it further vulnerable to the carcinoma of wall of heart. It is noticed in as many as four cases that the combination of Saturn

With that of Uranus in any zodiac in tenth house causes the carcinoma of heart muscles which otherwise a rare disease. This has created the onset of the disease in native in diagnosed on 15th September 2018 when in mahadasha of Jupiter with anterdasha also of Jupiter in prati antar dasha of Rahu in its advanced stage. The native himself is Doctor medical by profession and is practicing Endocrinologist specialized in diabetes; now bed ridden.   In this case noteworthy point is that the owner of zodiac in which Sun is placed in third house is Mars and is severely afflicted in Sagittarius with Neptune causing permanent damage to the cardiac muscles shortening the life span. Also it should be noted that owner of eighth cusp called as malefic cusp Mercury is conjoined with sun and also further afflicted by presence of Rahu. Therefore expectancy of life is limited till Mahadasha of Saturn in antardasha of i.e. till October 2022.

Planetary position

Sr,. No	Planet	Zodiac	Degrees: Minute: Second :	Lord zodiac	Lord star	Sub Lord
01	Ascendant	Aquarius	012 :32:50	Saturn	Rahu	Saturn
02	Sun	Aries	086 :13:15	Mars	Venus	Ketu
03	Moon	Taurus	107 :17:15	Venus	Mars	Saturn
04	Mars	Sagittarius	324 :43:02	Jupiter	Venus	Mercury
05	Mercury	Aries	072 :34:26	Mars	Ketu	Mercury
06	Jupiter	Aquarius	023 :25:39	Saturn	Jupiter	Saturn
07	Venus	Taurus	103 :25:10	Venus	Mars	Mars
08	Saturn ®	Scorpio	283 :59:41	Mars	Saturn	Rahu
09	Rahu	Aries	065 :16:56	Mars	Ketu	Mars
10	Ketu	Libra	245 :16:56	Venus	Mars	Sun
11	Uranus	Scorpio	297 :55:41	Mars	Mercury	Saturn
12	Neptune	Sagittarius	281 :51:26	Jupiter	Ketu	Mercury

Chapter10

An Eye on constellations

The defects or diseases related to eye or eyes may be temporary or of chronic type are caused by either infection or degenerative changes or sometimes by accident in general but also caused because of other diseases like hypertension or diabetes even sometimes due to continuous exposure to light or toxic compound. So also the eyes are the mirror of different ailments in body existed elsewhere in body. In fact ophthalmic diseases are mainly classified into four major types listed bellow as 1) Conjunctivitis:- This is most commonly occurred ailment of eye usually indicated by red eyes excessive watery even sometimes constant irritation followed by head ache. This is actually a Vitamin A deficiency disorder occurring in most of the tropical countries due to malnutrition syndrome. But the Horoscopic causes are Mars and Ketu afflicted in Aries. And also when in transition of Saturn these planets are severely afflicted. 2) Cataract:- This occurs in many people when the crystalline lens of eye becomes opaque due to development of certain cloud type condition which gradually diminishes the vision. The cause being planets Moon, Mars when gets severely afflicted by Saturn or Ketu in Aries in birth chart Affliction of Venus in twelfth cusp and Sun in second cusp give rise to this disorder. The remedial cause is only feco emulsification replacement of lens.

3) Astigmation:- This is caused due to loss of property of tissues which changes the focal length of lens in eye and movement of aperture with respect to light intensity making things visible clearly. Malefic planets afflicting house second and twelfth in birth chart causes this defect. Also in case of hypertension and uncontrolled diabetes the disorder is occurred.

4) Night blindness and color blindness: - This occurs when in second and/or twelfth cusp Aries or Leo falls with affliction due to Rahu, Mars, Ketu or even most often Neptune in birth chart creates this disease. Here are some traditional planetary combinations considered creating problems in eyes.

1) When mars occupies Ascendant and/or Aquarius in first house likely to create blindness in natal stages.

2) In case lord of second and twelfth cusp conjoins with Venus as lord of ascendant and occupy sixth, eighth or twelfth cusp give rise to blindness.

3) In case malefic occupy fifth and fourth cusp native is likely developing eye complications.

4) If Sun and Moon conjoin in twelfth cusp and are under aspect of malefic planet develop blindness.

5) If Moon be in Sixth cusp, Sun being in eighth and Saturn or Venus placed in twelfth cusp with Mars in second will make native loose his eyesight.

6) If Saturn and Mars conjoin in second or twelfth cusp is likely to produce permanent blindness.

7) If Saturn and Venus occupy Leo in ascendant the native is likely suffer from eye diseases.

8) Malefic planets in sixth, twelfth and eighth house may aggravate the eye defects and create blindness.

9) Association of Ketu in second cusp with Sun or in twelfth cusp creates cataract which needs surgery in early age of life.

10) Mercury either in fifth house or any where is afflicted produces temporary blindness.

11) If Venus occupies sixth house, eighth house or twelfth house with Moon night blindness may occur.

12) When Sun and Venus conjoin in Leo may lead to color blindness.

13) Sun conjoined with Saturn in first or If seventh house affects the right eye; while in conjoin with Mars and Rahu, the Sun create the defect in left eye.

14) Conjunction of lord of first house, second house, sixth house, eighth house, and/or twelfth house gives rise to loss of eye sight or cataract is developed.

15) Sun and Moon in eighth house while malefic in sixth, eighth, or twelfth house produces eye defects.

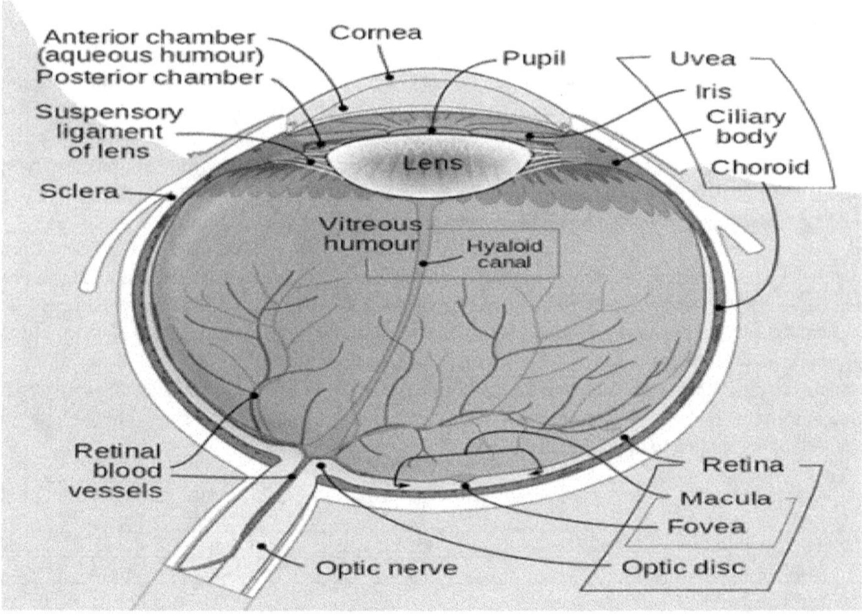

According to this postulate active vision or defective vision is caused by Moon, Sun, and Venus during their respective dasha period. Here the Venus is lord of Taurus the second house in natures chart Taurus rules over right eye.   Blindness at birth or natal period is a major defect and planets Sun, Moon, and Venus happen to be in sign/star/sub lord of eighth cusp are likely to create these defects. The house and their cusp to the eyes i.e. second and twelfth house and their sub lord be significator of twelfth house or connected to that house likely to create the defects.   The second house shows right eye and the twelfth denoting left eye and significator for right and left eye respectively. Venus is the significator of eye sight if afflicted by Rahu and Saturn give defects in vision. Any planet associated with constellation of the occupant or owner of second and twelfth house with sub-sub of the significator of twelfth house and connected with Sun, Moon, Venus, Rahu, and Saturn gives serious eye defects.   The sixth house indicator of disease and eighth house indicator of aggravation whilst twelfth house indicates hospitalization and hence the planets like Sun, Moon, and Venus any way connected to these houses by constellation or sub position they shall create defects in vision.

Case no 007

A female native having born on 26th August 1992 at 0100 am in Aurangabad Maharashtra

 The native female having horoscope; details as given here with, gives us the information for her permanently lost eye sight.

Here the ascendant house is occupied by Mars in Taurus which signifies the eye is with star lord Mars indicates some problems related to eye and owner of the ascendant Venus is placed in fourth house in Leo with again sub lord Mars creates complication in eye sight. Second house is occupied by Ketu in Gemini with star lord Mars makes further complications giving rise to irrecoverable disorder; so also Ketu under aspect of Uranus, Neptune and Rahu from eighth house which is said to be malefic house clearly denotes the difficulty in recovery. This further best can be explained sub lord of Uranus and Neptune being Venus which creates permanent blindness. Also we can understand it by observing the position of Moon in its own zodiac in third house with star lord Saturn in conjunction with Mercury defining the type of problem is associated with Choroid layer and makes ciliary body structure weak making expansion and contraction of Black aperture weak; also Sun in Leo with Ketu as star lord further complicates the very function of Fovea that gives sharp vision making it defective. In Choroid layer there are ruptured blood vessels creating the vision badly affected.   The occupant of ascendant i.e. Mars being lord of twelfth cusp permanently impairs the vision of Left eye; leaving no way for recovery. The onset of the vision blurring has started in the year 2001 December when Saturn mahadasha was active in antardasha Mars and prati antardasha of Rahu. This clears the impact of planets making defective vision; So also from birth the vision was may not be perfect but not this much deteriorated and only after onset of the disease in Saturn mahadasha and Mars antardasha here Mars being significator of vision defects has laid an impact that to in Rahu prati antardasha where Rahu is palced in malefic eighth house and aspects the second house with Uranus and Neptune leading to irrecoverable defects. Planetary position

Planes	Planet	Zodiac	Degrees: Minutes: Seconds	Lord of Zodiac	Star Lord	Sub Lord
01	Sun	Leo	099 :04 :01	Sun	Ketu	Jupiter
02	Moon	Cancer	066 :23 :45	Moon	Saturn	Mercury
03	Mars	Taurus	025 :50 :16	Venus	Mars	Jupiter
04	Mercury	Cancer	081 :42 :37	Moon	Mercury	Sun
05	Jupiter	Leo	116 :25 :10	Sun	Venus	Ketu
06	Venus	Leo	119 :02 :30	Sun	Sun	Mars

07	Saturn	Capricorn	260 :02 :10	Saturn	Moon	Ketu
08	Rahu	Sagittarius	213 :26 :54	Jupiter	Ketu	Sun
09	Ketu	Gemini	033:26:54	Mercury	Mars	Venus
10	Uranus	Sagittarius	230 :36:24	Jupiter	Venus	Jupiter
11	Neptune	Sagittarius	233 :42:19	Venus	Jupiter	Venus

Chapter 10

In Horoscope the second house rules the speech normally and planet Mercury is the factor that governs speaking skills; and as such affliction of any of these gives disturbed speech or even dumbness. The fifth house governs the intellect of native and if this house is afflicted the very speech gets affected; making native unintelligent or dumb who cannot speak or speaks with disturbance. The fifth, sixth, eighth, and twelfth cusps are important factors that defines the onset, intensity and details of the speech defects. So also during trauma of any type when occurs and Moon is either seriously afflicted or weak may create temporary dumbness.

If any malefic is present in second house or if second house or Mercury is severely afflicted anywhere in birth chart causes defective speech or even dumbness.

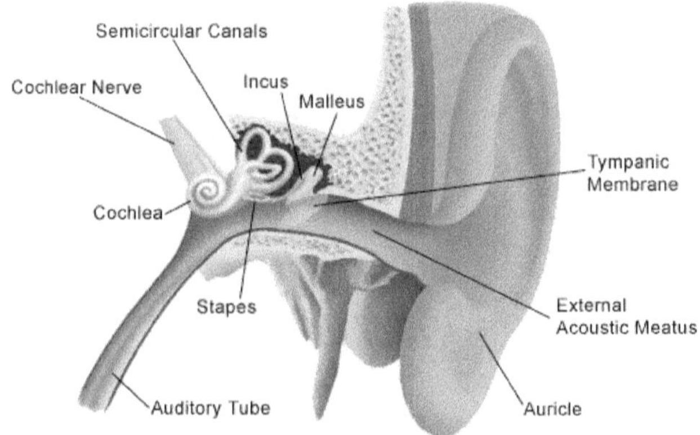

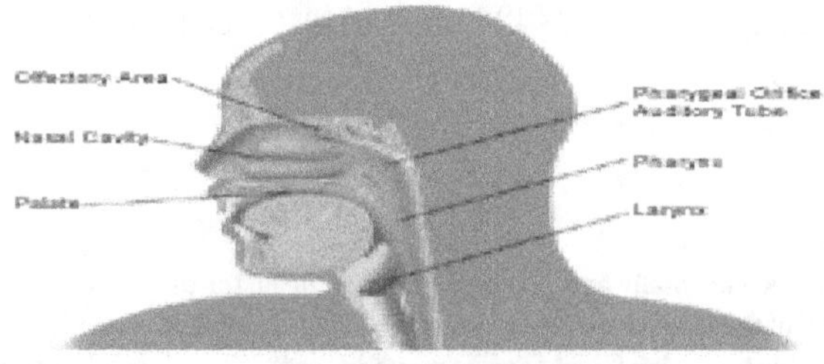

The defected speech only occurs when either second house is afflicted or Mercury is under aspect of malefic planets or connection of second house with any malefic star lord or Sub lord making it produce defects in speech or delayed speech or speech with disturbance and defective. If ascendant and second house both is afflicted and Mercury is free then the speech therapy works well and the native gets cured early; and if Mercury is afflicted then the native is likely to have permanent speech defect or problem in speaking. So also when Saturn is placed in Ascendant and Mercury is afflicted anywhere in chart and any malefic planet if placed in second house normally creates dumbness.

Following are the few points to be pondered to assess the root cause of the speech disorder. 1) When the lord of second cusp is associated with the lord of sixth cusp and under aspect from Saturn the native will be dumb. 2) If Mercury and lord of sixth cusp occupy the ascendant then native will be mute. 3) In case Jupiter and lord of sixth cusp occupy ascendant the native becomes mute. 4) In case Jupiter and lord of second cusp occupy the sixth, eighth, or twelfth house the native will become dumb.

5) In case Mercury occupies Cancer, Scorpio, or Pisces and is under aspect from the Moon which if positioned in day birth the native will be mute. 6) If Mercury is afflicted in ascendant or in seventh house the person becomes dumb. 7) If Mercury is in Cancer, Scorpio, and Pisces and is under aspect of Moon; and also occupy fourth cusp and under aspect of Sun or by malefic planet in sixth house the native is certain to be dumb.

8) In case Ketu occupies second house from the Lord of seventh cusp placed anywhere in chart give rise to dumbness. 9) In case Mercury occupies a sign owned by Saturn and under aspect form Saturn the native speaks with stammering or speech is faltering.

So also when there is dumbness it is normally associated with deafness and as such Third cusp and eleventh cusp are also considered respectively for right ear and left ear; and Gemini with Virgo which signs are owned by Mercury are considered to rule the function of hearing and speaking i.e. ear and Eustachian tube diseases.

1) If mercury occupies the fourth cusp from Saturn and lord of the sixth house is in sixth, eighth, or twelfth cusp from rising Sun the native becomes deaf due to irrecoverable defects in Tympanic membrane or Ossicles.
2) If Venus is conjoined with Mercury and occupy twelfth cusp the native develops defects in cochlea, Vestibule or semicircular canals of left ear.
3) If Venus and Mercury conjoin in third cusp the native becomes deaf by right ear.

4) If malefic are not under aspect from any benefic planet occupy third cusp,11th cusp, fifth cusp or eleventh cusp cause permanent defect in tympanic membrane and cavity leading to deafness. Also affliction of Mercury by Sun and Saturn in third or 11th cusp native develops defect in hearing.

We can have an example of female who is dumb and deaf as detailed here with for understanding of above rules.

Case no. 007

The native mentioned herewith is born on April 4th 1972 at 22:57 in Cuddalore in Tamilnadu having Lat. 011:42N and Long 079:48E.

As we have seen the second cusp and planets related to this cusp indicates defects in speech or fluency in speech; so also Mercury which is indicative of expression, when gets afflicted either by conjunction or by aspect or by association of any type with Uranus, Saturn, Neptune is known to create defects in speech. Cancer, Scorpio, and Pisces are known to be mute signs and dumbness is caused by affliction in these signs. Mute signs are supposed to cause impediments of speech specifically when Mercury is afflicted. Apart from these Taurus, Gemini are also considered as they rule the vocal cord, and cochlea with vestibule including semicircular canal which converts the sound waves into electrical signals to be send to Brain.
With respect to KP system Sub lord of the second cusp related to dumbness whilst third cusp is related to deafness and subdivision in Taurus i.e. Venus-Moon-Ketu at 019deg. 40min. 00sec. to 020deg .40min.00sec.gives the indication about defective or mute. And like this following subdivisions in the sign Gemini indicates the ear diseases and deafness.

1) Mercury-Rahu-Jupiter: 008deg 40min 00 sec. to 010deg 26min 40sec. Cochlear problems.
2) Mercury-Rahu-Mercury 012deg 33min20sec. to 014deg 26min 40sec. Tympanic membrane and Tympanic cavity.
3) Mercury-Rahu-Venus: 015deg 13min20sec to 017deg 26min 40sec Cochlear vestibule.
4) Mercury-Rahu-Moon: 018deg 06min40sec   to 019deg 13min 20sec Semicircular cannals.

If sub lord of second cusp is Mercury the native becomes over talkative and if it is Mars native becomes out spoken and blunt. If it is Saturn the native will be less talkative not ready to open up, if Ketu then native frequently use abusive words so also often defective speech and if these are in second house stammering occurs. In the above mentioned chart the ascendant considered to fall 00deg 00min 00sec in Sagittarius; while observing the chart it is seen that the ascendant is occupied by its owner Jupiter; a powerful benefic planet and its position in the ascendant greatly helps the matter connected with the health. But Jupiter in the star of Venus in sixth house creates the defects. According to KP the sub lord of the second cusp is Rahu and the second cusp is also falls in Sagittarius ruled by Jupiter. The constellation is ruled by the Sun and sub is ruled by Rahu ;a general malefic as positioned in second cusp itself. The sub lord of Rahu is also constellation Moon, lord of sign Gemini which is a mute sign. Rahu is also in the sub of Moon. Further the affliction of Saturn and Mars in Taurus, the second house of natural Zodiac ruling vocal organs i.e. throat etc.. The significater planet is also affected in Pisces which is again a mute sign. The above combination reveals the fact about defects in speech and dumbness.

The girl has been admitted in School for dumb and deaf in Chennai during July 1977 when in mahadasha of Mars and dasha lord was in sixth house; in the star of Moon in second cusp and Mars is in the sub of Jupiter which is lord of first cusp occupying sixth cusp. The child was dumb and deaf from birth.

Sr. No.	Planet	Zodiac	Degree : Min : Sec	Zodiac lord	Star lord	Sub lord
01	Sun	Pisces	141 : 34 : 01	Jupiter	Mercury	Sun
02	Moon	Scorpio	025 : 57 : 45	Mars	Mercury	Rahu
03	Mars	Taurus	192 : 05 : 42	Venus	Moon	Rahu
04	Mercury	Pisces	133 : 59 : 24	Jupiter	Saturn	Rahu
05	Jupiter	Sagittarius	044 : 12 : 42	Jupiter	Venus	Venus
06	Venus	Taurus	187 : 18 : 33	Venus	Sun	Ketu
07	Saturn	Taurus	189 : 40 : 06	Venus	Sun	Venus
08	Rahu	Capricorn	068 : 08 : 20	Saturn	Sun	Venus
09	Ketu	Cancer	248 : 08 : 20	Moon	Saturn	Venus
10	Uranus	Virgo	322 : 52 : 26	Mercury	Moon	Sun

In astrology Saturn is the most caustic planet and leaves behind the ailments for life time or prolonged diseases; it governs the worst and most chronic ailments. When Saturn afflicts fourth house from ascendant or from Leo the native suffers from pulmonary diseases, Moon in Gemini or in Leo also; in birth chart gives status asthmatics. This is practically incurable disease; the fourth cusp in birth chart rules the lungs and pulmonary function.   It is the Moon that rules the function of lungs and exchange of gases in lungs; so also fifth cusp of natures horoscope governs the heart and pulmonary artery that brings the impure blood to lung, plays great role in these ailments.

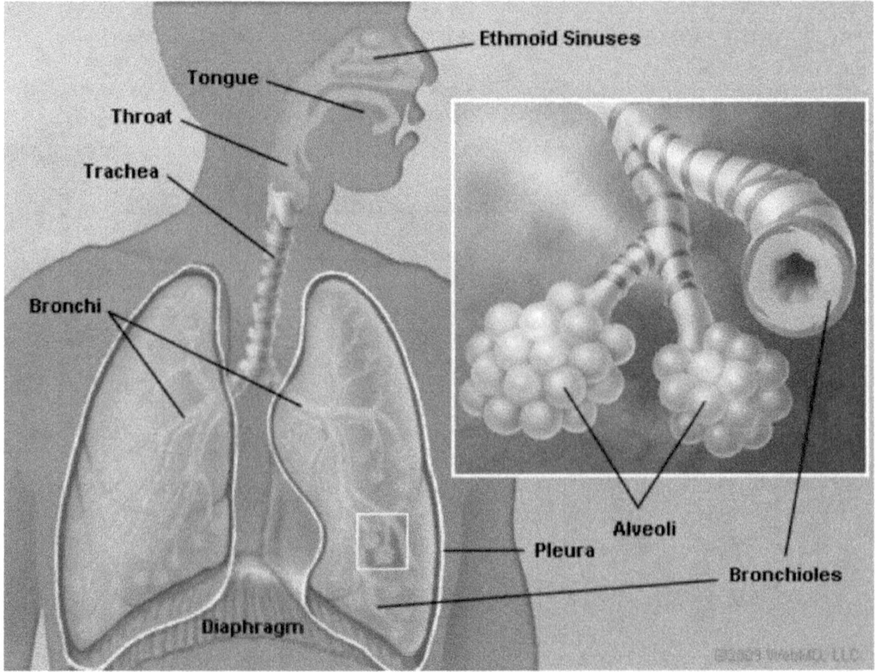

The pulmonary ailments so called are normally making human being suffer, are classified in four types i.e. 1) Asthma 2) Cold and cough 3) Allergic reaction 4) Lung Cancer.   1) Asthma: This is characterized by inflammation of bronchial tubes with secretion of histamines or phlegm which gives severe inflammation of wind pipe and creates obstruction in airways leading to coughing, wheezing, shortness of breath, chest tightness, pain in chest, pressure, sleepless nights. This usually caused when fiery sign Leo is occupied by planets with hot constitution the native suffers from Asthma; so also Mars, is afflicted in Leo it creates, and the native suffers from secretion of histamines. So also it creates inflammation of airways leading to asthmatic condition. Thus Sun, Jupiter, Mars, in Leo give rise to asthma; Saturn in Leo produces pleurisy. As such we can conclude that Saturn is major planet which if afflicts fifth cusp or Sign Leo, the native becomes status asthmatics; also Saturn is obstructive planet and when afflicts any planet in Leo acts as causative factor for Asthma condition. Symptoms are not same in all persons; varies with respect to the placement of Jupiter and Sun in the Horoscope. And sometimes the episodes or attacks may occur with delay or may occur frequently.   2) Cold and cough :- This occurs normally with cold climate or dusty climate, even sometimes due to pollen grains in air may cause these types of diseases; as per horoscope study the signs Gemini, Libra, and Aquarius govern the respiratory function i.e. exchange of gases in lungs, and therefore following planetary combination will cause the respiratory trouble.

1) When Cancer is in the rising sign with Mars occupied it; so also when Saturn occupies these signs the respiratory syndrome may occur.
2) When Ascendant is watery sign and the lord of ascendant cusp occupies malefic cusp respiratory diseases are produced.
3) When the lord of fourth cusp and sixth cusp exchange their cusp and if one of the sign so exchanged is watery sign respiratory diseases are occurred.
4) When Saturn which governs the very breath afflicts the fourth cusp the native is likely to suffer from respiratory diseases.
5)   If Mars and Saturn conjoin in the ascendant, and if ascendant is watery sign then respiratory syndrome is occurred.
6)   If lord of ascendant and Saturn conjoin in sixth cusp, eighth cusp or twelfth cusp then native suffers from respiratory diseases.

3) Allergic reactions:- In this type of allergic reaction normally sputum eosinophillia or eosinophillic asthma which occurs due to increase in white blood cells and also when fluid from blood vessels gets into air sacs in lungs while exchange of gases in lungs. This creates edema of lungs creating histamines and obstruction of airways. In these cases often it is noticed that sudden occurrence of these may sometimes create Cyanosis i.e. blue nails/ lips; or fainting, fatigue.   In these cases often emphysema is also seen. This is also related to smoking and exposure to chemical gases. This is the effect of sixth cusp and eighth house is occupied by

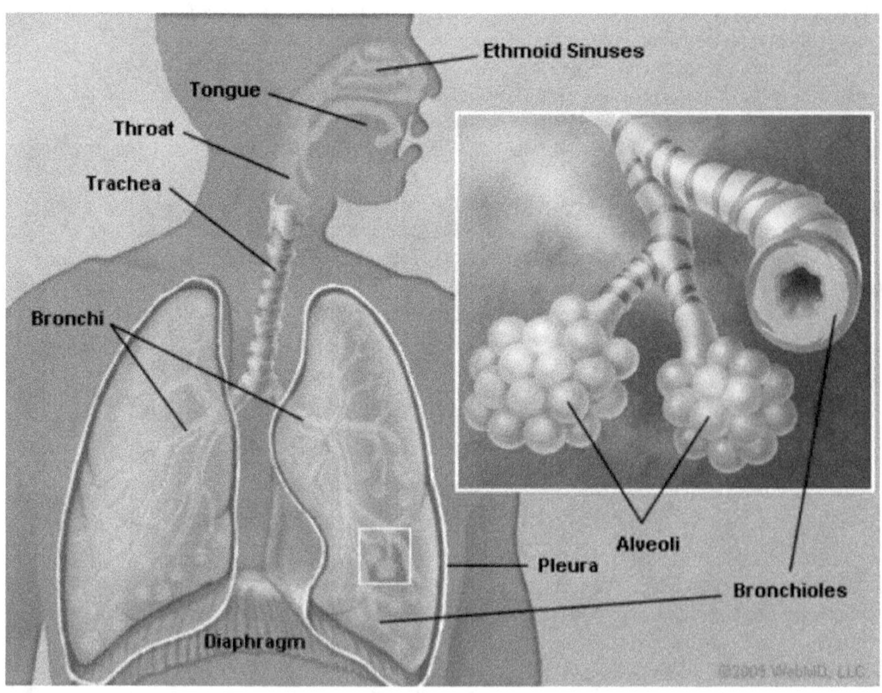

Trachea and major bronchi of the lungs

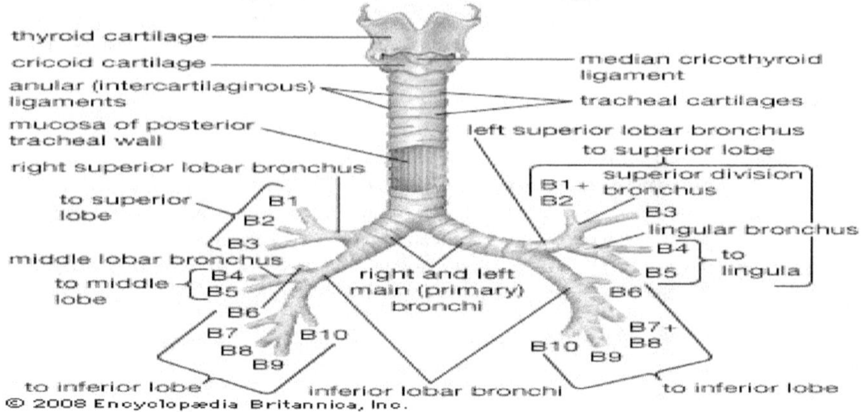

Mercury-Rahu-Moon   018deg: 06min: 40 sec. to 019deg:13min: 20 sec   Mercury-Jupiter-Mercury   023deg:53min: 20 sec. to 025deg:46min:20 sec

4) Lung cancer or Tuberculosis:- Acute respiratory distress syndrome is often noticed while in accident when

lungs are injured, so also when in advanced Tuberculosis or Lung cancer sometimes this is noticed. The disease Tuberculosis was very common few years back now due to availability of new drug combination it is very much reduced. The cancer of lungs is occurred in mostly smokers and as such referred as smoker's syndrome. In both the above types the lung function is severely affected due to damage of tissue of small clusters in lungs where the exchange of gases takes place and thereby creating obstruction in exchange. So also when because of these diseases the deoxygenated does not get purified leading to short of oxygen in tissues fatigue is observed. The cause of this syndrome can be explained better by Astrology as discussed bellow. According to KP system the sub lord of sixth house is either Saturn or connected to fixed sign like Taurus, Leo, Scorpio, or Aquarius the native suffers from Tuberculosis; if the lord of sixth cusp is Mercury or Saturn and in any way connected to fourth or fifth cusp and also signs like Gemini, Leo the native will suffer from lung cancer. If the same is connected to eighth cusp and fixed sign then death certainly occurs. Hence for diagnosis of this disease we have to study the sub lord of sixth cusp, planets Mercury, Saturn, Moon and Jupiter along with signs Gemini, and Leo. Also the cusps fourth and fifth are also required to be scrutinized.

We can study further with this example as stated.

Case no 007   This male native is born on 19th September 1953 at Dadar/Mumbai with Lat. 019:19 N Long 072:50

With this case the ascendant falls in Taurus 020 deg—00min—24sec, Venus as sign lord, Moon as Star lord and Ketu as Sub lord. The sign lord Venus is in Leo; the fifth sign of natural zodiac. Venus is in constellation of Ketu an occupant of Cancer, signifying the respiratory problems

Sign Leo also represents pulmonary disorders; Venus is in its own sub and also lord of sixth house, occupied by Saturn. The star lord of Ascendant, Moon is placed in ninth cusp afflicted by conjoining with Rahu; and Cancer in third malefic house afflicted by Ketu giving rise to debilitate Moon which is certain to produce respiratory diseases with complications. The sub lord of Moon i.e. Jupiter is in Gemini and also being lord of eighth cusp causes the irrecoverable respiratory diseases. The sub lord of ascendant is Ketu placed in sign Cancer in third cusp with star lord being Saturn; being known to cause chronic ailments and severe obstructions in airways also increases the severity of the disease. Saturn is placed in sign Libra which governs the function of exchange of gases in lungs produces obstruction leading to state called Asthma. So also Ketu is in Sub of Mercury a significator of the disease Asthma.   The sixth cusp is owned by Libra i.e. Venus as sign lord and Rahu as Star lord with Venus as sub lord; interesting to note here is that the Venus is placed in sign Leo which is an important sign for respiratory diseases. The sixth cusp is under aspect of Jupiter; lord of eighth cusp and planet of breathing disorders, when placed in Gemini that produces histamines in body creating allergic reactions is also afflicted by Uranus. The star lord of sixth cusp is Rahu with star lord Sun which owns the zodiac Leo causing Acute Respiratory Distress Syndrome is placed in fifth cusp indicating respiratory disorders with significator Rahu confirms the onset of disease. Further we can confirm by understanding that planet i.e. sub lord of sixth cusp is Venus and as lord of ascendant and sixth house is placed in sign Leo in fourth cusp which is governor of function of

Lungs and indicator of Asthma; with star lord Ketu , a significator of sixth cusp and in its own sub lord making the disease severe and difficulty in recovery.

The fourth cusp related to chest diseases, fifth cusp which is further indicator of function of lungs also needs to be studied further for accuracy in diagnosis of this disease; as here we see the fourth house is afflicted by Mars, the lord of this cusp Sun is also afflicted by Neptune in fifth cusp. The sub lord of fourth cusp is Jupiter which is lord of eighth cusp; a malefic house and is in sign of Gemini producing the obstruction in lungs and airways. Jupiter is with star lord Mars placed in fourth cusp and in sign Leo making disease further complicated and weakening the native. As the sixth cusp is afflicted by Saturn; a planet of chronic and prolonged type of nature of disease and the sub lord of sixth cusp Venus is placed in fixed sign Leo in fifth cusp, the native will have to suffer through out of her life. The diseases of respiratory organs made its first appearance in Mahadasha of Rahu in antardasha of Ketu in June 1978 at the age 24, and we can ascertain here that Rahu is in ninth cusp afflicting Moon; the planet again concerned with respiratory or allergic types of diseases. Rahu is with star lord Sun which in turn is owner of fourth cusp Leo. Rahu represents as star lord of sixth cusp and hence onset of the disease in Rahu Mahadasha giving chronic type of disease. The native will suffer from this ailment through entire next Mahadasha of Jupiter for 16 years followed by next Mahadasha of Saturn for 19 yrs i.e. for prolonged period. The nature of death can be found from significators of eighth cusp as the sub lord of eighth cusp is Venus which is lord of ascendant and sixth cusp and sub lord of sixth cusp placed in sign Leo, a fixed sign and hence the death due to ailment of respiratory function clearly indicated. As such the death occurred on 22nd May 2017 due to multiple organ failure.

5) Planetary position in birth chart.

Sr. No	Planet Name	Name of zodiac	Deg. : Min: Sec	Lord of Zodiac	Star Lord	Sub Lord
01	Sun	Leo	123 : 15 :24	Mercury	Sun	Saturn
02	Moon	Capricorn	255 : 03 :45	Saturn	Moon	Jupiter
03	Mars	Leo	099 : 55 :55	Sun	Ketu	Saturn
04	Mercury	Virgo	133 : 20 :54	Mercury	Moon	Rahu
05	Jupiter	Gemini	032 : 13 :05	Mercury	Mars	Ketu
06	Venus	Leo	091 : 25 :45	Sun	Ketu	Venus
07	Saturn	Libra	152 : 55 :00	Venus	Mars	Venus
08	Rahu	Capricorn	247 : 00 :03	Saturn	Sun	Ketu
09	Ketu	Cancer	037 : 00 :03	Moon	Saturn	Mercury
10	Uranus	Gemini	059 : 11 :38	Mercury	Jupiter	Sun
11	Neptune	Virgo	149 : 24 :36	Mercury	Mars	Saturn

Chapter 13

Cancer and Planets

The term Cancer is considered as certainty of death in near future with pains and sufferings. There are various verities of Cancer with even different terminology and aspects. Cancer cell differ from normal cells in body in many ways; normal cells become cancerous when series of mutation leads the cell to continue grow and divide out of control. Cancer cell is a cell that achieves state of immortality. These cells remain in the region where they began to grow. They have ability to both invade nearby tissues and spread to distant region of the body. Body may not recognize the cancer cells and as such our immune system cells called natural killer cells which have job of finding cells that have become abnormal and remove them; cannot remove them. There are many types of cancer cells as there are types of cancer; most are named after the tissue where they have began to grow. Carcinomas are cancer cells that arise in epithelial cells; Sarcomas are cancer cells that arise in mesenchymal cells in bone, muscles, blood vessels, tissues. Leukemia's, Lymphomas and myelomas are blood related cancers; they are fed by nutrients from blood stream, and Lymph fluid; such that they don't need to form tumors. Various cancer cells behave differently; they appear through a series of genetic and epigenetic changes. Some of which are inherited and some are caused by carcinomas in environment like asbestos or other irritants. These are solid tumors and thus form by multiple mutations. Interestingly by the metastatic process and this is the main culprit for high mortality rate in advanced cancer is thought to be caused mostly by epigenetic changes as no specific genetic alteration have been formed in

metastasis. Now if we look into the horoscope reference it is found that following conditions are necessary to allow cancer cells form or epigenetic metastatic mutation to take place are--

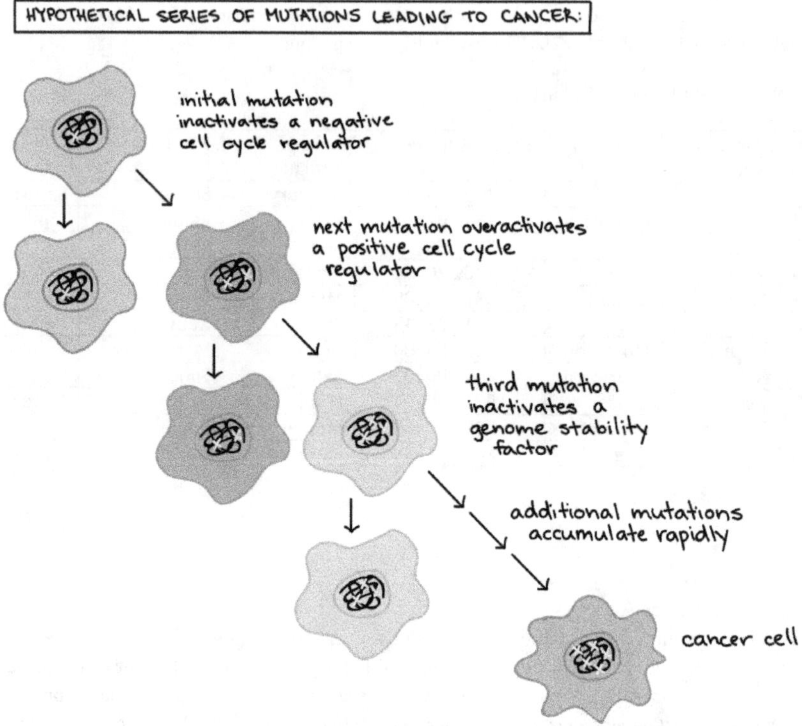

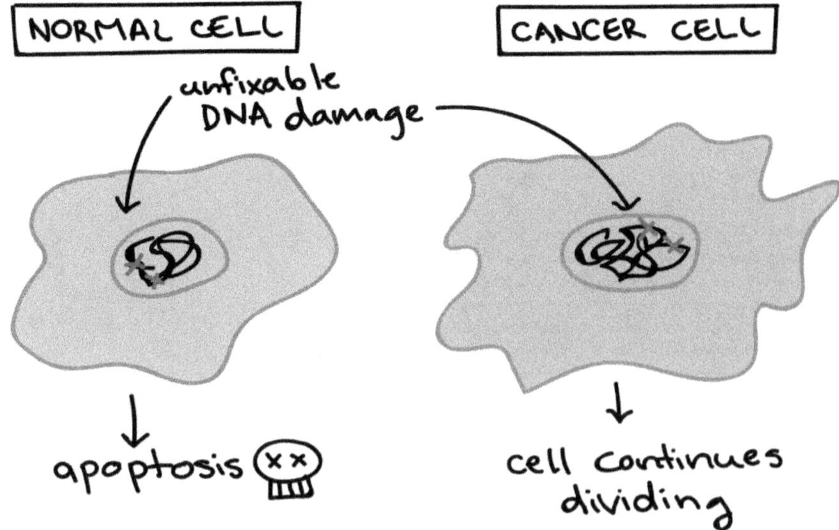

1) If Moon is afflicted by three malefic in any sign the epigenetic metastasis start and cancer cells start growing.

2) If Saturn and Mars in sixth cusp are under aspect from Rahu and Sun, Cancer cells are formed.

3) Malefic in fifth and Sun in sixth, eighth or twelfth cusp or Sun is severely afflicted the metastatic mutation start anywhere in body.

4) If Mars joins the lord of sixth cusp in ascendant, sixth house, seventh house and tenth house may start metastatic mutation in body.

5) Saturn in fourth cusp with Venus and Mercury, and when Sun is also afflicted severely affects the mutation leading to growth of cancer cells.

It is also customary to note that genetic predisposition does not mean the native will get cancer, but simply if few mutations are already in place will likely take few more acquired mutations to become cancer cells. This better can be explained by following conditions in birth chart.

1) Combination of Rahu Saturn under aspect of other malefic may allow cells for further mutations to become cancerous.

2) Saturn, Mars combination in sixth cusp, eighth cusp, twelfth cusp or in seventh cusp may cause cancer cells to grow further.

3) Conjunction of Saturn, Ketu, and Jupiter in any sign may help these cells with acquired mutation to get converted into cancerous cells.

The process of normal cells become cancer cells often goes through different stages of epigenetic changes making it progressively more abnormal in appearance. These stages may include Hyperplasia, Dysplasia and finally come to mutation which results in the growth of cancerous cells. These cancer cells are called as driver mutation causing cells and others called as passenger; normal genes called proto-oncogenes can become oncogens when mutated. Code for protein that drives the growth of cancer and give cancer its immortality. Tumor suppressor genes in contrast are genes within cells which tell the cell to slow down and stop growing; repair damaged DNA, or tell cells to die. Most cancer cells have mutation in both oncogens and tumor suppressors which lead their behavior as such most cancer cells are detected and removed from body system, these in our immune system cells called as Natural killers. They have job to find out the abnormal cells and to remove them. In some conditions which confuse these cells is called CIS; that is Carcinoma in Situ cells have abnormal changes and confuse immune system or killer cells to find them. These conditions are again ruled by following horoscope condition,

1) Conjunction of Jupiter, Ketu and Venus in any sign may cause development of Oncogens.
2) Conjunction of Moon-Ketu, Saturn-Moon, Ketu-Mars, Mars-Moon, and Moon-Rahu-Saturn may cause the stage called Hyperplasia, Dysplasia to take place and reduces effect of Tumor suppressant cells.
3) Mars if placed in sixth cusp in fixed sign may give rise to growth of tumors in body.
4) Saturn if placed in sixth cusp in dual sign may help grow oncogens.

The Rahu and Saturn and Mars are the planets which cause malignant growth anywhere in body. The lords of sixth, eighth cusp, and twelfth cusp are responsible for cancerous growth anywhere in body. So also when the lord of the sixth house joins the ascendant, eighth or tenth house and afflicted Rahu cancerous growth takes place in respective part of body. So also Saturn and Moon if afflicted or planes Neptune and Saturn are considered cause of the disease. The midpoint of Saturn and Neptune in natal chart are normally considered for confirming this disease; where this point denotes chronic type of the disease, in case this point is afflicted severely the cancer becomes cause of death

The sixth cusp is called as house of disease and eighth gives intensity of the disease whilst twelfth house indicates hospitalization and isolation. The sixth house is responsible for onset of the disease; but all natives with malefic planet in sixth house do not suffer because the same significator of sixth house may not become also significator of ascendant. The sixth cusp reveals the type of disease that native may suffer; sixth cusp is ruled by three planets as the lord of the sign in sixth cusp, lord of the star of sixth cusp and lord of sub; where this sixth cusp falls, if it is Venus ruled sign Moon star and Venus as sub lord then the native is likely to be diabetic. The disease cancer is indicated when the significator of sixth cusp, eighth cusp or twelfth cusp conjoins with Rahu.

1) If the sub lord of sixth cusp is Sun and signifies sixth, eighth and twelfth houses with reference to Rahu then growth of tumor specifically in stomach and or intestine.
2) If the sub lord of sixth cusp is Moon then likely hood of breast cancer and afflicted by Mars then blood cancer may occur.
3) If Mars is the sub lord of sixth house then it may be cancer in neck, head and if Uranus is present in sixth cusp then cancer of ovaries may occur.
4) If Mercury is sub lord of sixth cusp then cancer may occur in mouth or navel.
5) If Jupiter is sub lord of sixth cusp then cancer may occur in liver, tongue, or ears.
6) If Venus is sub lord of sixth house then it may occur in Throat, Prostate, or Uterus.
7) If Saturn is sub lord of sixth house then cancer may occur in hands, legs, or mouth.
8) If Rahu is sub lord of sixth cusp then cancer may occur in cervix of uterus, veginal vault or tissues of penis.
9) If Ketu be the sub lord of sixth house then cancer may occur in feet.

There are two rules as per KP system of diagnosis and these are 1) the cusp rule and 2) the significator rule.

The cusp rule states the nature of the disease and part of body affected where as the significator rule states us the exact time of onset of the disease.

a) The cusp Rule i.e. the nature of the disease

To predict the nature of the disease we can follow these steps

1) The sub lord of sixth cusp to be noted
2) The constellation in which the sub lord is placed
3) The sign where the lord of the constellation is placed
4) The sign where the sub lord is placed.

Then study both the signs as in 3 and 4 as well both the plan

5) The houses signify the planet as in 1 and 2 or connected in broad sense for exact location of growth of cancer cells.
6) Lastly combine the 5 and 6 together and considering all predict the nature of disease and part affected. Here the nature of the disease can be predicted by the nature of the planet involved in all respect and nature of zodiac as per Natures chart will indicate the part of the anatomy affected. This is called as cusp rule as per KP system.

b) Significator rule to assess the exact period / time of the disease.

    1) First find out the Significators of the houses ascendant and sixth

    2) Take common significator as in 1 if no common significator then find out the strong significator and look at the connection of planets with house of malefic or eighth house.

    3) Take the planet which is under aspect of or conjoined with strong significators, then make list of significators and in case if significators are connected either with ascendant or sixth house or eighth house.

    4) Take all above notes into consideration i.e. sub lord also be the significator of ascendant or sixth cusp or eighth cusp and its relation with part of the body; the significator thus obtained are strong significators.

    5) Lastly predict the time of onset according to Mahadasha, with strong significator when their conjoined period, the transit of the dasha lord which is phase with period of disease. That means until sub position synchronizes with significator for that event is considered as strong significator.

    Case no. 008 A female native   Birth date 16th May 1952 at 1645 hrs in Ahemdnagar of Maharashtra   With Lat: 019: 05N Long: 074: 44 E

If we study this chart following points we can seat first glance that the ascendant falls in sign of zodiac Libra owned by Lord Venus which is also a lord of eighth cusp Taurus, the ascendant star lord is Mars; and Sub lord is Mercury which again is sub lord of eighth cusp. The sign Libra is stable sign and earthy also. The ascendant lord is Venus represents the body is also significator of uterus, the prevailing reproductive system. It is with Jupiter the lord of sixth cusp placed in seventh house indicating the part of body that may get affected i.e. again Uterus; and with the lord of eighth cusp i.e. again Venus, here the Jupiter and Venus are under aspect of Mars from ascendant house also aspects Mercury sub lord of ascendant and eighth cusp. The sixth cusp is under aspect of Saturn from twelfth house so also from Neptune; Saturn being sub lord of Jupiter and Mars has become the cause of the disease which existed for long period. Mars placed in the sign Libra with zodiac lord Venus and aspect Venus in seventh house and sub lord of Mars i.e. Rahu is placed in fifth house indicates the growth of tumor in Uterus. Saturn as sub lord of Mars and as sub lord of Jupiter is also sub-sub lord of Ascendant creates the onset of disease and aggravates the disease. The Rahu placed in fifth house is afflicting Moon, which

Governs the production of Carcinoma In situ i.e. cells with abnormal changes in them; and presence of Rahu in zodiac owned by Saturn i.e. Aquarius creates conditions for growth of mutagenic virus called Human Pappiloma Virus which brings about the series of mutation in endometrial cells causing onset of the disease. Saturn being placed in twelfth house is further afflicted by Neptune in the same house and the lord of the zodiac of this house is placed in seventh cusp conjoined with the lords of sixth and eighth houses making hospitalization several times during disease; Saturn is also sub lord of Jupiter owner of sixth house and Mars owner of seventh house placed in ascendant creates further complications in native making suffered from other ailments such as cardiac problems. The lord of ascendant is also a lord of eighth house and sub lord of Rahu placed in fifth house; where the house represents Kidney and Reproductive system is afflicted severely denoting the gradual growth of disease which goes uninterrupted even with invading by drugs. Here we can note that sub lord of Rahu is again Venus owner of eighth cusp making the case more vulnerable and incurable. Mars the star lord of Rahu is zodiac lord of Venus and Jupiter the owners of Eighth and sixth house respectively aspects them making the disease severe. The Sun placed in eighth cusp owns the eleventh house occupied by Ketu aspects in its turn Rahu and Moon in fifth house and so also Sun making native suffer psycho somatically also. Neptune in twelfth house in Virgo indicates the persistence of disease even after Hysterectomy and reoccurs eventually. The sub lord of Sun i.e. Jupiter owner of sixth house is also sub lord of Venus and zodiac lord of Mars is star lord of Venus indicating the growth of cancer repeatedly occur even after total removal by surgery.

As such this becomes the classic case of invasion of cusps sixth eighth and ascendant with planets Mars, Jupiter and Venus indicating onset, growth and causing serious complications beyond the realms of recovery. Here we can see the onset of disease as on 16th Nov. 2005 when in Mahadasha of Saturn and was required to undergo surgery on 18th Dec 2005 in antardasha of Rahu and prati antar dasha of Mars, in this period the native also had suffered from heart problem which resulted in delay of surgery. The native got cured as then Maha dasha of Saturn was over and Mercury mahadasha was started. Important to note here is that the growth of cancer cells i.e. driver cells and passenger cells was triggered at the moment when in Mahadasha of Saturn and antardasha of Rahu prati antar dasha of Mars just started giving rise to pre developed tumor started bleeding and was noticed till there were no symptoms or abnormal changes in body noticed. Distinguished is that because of presence of lord of fourth house in twelfth cusp with Sub lord Jupiter; a lord of eighth cusp and afflicted with Neptune also created cardiac troubles which were settled later on in anter dasha of Jupiter leaving behind hypertension for life time. This actually also appears to be the blurred sign of onset of tumor went unnoticed.

In February 2013 when Jupiter lord of eighth house was transiting into Leo from Gemini the recurrence of the disease occurred noticed by bleeding and confirmed by MRI on 19th February 2013 and from this date the last journey was started leading to death on August 07th 2016 when in Mercury Mahadasha and Moon antardasha the prati antardasha of Mercury was just starting. Here note worthy point is that Mercury lord of twelfth cusp present in seventh house in conjunction with the lord of eighth cusp and lord of sixth cusp in the zodiac owned by Mars and under aspect of Mars which caused the death with multiple organ failure due to septicemia and the causative factor for this being Mercury which is lord of twelfth cusp and sub lord of ascendant where Mars is placed.

Case no 009

A female native born on June 25th 1958 at 0815hrs in Kolkata with Lat: 022:35N and Long. 088: 23 E

In this case the ascendant falls in sign of Cancer ruled by Moon, star lord being Mercury and the ascendant sub lord is Mars. The sign Cancer is movable and watery sign. The ascendant lord Moon represents the body and Moon being significator of Blood and blood circulation, the prevailing fluid of the body; Moon is also afflicted by Jupiter the lord of sixth cusp in the sign Virgo again sixth sign in Natures own chart, Jupiter also ruler of Blood as tissue. Moon is under aspect of Mars from ninth cusp; again a planet rules the function of blood and exchange of

Nutrients. Rahu under aspect from Mars is a planet responsible for growth of Oncogens i.e. basic cancer cells having undergone series of mutations. The native was suffering from the dreaded disease called LEUKEMIA or a type of blood cancer. The fourth, eighth, and twelfth houses are afflicted by Rahu, Saturn, and Mars indicating blood cancer. In this chart sign lord Moon in Virgo and in third cusp with Jupiter which is lord of sixth house; Moon is also in its own star and is sub lord of Mercury in twelfth cusp, which rules the composition of blood. The Star lord of the ascendant is ruled by Mercury, and Mercury as lord of third and twelfth house is placed in Gemini in twelfth cusp with star lord of Rahu in fourth cusp. Here fourth cusp indicates blood apart from other. The Rahu and Neptune in fourth indicate the stages called hyperplasia and dysplasia leading to cancerous growth in blood cells; this also causes clotting of blood in arteries and Veins. Mercury is also with sub lord of Sun and in twelfth cusp. The ascendant sub lord is Mars, another significator of flowing blood in Arteries and Vein. Mars in the sign Pisces and aspects Moon and Jupiter which is lord of sixth cusp, Mars is in the star of Mercury again lord of twelfth cusp. Mars as lord of fifth and tenth cusp is in the sub of Venus, the lord of fourth cusp and placed in ninth house. Now if we see the important cusp of the disease i.e. sixth cusp for deciding the nature of disease; the sub lord of this cusp and its significators indicate the nature of ailments. If the sub lord of the sixth cusp either Moon or Mars and connected to houses fourth, sixth or twelfth and also a watery sign there will be the disease related to the blood called fluid of life. In the chart the sixth sign is falls in Sagittarius 024deg: 16min: 26sec. with sign lord Jupiter star lord Venus and sub lord Mercury.   The sign lord Jupiter is also planet responsible for blood and blood disorders; also significator planet for this disease. Jupiter placed in sign Virgo the sixth sign in natural chart, along with Moon which is lord of ascendant indicating growth of abnormal cells in body fluid i.e. blood. Jupiter is in third cusp and in the constellation of Mars, another planet causing blood disorders and growth of cancerous cells in tissues. Jupiter also is under aspect of Mars; Jupiter is in the sub of Saturn; a planet that creates obstruction and enhances growth of malignant type of cancer. Saturn is also lord of eighth cusp causing blood cells behave abnormally, and is placed in Scorpio, the eighth sign in natural zodiac and a Martian sign. The star lord of sixth cusp is Venus; as lord of fourth cusp which is related to blood, Venus is in the star of Sun in Gemini i.e. twelfth cusp, so also Venus is in the sub of Saturn which is significator of eighth and twelfth cusps. In fact the key planet that had triggered very series of mutations in blood cells is sub lord of sixth house Mercury which rules the generation of new cells and helps bringing old cells to death. Mercury is lord of third and twelfth cusps in the star of Rahu which is an occupant of Libra i.e. fourth cusp again which controls the replication of cells by undergoing changes in its DNA molecule making it prone to produce cancer cells or making them prevent the formation of onco genes or cancer cells. Rahu is also a planet that helps producing chronic diseases like cancer and hence the sub lord of sixth cusp Mercury is well connected to houses fourth, eighth, and twelfth cusps. Saturn, Rahu, Jupiter, and Moon are also well connected to fourth, eighth, and twelfth cusps and watery sign indicates the disease type as malignant, and related to body fluid i.e. blood to the native. The Mercury also aspects sixth cusp and makes it further malefic as lord of twelfth house.   The disease occurred or appeared at the end of December 1981, when the native was passing through Rahu mahadasha and Venus antardasha;Rahu is significator of fourth house and Venus is lord of fourth house, during this period there was profuse bllod discharge which was mistaken as menstrual discharge at first instance, and native was hospitalized. Here mahadasha of Rahu in Venus in sign; where Rahu is with Star lord Mars indicating the confused and delayed diagnosis of the disease cancer and as such aggravated it. Naturally the native was driven to death bed unknowingly.

The nature of death can be found from the sub lord of eighth house and its significators; the eighth cusp sub lord is Mars, a planet for blood disorders and is with star of Mercury which is significator of fourth and twelfth cusp. Mars is in the sub lord of Venus and twelfth cusp is also under aspect of Mars. And hence the death was due to due to chronic and painful dreaded blood cancer that too in hospital. The native died on 30th August 1982 when in middle of Rahu mahadasha and Venus antardasha both well connected to eighth cusp.

Planet position in the chart

Sr. No.	Name of planet	Nirayan Sec	Deg.: Min :	Lord of zodiac	Star lord	Sub lord
01	Sun		069 : 52 : 27	Mercury	Rahu	Jupiter
02	Moon		169 : 13 : 49	Mercury	Moon	Mercury
03	Mars		349 : 24 : 14	Jupiter	Mercury	Venus
04	Mercury		077 : 36 : 52	Mercury	Rahu	Sun
05	Jupiter		178 : 38 : 02	Mercury	Mars	Saturn
06	Venus		034 : 39 : 27	Venus	Sun	Saturn

07	Saturn		238 : 25 : 22	Mars	Mercury	Saturn
08	Rahu		184 : 55 : 36	Venus	Mars	Sun
09	Ketu		004 : 55 : 36	Mars	Ketu	Mars
10	Uranus		106 : 25 : 16	Moon	Saturn	Jupiter
11	Neptune		188 : 55 : 50	Venus	Rahu	Jpiter
12	Pluto		336 : 49 : 26	Jupiter	Saturn	Mercury

Case no 010

A female native born on December 17th 1955 in Nangnallur Chennai at 0731 hrs
Lat: 013: 04 N and Long. 080: E

Again this is classical case to understand the relation between Cancerous growth and planetary set up in birth chart; where in ascendant falls in the sign Sagittarius ruled by Jupiter as lord of zodiac and Venus as star lord with Sun as sub lord. The lord of ascendant Jupiter; a planet of growth is placed in ninth cusp with zodiac lord Sun star lord ketu, and sub lord Jupiter under aspect from Saturn from twelfth cusp; the lord of the zodiac being Mars afflicted by Neptune and causative of growth of malignant type of tumors. This afflicted Jupiter with star lord Ketu and sub lord again Jupiter helps genetic predisposition to cancer here as fact genetic predisposition doesn't mean that Cancer will occur but increases probability of having some cells in chest area specifically in mammary tissues having undergone few mutations on the way and with another few the native may develop into malignant tumor. The zodiac lord of the sixth cusp Venus; is also the star lord of Ascendant and also sub lord of ascendant significator of the mammary tissue/gland and clearly denotes the onset of the cancer certain. The ascendant sub lord Venus is in first cusp and lord of sixth cusp triggers the process of normal stage undergo progressively abnormal stage resulting into growth of cancerous tissue in mammary gland. So also Ketu placed in Sixth house with star lord and sub lord increases the chances of growing tumor which goes undetected for even months. The Moon placed in second cusp i.e. Capricorn owned by Saturn which occupies the twelfth cusp afflicts own house as it is in its third aspect as such the afflicted Moon also under aspect of Mars from eleventh cusp which in its turn is afflicted by Neptune present in the same cusp; makes Moon cause the lymphatic glands disorder i.e. breast cancer. As this Moon is also lord of eighth cusp and under aspect from Uranus from eighth cusp making the native vulnerable to the disease which cannot be diagnosed for long time till becomes severe. Here the star lord of the eighth cusp is Mars and the sub lord being Moon significator of epigenetic changes in cells of mammary gland and these metastatic changes then become the disease dreaded. So also the Mars being lord of eighth cusp is also star lord of Rahu placed in twelfth house and Sub lord of Rahu leads hospitalization. This Mars is also lord of eighth house with star lord Saturn aspects the sixth cusp and Ketu which occupied the house causing profuse bleeding with no certain clue to assess the type of disease. The sub lord of ketu Saturn is placed with Rahu;is the sub lord of Moon placed in second cusp, causing un obstructed growth of Tumor in breast. The lord of fourth cusp is Jupiter, placed in ninth cusp with star lord Ketu which is placed in sixth cusp also causes abnormal changes in blood supply to breast and mammary gland leading to cancer. And hence all the significators of sixth cusp are well connected to eighth house, twelfth house and fourth house including planets like Moon, Ketu, Mars, and Saturn indicating clearly the onset of disease, further deterioration and death of native caused by breast cancer.

Planetary disposition

Sr. No.	Planet Name	Name of Zodiac	Deg : Min : Sec	Lord of Zodiac	Star lord	Sub Lord
01	Sun	Sagittarius	001 : 06 : 01	Jupiter	Ketu	Venus
02	Moon	Capricorn	031 : 08 : 21	Saturn	Sun	Rahu
03	Mars	Libra	318 : 27 : 22	Venus	Rahu	Moon
04	Mercury	Sagittarius	008 : 03 : 43	Jupiter	Ketu	Jupiter
05	Jupiter	Leo	248 : 15 : 32	Sun	Ketu	Jupiter
06	Venus	Sagittarius	027 : 48 : 41	Jupiter	Sun	Moon
07	Saturn	Scorpio	334 : 03 : 52	Mars	Saturn	Saturn
08	Rahu	Scorpio	353 : 38 : 03	Mars	Mercury	Mars
09	Ketu	Taurus	173 : 38 : 03	Venus	Mars	Mars
10	Uranus	Cancer	218 : 26 : 28	Moon	Saturn	Venus
11	Neptune	Libra	306 : 34 : 50	Venus	Mars	Moon
12	Pluto	Leo	245 : 18 : 12	Sun	Ketu	Mars

Chapter 14

Tuberculosis and Birth chart

Tuberculosis is disease mostly caused due to Mycobacterium Tuberculosis and it is infectious usually occurred in lungs but May sometimes in other parts or organs of Body. Total of 1.5 million people died of Tuberculosis in 2018 and is one of the top ten diseases which cause death due to single infectious agent even more than HIV/AIDS.

In general when Sun and Moon conjoin in watery sign, the lung diseases are produced and if there is malefic aspect to such combination further complications occur and the disease becomes chronic. Although the disease Tuberculosis is fully recoverable and the rate of mortality has gone down drastically since last few years due to medical science has invented cure even for resistant strain of Tuberculosis; the Astrological explanation and detailed planetary effect can help in finding whether the native is susceptible for the disease or not. Tuberculosis is caused by tubercle bacilli and once it enters the body it can get settled anywhere in body parts like Bones, Joints, Bladder, Spine, Lungs Kidneys, or glands in body causing infection of the organ. Most commonly it is noticed that the affected organs are Lungs. The essential medical treatment advised by doctors is total bed rest with different combinations and permutations of antibiotics.

Tuberculosis also called as phthisis and in astrology the fourth cusp from ascendant in birth chart and fifth cusp i.e. Leo in natures chart rules the disease, where Moon is significator for fourth cusp if afflicted by Saturn and or Rahu in fourth house, the native is likely to suffer from this infectious disease. So also lord of ascendant in eighth cusp may cause the native to suffer from this disease; as well as Saturn and Jupiter in eighth house may also cause the said disease.   The sign Gemini, Libra, and Aquarius governs the respiratory function and Cancer, Scorpio, Pisces (watery) signs control the circulatory system, and total immunity system. This can be summarized as given under.

1) If Sun and Moon conjoin in the sign cancer or Leo and under aspect from tenth cusp by any malefic planet leads to reduce immunity level and make native suffer from infectious diseases.
2) If Moon and Saturn in conjunction are under aspect fully by Mars the immunity towards bacterial infection goes down causing immediate infection.
3) If Sun and Jupiter are conjoined in sixth cusp connecting with watery sign may cause the infection by Tuberculosis.
4) If Moon and Sun conjoin in Scorpio and are under aspect by Mars and Saturn causes the infection.
5) If Mars and Mercury conjoins in sixth cusp and are under aspect from Moon or Venus this disease is caused.
6) The placement of cusp lord of sixth cusp sub lord in sixth while Sun and Moon in tenth house reduces the immunity level making native prone for the disease.

We can see some other combinations also in addition to above as listed under,

1) Affliction of Moon, Mars, weak fourth house and in case Sun is also afflicted by Saturn makes native suffer from Pulmonary Tuberculosis.
2) If Moon is weak or debilitated and malefic planet conjoins with them in watery sign the native is sure to suffer from obstructive respiratory infectious diseases.
3) If Mars and Saturn in sixth cusp under aspect of Venus and Moon also produces infection in lungs.

4) If Saturn and Jupiter are in seventh cusp or eighth cusp from rising Sun the native is likely get infection from Tuberculosis.
5) If Rahu is in sixth cusp and lord of ascendant in twelfth house are prone to diminished immunity leading to infection mainly Tuberculosis.
6) If Mercury owns third cusp and if placed in ascendant and connected with Moon and Sun there will be loss of immunity towards bacteria leading to Tuberculosis.
7) Rahu in sixth cusp and lord of ascendant occupies eighth cusp certainly gives rise to Tuberculosis followed by death.
8) Mere presence of Rahu or Ketu in sixth house or eighth cusp predisposes the native for the infection leading to Tuberculosis.
9) If Saturn, the planet of respiratory obstruction placed in sign Gemini, the sign that rules lung function influences the infection.

Tubercle Bacilli are found in sputum and Mars, Venus and Saturn, denotes the generation of histamines and enhance the growth of Tuberculosis. These natives inhaling the contaminated air are likely to suffer from Tuberculosis; due to reduced level of immunity and this lowering of immunity is caused due to any of above mentioned combinations. So also Jupiter also is required to be considered to lower the immunity, subjecting the native to suffer from Tuberculosis. Jupiter rules over twelfth cusp; and represents lungs indicates isolation and or hospitalization. Mercury rules the soft tissues and fibers and is dual planet, rules the Gemini governing exchange of gases in lungs and if afflicted cause pulmonary diseases. The Gemini being the third sign in natures chart and rules lungs and pulmonary functions; as such if Mercury, Jupiter, or Moon is afflicted in Gemini by any malefic planet reduces the body immunity capacity leading to infection by Tubercle Bacilli. So also Rahu denotes the breathing and afflicts the planets mentioned above produces Tuberculosis. Further Moon rules the function of colon, and sign Cancer rules the process of absorption of nutrients from food while Virgo governs the function of intestine also lead to the loss of immunity syndrome may cause Tuberculosis anywhere in body. In tropical countries if the natal chart of native shows Moon Are afflicted by Saturn causes reduction in immunity leading to Tuberculosis of bones, tissues, spine and also in case of female natives if the Mercury is afflicted by Saturn and Moon is very weak immunity of any organ in the body is infected.

1) Native suffers from Tuberculosis of spine specifically, the onset occurs after child birth or even during pregnancy. When Moon and Mercury are weak or severely afflicted by Saturn the native shows loss of vitality, loss of weight, and proneness to Tuberculosis. The bovine type of bacilli causes tuberculosis of any organ especially in children. Here the birth chart clearly depicts the financial set up of native and his family shows or indicates malnutrition leading to suffer from this disease. Important to note is that the tuberculosis is not genetically transmitted disease. The onset of

the disease initially indicated by simple flue type fever which then persists for prolonged period and gets converted to tuberculosis. The fever may be mild or may it be pyrexia weakens the native with constant reduction in immunity; occasionally pains in chest and body or symptoms related to pneumonia may occur, may these symptoms sometime show little blood in sputum. All these symptoms that manifests in case of tuberculosis can be studied and observed during that specific period individually or collectively and can be summarized as
Cancer

01deg –20min—00sec.to 03deg—20min—00sec	Moon/Jupiter/Rahu
03deg—20min—00sec to 05deg—26min—40sec	Moon/Saturn/Saturn
07deg—20min—00sec to 08deg—06min—40sec	Moon/Saturn/Ketu
11deg—00min—00sec to 12deg—12min—40sec	Moon/Saturn/Moon
16deg—40min—00sec to 18deg—33min—20sec	Moon/Mercury/Mercury

If sixth cusp sub lord is placed in above sensitive segment of constellations and afflicted by sign Gemini, Cancer, and also in watery signs like Scorpio and Pisces the disease tuberculosis certainly occurs.

A case study No 014 : - Female native born on 11June 1981 at 1752 hrs in Ahmed nagar Maharashtra Lat. 019:05N Long 074:44E

The female native mentioned above born with Scorpio ascendant and if we see the birth chart it is clear that the ascendant is under aspect of Saturn from eleventh cusp afflicting Moon as they are conjoined making ascendant cusp weak which governs the health and specifically immunity. Further we can see the lord of eleventh house occupied by Saturn, Moon and Jupiter is placed in eighth house; a malefic house with lord of twelfth cusp Venus. The lord of sixth cusp Mars is placed in the cusp Taurus owned by Venus a lord of twelfth cusp and placed in eighth house with Mercury in its own zodiac; the lords of twelfth and eighth cusp are under aspect of Saturn from eleventh cusp making sudden loss of immunity and causing the infection, as it is clear from the chart that the lord of sixth house is under aspect of Uranus and Neptune so called planets of uncertainty gives rise the outbreak of the disease in the period of Mars mahadasha with delayed and difficult diagnosis. The star lord of Mars i.e. Moon which is

also a sub lord is afflicted in Virgo with conjoined Saturn making the diagnosis further difficult. The star lord of Mercury which is lord of eighth house; is also a star lord of Venus which again is lord of twelfth house is placed in ninth cusp in Cancer with star lord Saturn reduces the immunity to great extent making room for the disease to appear and become resistant to the drugs. Here noteworthy is that, Rahu aspects the ascendant with lord of ascendant placed in seventh house with star lord Moon which is weak planet causing the severity of disease to increase.

Another fact that the Moon is very weak and afflicted by Saturn, the lord of zodiac where Moon is placed is also owned by Mercury i.e. eighth house and as such making Moon a weak planet that governs the respiratory function with decrease in immunity level. The Rahu being placed in Cancer, and sub lord of Rahu placed in seventh house conjoined with Mars, owner if sixth house affects the metabolism of the body to great extent with appreciable decrease in immunity level and also affecting the function of lungs making the native pray to the disease Tuberculosis. Noteworthy is that the onset of the disease occurs in the Mahadasha period of Mars which is lord of ascendant too at end of mahadasha in antardasha of Rahu which had afflicted the ascendant with delayed and difficult diagnosis; the onset occurs on 28th February 1991, also interesting is that the recovery starts in the period of Rahu mahadasha when Jupiter antardasha starts.

Planetary disposition

Sr. No	Planet name	Name of Zodiac	Degrees: Minutes : Second	Lord of zodiac	Star Lord	Sub lord
01	Sun	Taurus	206 : 53 : 09	Venus	Mars	Jupiter
02	Moon	Virgo	319 : 44 : 19	Mercury	Moon	Ketu
03	Mars	Taurus	190 : 53 : 04	Venus	Moon	Moon
04	Mercury	Gemini	164 : 02 : 50	Mercury	Rahu	Mercury
05	Jupiter	Virgo	307 : 10 : 31	Mercury	Sun	Ketu
06	Venus	Gemini	164 : 02 : 50	Mercury	Rahu	Mercury
07	Saturn	Virgo	309 : 26 : 06	Mercury	Sun	Venus
08	Rahu	Cancer	250 : 22 : 11	Moon	Saturn	Sun
09	Ketu	Capricorn	070 : 22 : 11	Saturn	Moon	Moon
10	Uranus	Scorpio	003 : 34 : 24	,Mars	Saturn	Saturn
11	Neptune	Scorpio	029 : 58 : 28	Mars	Mercury	Saturn
12	Pluto	Virgo	328 : 03 : 03	Mercury	Mars	Saturn

Chapter15

Appendicitis and Horoscope

The appendix is small finger shaped tube projecting from the large intestine near the point where it joins the small intestine and likely to have some immune related function but still not essential organ. It is most common cause of sudden severe abdominal pain and leads to abdominal surgery; world over 5% of the population develops appendicitis at some or the other point. It most commonly occurs during adolescence till the age of 20th. The exact cause of appendix is not known fully however in most cases a blockage inside the appendix probably starts the process. The blockages may be of fecal mass or foreign body or rarely even worms. As a result of blockage the appendix becomes inflamed and infected and if inflammation persists without treatment, the appendix can rupture and may cause pus filled pockets of infection i.e. abscess to form. This leads to peritonitis i.e. infection and inflammation in abdominal cavity which may sometimes results in life threatening. In women the ovaries and fallopian tubes may become infected resulting in scaring and even may block fallopian tubes causing infertility. Ruptured appendix may also allow stream of bacteria to infect blood. The symptoms in which pain begins in upper abdomen or around navel, followed by nausea, vomiting then after few hours nausea passes away and pain shifts to right lower portion of abdomen when doctor presses on this area it is tender and when pressure released pain may increase sharply. Fever 100 deg. To 101 deg f. is common; moving and coughing with increase in pain. In many patients particularly infants and children, the pain may wide spread rather than confined to right lower portion of abdomen. In older patients and pregnant woman, the pain may be less severe and the area is less tender. If appendix ruptures pain may lessen for several hours then peritonitis occurs and pains with fever may become severe worsening which may lead to trauma.

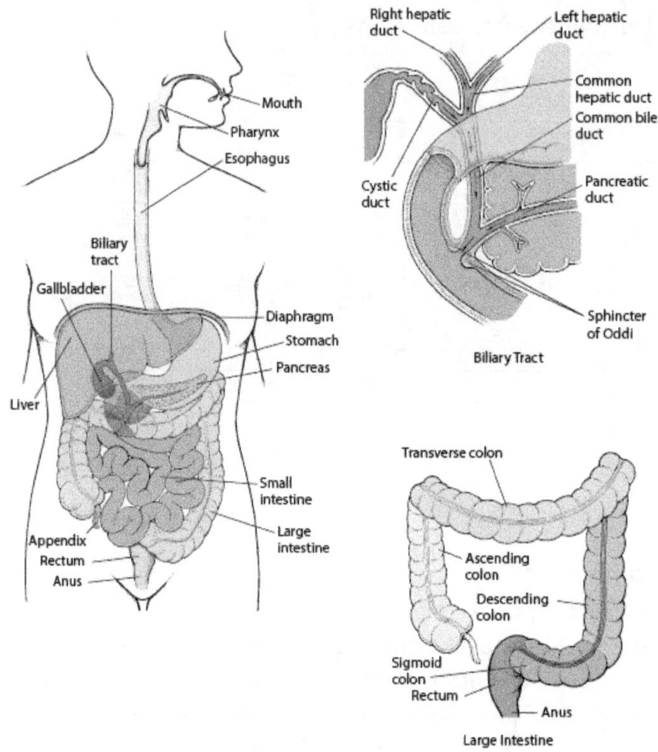

The location of this part of body is ruled by sixth cusp of birth chart and sixth sign in natures chart. Mars the major causative planet for appendicitis; and if Mars is afflicted by Saturn may give rise to the appendicitis. Mars is responsible for elimination of wate and injurious substances fro body by creating either inflammation or fever. Mercury is

concerned with those parts of body which carry outward byproducts within body and tries
to retain them without any consideration of their beneficial or injurious effects.

Uranus is concerned with glands and growth of any ailment injurious to heath in them.
Neptune deals with spine and any traumatic condition that may occur due to outburst of
the appendix inside the body. All these can be summarized as bellow,

1) The sign Gemini, Virgo, Scorpio, and Pisces are prominent signs that are
   concerned with disease Appendix.
2) The sixth, eighth, 12th, cusps are related to the occurrence of this ailment.
3) Uranus, Mercury, Mars, and Neptune, are important planets to be considered to
   study the onset of Appendicitis.
4) Aspects, applying, or separating between planets or planets and houses must be
   inharmonious i.e. semi square, square, Quincunx, or opposition.
5) The Saturn in fifth house makes a person voracious eater with consequent
   disease of over eating, the disease like appendicitis is caused.

As the appendix is attached to the caecum near its junction with the large intestine shown
by star Hastham related to bowels and large intestine, Chitra related to disorders of
bowels, abnormal growth of any part in intestine or lower abdomen, and any malefic planet
in these Stars will cause the occurrence of this disease. So also as function of Appendix is
more or less similar to tonsils the planet in Rohini star at time contributes the disease.
Mars is the causative for all ruptures, inflammation, tumors, abscess, boils etc. Its concern
is to eliminate waste and injurious substances from body by above process. Therefore in
the case of appendicitis irrespective of presence of Mars in specific house or not the, the
inflammation of appendix, fever, pain besides the surgical treatment.
Mercury rules ulcers besides tissue and intestine. Uranus causes affliction of colon, the
most of the diseases caused are sudden and unexpected including death. As such Uranus
concerns Appendix and its function and also if in Virgo or Libra and in constellation of
Hatham and chitra causes sudden disorder of bowels or colon. In several cases the
inflammation is caused by Mars may lead to abscess formation and abscess that may burst
into lower abdominal cavity called peritonitis; sixth cusp cause acute prerogative
peritonitis in case Mercury and Uranus conjoined in this house. This may lead to severe
toxemia usually driving to death. As Sun is the causative of digestive system especially
small and large intestine and moon denotes colon or removal of body waste if connected
lead to the Appendicitis. Venus being again rules the organs those responsible for
segregation and removal of waste from body like tonsils; is also responsible for function of
appendicitis is no wonder if occurs as the cause of appendix inflammation and infection or
even growth of any worms in it. Generally sixth, eighth, twelfth houses or lords of these
houses are relevant to this disorder; sixth cusp denotes disease besides the location of the
diseased part, eighth house is the house of intensity of the disorder; whilst the twelfth

house denotes the hospitalization/ isolation including surgical treatment. Therefore zodiacs Pisces, Scorpio, Virgo, besides Gemini are prominent signs required to be assessed for appendicitis. If the sixth cusp in any of the above signs or ruler of the sixth cusp including sub lord of sixth cusp and lord of constellation where the lord of constellation is placed; the native may suffer from appendicitis. Also it is noticed that Jupiter, Mars, Mercury, Uranus, besides Venus are relevant.

Case No 015

A male native Born on 27th June 1981; 0822 hrs. Pune Lat. 018: 30 N, Long 073:48E

This native with sudden onset of Appendicitis reported pain in stomach around navel region which in few hours followed by nausea and vomiting. This persisted for few days then the pain persisted but nausea and vomiting disappeared and pain shifted to lower abdomen on right side so also the lower abdomen appear tender and pain becoming severe after releasing the pressure on stomach. Ultimately the native was shifted to hospital for surgical treatment and removal of appendix was carried out.

The sequential analysis of the case shows that as we see in the birth chart of the native we find the ascendant is Aquarius occupied by Mercury denoting the disease related to stomach may occur. The sixth house is occupied by Rahu in Cancer with star lord and sub lord Mercury which denotes the disease related to abdomen with high intensity and connecting this house to ascendant; the Mercury is also lord of eighth house giving the indication of seriousness of the disease with sudden onset, so also the lord of ascendant Saturn is placed in eighth cusp further indicates the obstruction or growth of appendix. Again if we see the Saturn is also a lord of twelfth house requiring urgent hospitalization followed by surgery. This Saturn is sub lord of Jupiter and Jupiter is placed in Eighth cusp conjoined with Saturn making the native suffer with huge pains and rupture of the part is indicated. Mercury being lord of eighth cusp is placed in ascendant afflicting the house; further star lord of the ascendant is Mars placed in eighth cusp creating complication in the disease, as such the diagnosis was delayed causing traumatic conditions leading to surgery. Lord of sixth house is Moon and is placed in ninth house owned by Venus which is afflicted by conjoined with Neptune; here note worthy is that Neptune being planet of mysterious disease; is associated with lord of sixth house and sub lord and star lord of sixth house is Ketu which is placed in twelfth house aspects the sixth house and Rahu making the growth of worms in appendix, later on requiring surgical operation and removal of the appendix.

We can also note here that Saturn placed in sixth house makes the native fond of food leading to faulty food habits and as result the blockage of appendix. So also afflicted and retrograde Jupiter causative of abscess and complicated inflammation; along with Mars placed in twelfth cusp in Capricorn leaves no treatment other than surgical removal of the part makes native compelled to get hospitalized and undergo surgery. So also Mars is lord of tenth house occupied by Uranus which aspects the fourth house causative of disease related to bowel disorder and growth of foreign body in intestine which was confirmed by occurrence of worms in appendix. Planetary disposition as tabled below

Sr. No	Planet Name	Name of zodiac	Degree : Min : Sec	Lord of Zodiac	Star Lord	Sub lord
01	Sun	Capricorn	343 : 29 : 48	Saturn	Moon	Rahu
02	Moon	Libra	241 : 58 : 58	Venus	Mars	Ketu
03	Mars	Capricorn	357 : 50 : 33	Saturn	Mars	Jupiter
04	Mercury	Aquarius	000 : 12 : 48	Saturn	Mars	Mercury
05	Jupiter	Virgo	226 : 47 : 23	Mercury	Moon	Saturn
06	Venus	Sagittarius	326 : 13 : 40	Jupiter	Venus	Ketu
07	Saturn	Virgo	226 : 07 : 41	Mercury	Moon	Saturn
08	Rahu	Cancer	167 : 32 : 37	Moon	Mercury	Mercury
09	Ketu	Capricorn	347 : 32 : 37	Saturn	Moon	Saturn
10	Uranus	Scorpio	275 : 54 : 42	Mars	Saturn	Mercury
11	Neptune	Sagittarius	300 : 20 : 14	Jupiter	Ketu	Ketu
12	Pluto	Libra	240 : 45 : 21	Venus	Mars	Mercury

Chapter 16

Renal dysfunction and KP sub lords

Kidneys filters blood in three steps

1) Nephrons filter blood that runs through the capillaries; that network in glomerules by a process called Glomerular filtration.
2) Secondly the filtrate is collected in renal tubules; most of the solutes get reabsorbed in PCT by process called tubular re absorption. In the loop of Henle

filtrate continues to exchange solutes and water with renal medulla and the Peri tubular capillary network. Water is also reabsorbed during this step.

3) The additional solutes and wastes are secreted into the tubules during tubular secretion which is in essence, the opposite process to tubular re absorption. The collecting ducts collect the filtrate coming from the nephron and fuse into medullar papillae, from the papillae deliver the filtrate now called Urine into minor cycles that eventually connect to the urethras through renal pelvic.

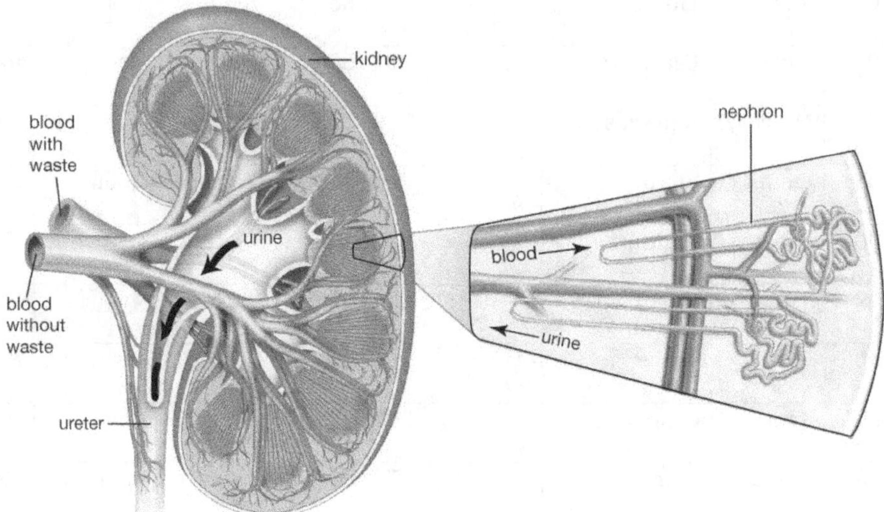

© Encyclopædia Britannica, Inc.

The disease Kidney trouble is mainly associated three planets Venus, Jupiter, and Moon   the seventh house rules over the function of Kidneys, so also seventh zodiac in natures own chart that is Libra governs the function and anomalies in function. And as such if seventh cusp is afflicted by any malefic planet the native is likely to suffer from kidney trouble; also if any malefic occupies Libra may lead to the renal dysfunction. Mars is major malefic that affect the kidney and disorder appears. If Mars and Venus are afflicted by malefic in watery sign the native may suffer from urinary disorder and disturbed kidney function. Moon in watery sign like Cancer, Scorpio, Pisces and falls in sixth cusp while lord is under aspect from Mercury placed in watery sign may indicate the malfunction of kidneys. Nephritis is a common disease which affects both adult and children. The combinations for renal dysfunction to occur are summarized as given as

1) If Saturn, Sun, and Venus are in fifth cusp the native will suffer from the Nephritis.
2) Mars in tenth cusp conjoined with or under aspect from Saturn causes nephritis.
3) If Sun and Mars occupy ascendant and seventh respectively the native may suffer from Nephritis.
4) When Moon is in a watery sign and its lord is in sixth cusp and under aspect from Mercury which in its turn if placed in watery sign the native suffers from glomerular filtration or re absorption syndrome.
5) If any malefic occupy sixth cusp or seventh cusp the native will suffer from cysts in either urethra or tubules.
6) When Mars and Venus conjoin in seventh sign i.e. Libra the native is likely to suffer from burning sensation in urethra or painful urination.
7) When Mars, Rahu aspect each other chyle urea or poly urea occurs.
8) If the lord of ascendant associates with lord of seventh in eighth cusp renal dysfunction occurs; sometimes is related to auto immune type of disorder.
   In Astrological arena the sixth cusp is responsible for disease or dysfunction of any organ in body and as such any affliction to sixth cusp causes disease to occur as such needs to be studied for----
   1) The cusp and 2) Significators. 3) Lord of the cusp, 4) occupants of the cusp 5) Sixth cusp from Moon or Ascendant and 6) Planets that aspect sixth cusp.

Accordingly the sub lord of the sixth cusp, if it is in any way connected with ascendant or its lord; then upset of the renal function may occur. If we note which planet will cause the disease in which sign it is placed and the significator of both the first and sixth cusp considering all these we can predict the nature of the disease from which one the native will suffer; then calculating the time when the significator of ascendant, sixth, eighth, and twelfth will operate in their dashas. If the sub lord of ascendant or sixth cusp happens to be the Venus and connected to Libra kidney failure may occur. Venus governs kidney and if placed in sixth with spasmodic attack may occur. Venus governs the Renal function and if in Libra in the star of Mars may cause inflammation of glomerules or rupture of the Henle's loop leading to kidney failure. Nephritis called Bright's disease marked by albumin in urine and swelling of body tissues is generally appeared when Venus becomes a significator of sixth cusp and connected to Libra; so also Venus in Libra if afflicted by malefic affects the functional activity of second and third stage of filtration and secretion of urine causing protein in urine and or polyurea. This also causes suppression of urine leading to inflammation of urethra when Saturn occupies Scorpio or eighth causative of obstruction leads to this disease. When Libra, Scorpio, and sixth and seventh cusp and or their lords with significators are afflicted by association or aspect or placed in malefic house or by conjunction with malefic give rise to renal function disorders. Here it is noteworthy that twelfth cusp or eighth cusp significators are connected with each other or with sub lord of eighth cusp and its significators certainly cause the Bright's diseases.

This further can be explained by following cases individually studied.

Case no 016

Male native born on 29th October 2014 at 1029hrs Pune Maharashtra

       Lat. 018: 30 ----N   Long 073: 48----E

The chart clearly shows at first instance Venus placed in Libra afflicted by Saturn conjoined with Venus in Libra which denotes the severe swelling of the native with passage of albumin in urine causing serious Nephritis. In this case if we take sixth cusp into consideration, the lord of which is Venus; and star lord Rahu of the same is placed in tenth house creating semi quadrant with seventh cusp and as such afflicting the same, so also the lord of seventh house Mercury is conjoined with Rahu in tenth cusp further deteriorating the function of renal tubules in PCT by process called tubular re absorption. Here important to note that the ascendant lord is Jupiter is placed in eighth cusp in Cancer, the lord of the cusp being placed in Ascendant causes affliction of both cusps and also makes exchange of solutes in renal medulla and the affliction of both cusps and also makes exchange of solutes in renal medulla and the peri tubular capillary network; that leads to secreting protein in the urine and giving swelling of body due to retention of cellular fluid.

We further can note that the star lord of Moon is Venus, placed conjoined with Saturn in Libra; also Star lord of Jupiter is Mercury the lord of seventh house; as we have discussed earlier causes collecting of filtrate coming from nephrons which further fused in medullar papillae. This carries the albumin which secreted in glomerular filtration and escaped the re absorption process in peri tubular network causing loss in urine that leads to less absorption of cellular fluid which re circulates in tissues causing swelling of tissues that causes the disease called Nephritis.

Also here we further can note that sub lord of Jupiter placed in sixth house is placed in conjoined with Mercury, lord of seventh cusp confirming the onset of the disease in Antar dasha of Rahu and Mahadasha of Venus. Further it can be seen that the lord of twelfth cusp occupies the ascendant with lord of eighth cusp and thus connecting eighth and twelfth cusp causing repeated episodes of the disease as also the sub lord of mars placed in fourth cusp aspects the Mercury in tenth house which is lord of seventh cusp and leads to malfunctioning of renal function. Interestingly Ketu is star lord of ascendant aspects the lord of seventh house Mercury conjoined with Rahu which is sub lord of the tenth cusp and sub sub of eighth cusp creating obstructions in renal filtration as well as inappropriate secretion of cellular fluid in urine causing swelling all tissues all over the body. So also the lord of sixth cusp Venus is also sub lord of seventh house and is placed in eleventh house conjoined wit malefic planet Saturn which further is also sub sub of seventh house and known planet causative of obstruction in physiological functions in body. Saturn is also star lord of eighth cusp sub sub of sixth house is responsible for the occurrence of the disease that recur repeatedly for prolonged period.

Here period in which the occurrence of disease is denoted can be predicted with respect to the Mahadasha of Venus; main planet and lord of Libra main zodiac which had triggered the onset of the disease. That is in Mahadasha of Venus and antardasha of Rahu which afflicted the lord of seventh cusp and also sub lord of eleventh cusp where Venus is placed. It can be seen the occurrence had took place on July 2017 when Venus mahadasha and Rahu antar dasha with Rahu prati antardasha period confirming the above. This also can be predicted that till 14th of 2019 the episode of Nephritis will reoccur and then the disease will pass away as after 14th October 2019 Jupiter antar dasha starts and then after the Venus Mahadasha is over Mahadasha of Sun starts giving perfect health to the native.

Planetary disposition is given as under

Sr. No.	Planet	Zodiac	Degrees : Min : Sec	Lord Zodiac	Star Lord	Sub Lord
01	Sun	Libra	311 : 47 : 46	Venus	Rahu	Saturn
02	Moon	Sagittarius	016 : 48 : 18	Jupiter	Venus	Moon

03	Mars	Sagittarius	007 : 58 : 43	Jupiter	Ketu	Jupiter
04	Mercury	Virgo	293 : 43 : 31	Mercury	Mars	Mars
05	Jupiter	Cancer	236 : 01 : 39	Moon	Mercury	Rahu
06	Venus	Libra	312 : 37 : 30	Venus	Rahu	Mercury
07	Saturn	Libra	329 : 29 : 01	Venus	Jupiter	Moon
08	Rahu	Virgo	294 : 14 : 55	Mercury	Mars	Rahu
09	Ketu	Pisces	114 : 14 : 55	Jupiter	Mercury	Rahu
10	Uranus	Pisces	109 : 37 : 23	Jupiter	Mercury	Venus
11	Neptune	Aquarius	070 : 49 : 35	Saturn	Rahu	Saturn

Case no 017   this is classic case of Kidney failure at the onset of old age

This is world renowned personality born on   12th October 1902 in Munger Bihar at 00:42 hrs

Lat   025:23 N and   Long 086:30 E

This native had suffered from renal function failure and was on dialysis till life. In this chart ascendant falls in Cancer sign 14deg: 15min: 51sec ruled by Moon, a lord of watery sign; the star lord of ascendant is Saturn, a planet of obstruction. Ascendant sub lord is Rahu and ascendant lord Moon is in its own star lord in seventh along with Jupiter, lord of sixth cusp and Pisces; which is watery sign. The star lord of ascendant Saturn; a planet of obstruction is placed in sixth cusp itself with no other planets and is also a lord of seventh and eighth cusp. The ascendant sub lord is Mercury, placed in Libra with Rahu which is an important sign to be considered for kidney related diseases, is in star of Mars which again is lord of Scorpio, a watery sign. Hence as all significators of Ascendant are well connected with sixth cusp, the planet Venus, the sign Libra, and also seventh and eighth cusp with watery signs like Cancer, Scorpio and Pisces the native had suffered from renal failure.

The sixth cusp falls in the sign Sagittarius 14degrees: 40 minutes: 51 seconds is ruled by Jupiter a planet known to cause swelling and inflammation; the star lord and sub lord of the sixth cusp is ruled by Venus also leads to the kidney failure. The sign Sagittarius rules thighs, hips, femur, ileum, occeygeal vertebrae, sacral region, sciatic nerve, and ischium. Also governs or causes loco motor ataxia, sciatica, Lumbago, Rheumatism, hip diseases, and accidents to thighs. The star lord and sub lord Venus; which is lord of the sign Libra denotes the Renal function dis- order, Adrenal dysfunction, Lumbar region diseases, urethra related disorder, and diseases related to vasomotor system, also indicates the occurrence of diabetes, Nephritis. In the chart under discussion the sixth cusp sign lord Jupiter is in seventh house which is related to kidneys, is conjoined with Moon; and Moons constellations, ascendant being Cancer a watery sign is under aspect from Jupiter which owns the Pisces again a watery sign. The star lord and sub lord of sixth cusp Venus, a significator of   renal dysfunction and lord of Libra which again a sign indicating the kidney diseases, is in the star of Moon in seventh house. Venus is in the sub of Rahu an occupant of Libra so also Venus placed in Virgo the sixth sign in natures chart and aspects sign Pisces, a watery sign.

Another important sign to be considered is seventh sign and eighth sign; both are ruled by Saturn, a planet indicative of obstruction and inflammation is placed in sixth cusp. The sub lords of seventh and eighth cusp, both are ruled by Saturn is placed in sixth house having no planet in its star. The Disease of renal function made its appearance in Maha dasha of Mercury, lord of fourth and twelfth cusp and placed in Libra, also afflicted by Rahu; is in sub of Saturn, a occupant of sixth cusp and lord of seventh and seventh and eighth cusp. The native suffered a serious renal function disorder for prolonged period and was on dialysis till death on 8th August 1979, when he was running through Mercury Maha dasha Jupiter antar dasha and Venus prati antar dasha i.e. with effect from 2nd September 1979 till 18th January 1980. The nature of death as described by sub lord of eighth cusp and lord of sixth cusp Jupiter is multiple organ failure due to diseased kidney.

Planetary disposition of case no 12

Sr. No	Name of Planet	Name of Zodiac	Degrees: Min: Sec.	Lord of Zodiac	Star Lord	Sub lord
01	Sun	Virgo	085 : 01 : 50	Mercury	Mars	Rahu
02	Moon	Capricorn	198 : 09 : 03	Saturn	Moon	Mercury
03	Mars	Leo	030 : 21 : 50	Sun	Ketu	Ketu
04	Mercury	Libra	100 : 51 : 37	Venus	Rahu	Saturn
05	Jupiter	Capricorn	195 : 00 : 01	Saturn	Moon	Jupiter
06	Venus	Virgo	072 : 51 : 23	Mercury	Moon	Rahu
07	Saturn	Sagittarius	178 : 52 : 48	Jupiter	Sun	Mars
08	Rahu	Libra	092 : 58 : 15	Venus	Mars	Venus
09	Ketu	Aries	272 : 58 : 15	Mars	Ketu	Venus
10	Uranus	Scorpio	145 : 37 : 30	Mars	Mercury	Rahu
11	Neptune	Gemini	341 : 14 : 14	Mercury	Rahu	Saturn
12	Pluto	Taurus	357 : 05 : 12	Venus	Mars	Jupiter

Chapter No 17

Human Reproductive system and Horoscope

The ailments related to reproductive system are divided in to two major types 1) Female Reproductive System Disorders and 2) Male Reproductive system disorder.

1) Female reproductive system disorders are further caused by two different causes, first being the malfunctioning of organs or some tumor likes growth and secondly

infectious disease caused mainly fungal infection or bacterial infection.

The malfunctioning of organ mostly occurs in females after the onset of adolescence indicated by Amenorrhea, dysmenorrhoea, Dysfunctional bleeding, PCOS, Scanty discharge, Endometriosis, and many more related to uterine bleeding. The most important organ in females related to human reproduction is Uterus and is connected to Ovaries, Fallopian tubes   which are ruled by fifth cusp in natal chart and sixth, eighth house relations so also zodiacs owned by Mercury, Mars, Saturn, normally causes the diseases related to female reproductive system so also combinations given bellow may lead to the problems mentioned here before or even next chapters,

1) When Saturn becomes the Lord of ascendant and under aspect by Ketu.
2) When the ascendant is afflicted with Rahu and Saturn.
3) When the lord of the eighth house is hemmed in between Rahu and Saturn and is devoid of benefic aspect of Jupiter.
4) When both Rahu and Saturn combine with Moon in fifth cusp.
5) Rahu and Saturn in second cusp and Mercury in eighth with Moon in twelfth cusp leads to infertility and diseases related to Uterus.
6) If Mercury is combined with Saturn in eighth cusp and if the Moon is afflicted by Rahu then PCOS, PID occurs.
7) If Moon be hemmed in between malefic and if the eighth cusp be as the same time be occupied by Ketu or Mercury or even Mercury in eighth cusp leads to Endometriosis.
8) If Venus and Mars occupy a sign of Mars, then also the native will suffer from uterine fibroids.
9) If Venus and Mars occupy seventh cusp the native will have sexually transmitted disease.
10) If Mars, Saturn, Sun and Moon placed in second, sixth, eighth and twelfth cusp the native will suffer from Gonorrhea, Chlamydia, even pelvic inflammation.
11) Malefic in eighth cusp cause primary ovarian insufficiency leading to cranky mood, trouble concentrating.
12) If Jupiter is placed in twelfth cusp and Uranus with or without Ketu in fifth cusp causes the prolapsed uterus leading to herniated syndrome.
13) If seventh house is occupied by ketu or under aspect from ketu the native suffers from oligomenorrhea a symptom where in the menstruation cycle is disturbed.
14) When Mars occupies sixth cusp and Moon is placed in seventh or eighth cusp the Amenorrhea is occurred
15) When Saturn, Rahu, Ketu or placed in fifth cusp and afflicted by Mars or Uranus, Neptune the Dysmenorrhea is occurred or irregular menstruation is caused. So also if Saturn in fifth cusp is under aspect from Ketu or Neptune then uterine

fibroid is occurred.

It is generally considered that the seventh and eighth cusps deals with reproductive organ and sign Libra owned by Venus and Scorpio owned by Mars indicates that the disease related to reproductive organ even may lead to infertility. The combination of lord of ascendant, Mars, and Mercury in fourth cusp, twelfth cusp, or their combined aspects on sixth cusp shows the disease related to uterus, skin, or rectum. If the sixth cusp, sub lord is Venus, Mars, Mercury, Saturn and signifying seventh, eighth cusp with Libra, Scorpio the native will suffer from infectious diseases like gonorrhea, syphilis. Again as we study further with reference to the KP system of diagnosis in this type can be predicted as referred bellow.

1) If the sub lord of seventh cusp is Mars and signifies seventh cusp the native will suffers from uterus related ailments.

2) If the sub lord of the seventh cusp is Jupiter and signifies seventh cusp the native will suffer from ovaries related disorder.

3) If the sub lord of seventh cusp is Saturn and signifies seventh cusp the native will suffer from blockages in fallopian tubes.

4) If the sub lord of seventh cusp is Rahu and signifies seventh cusp, then native suffers from ectopic pregnancy.

5) If the sub lord of seventh cusp is Ketu and signifies seventh house the native will suffer from pelvic inflammatory disease.

6) If the sub lord of seventh house is Venus and signifies seventh house then native will suffer from Endometriosis.

7) If the sub lord of seventh cusp is Mercury and signifies seventh house then native will suffer from fibroid in uterus leading to cancerous disease.

8) If the sub lord of seventh cusp is Moon and signifies the seventh house then native will suffer from cervical cancer.

9) If the sub lord of the seventh house is Sun and signifies the seventh cusp then the native will suffer from irregular menstruation cycle.

To clarify this we can study following case as an example

Case no 017

Female native Born on 31st July 1979 at Mumbai Santacruz,

Lat. : 019: 05 N   Long : 072: 50 E

If we study this chart it is clear at first instance that the Star lord of Seventh cusp is lord of zodiac Capricorn and Aquarius falls in fifth and sixth cusp and star lord of the sixth cusp is Rahu and placed in twelfth cusp aspects the sixth cusp so also the lord of fifth house is Saturn placed in twelfth house and afflicted with Rahu and under aspect from Ketu. This Saturn causes the inflammation of the female reproductive tract even traverse the uterine tubes. Inflammation of these results into PID referred as pelvic inflammation disease. This caused infertility and irregular menstruation cycle leading to inflammation of uterine tubes which occludes resulting into infertility. So also as we observe here in chart the lord of seventh cusp Jupiter is placed in Cancer in eleventh cusp and aspects the fifth house causative of normal uterine function leading to healthy conception. The lord of eleventh house is Moon is placed in second cusp and is afflicted by Uranus; so also lord of second cusp is Venus occupies eleventh house with sub lord Saturn causative of obstructions and inflammation of uterine tubes. Sub lord of Jupiter Mars is placed in tenth cusp aspecting fifth house responsible for ovaries function; which is also star lord of Moon Causative of Hormonal imbalance with sub lord Ketu placed in sixth cusp with star lord Rahu afflicting Saturn lord of sixth and fifth cusps. This causes dysfunctional uterine bleeding and results into infertility. Mars is also lord of eighth cusp and third cusp; placed in tenth house, is sub lord of seventh house sub lord of Jupiter placed in Cancer responsible for pregnancy making Jupiter afflicted. Here noteworthy is that the sixth house and eighth house are well connected with twelfth house so also their star lord and sub lord are connected causing prolonged dysfunctional uterine bleeding. The onset of the disease as we can see has occurred in the Maha dasha of Rahu and antardasha Venus and prati antar dasha of Rahu on 20th February 1995 persisted till 20th October 2015 when Jupiter mahadasha was due and Rahu antardasha was passing through Moon prati antar dasha.

Planetary disposition

Sr. No	Planet name	Zodiac	Degrees	Lord of Zodiac	Star lord	Sub lord
01	Sun	Cancer	313 : 50 : 42	Moon	Saturn	Rahu
02	Moon	Libra	031 : 56 : 01	Venus	Mars	Ketu
03	Mars	Gemini	270 : 49 : 01	Mercury	Mars	Mercury
04	Mercury	Cancer	313 : 43 : 48	Moon	Saturn	Venus
05	Jupiter	Cancer	314 : 43 : 48	Moon	Mercury	Mars
06	Venus	Leo	336 : 53 : 10	Sun	Saturn	Mercury
07	Saturn	Leo	346 : 28 : 15	Sun	Venus	Rahu
08	Rahu	Leo	166 : 28 : 15	Sun	Venus	Moon
09	Ketu	Aquarius	053 : 21 : 35	Saturn	Rahu	Venus

Also we can further study that lord of twelfth cusp is Sun placed in tenth cusp afflicted with Saturn the lord of sixth and fifth cusp and Mercury causative of abdominal disorder and as such making the infection serious. So also lord of eighth cusp is Mars placed in eighth cusp in Aries which controls the function of area of brain i.e. nerve centre connected with function of hormones and steroids in body and as such causes diseases related to functional disorder of hormonal imbalance, the star lord and sub lord of Mars Venus is associated with Moon in twelfth house, a malefic house and afflicted with Moon in Leo; and under aspect of Saturn from tenth house causing hospitalization. The onset of the infection started in Mahadasha of Mars and antardasha of Saturn the lord of sixth cusp and pronged till the Rahu mahadasha was due and antardasha of Venus completed and antardasha of Sun starts on 12th Sept 2019. The disease was totally recovered but leaving behind the mark of permanent infertility.

Case no 018

Male native born on 29th April 1974 at 1915 hrs in Pune/Pimpri Lat 018:30 N Long 073:52E

The Birth chart of this native shows typically few prominent signs that led to the infertility. The Virgo ascendant with Mercury being lord of ascendant occupied in sixth house conjoined with Jupiter which is lord of seventh house; the sign Aquarius that denotes the disease related to male hormonal disorder. Further the lord of fifth house that rules the male reproductive organs falls Capricorn denoting the disease related to degenerative type of disorder, and also indicate the dysfunctional male hormone testosterone. The ascendant Mercury rules the testicular function leading to testicular torsion, also which may cause hypogonadism. This particular rare degenerative disease leads to deformed sperms associated with chronic azoospermia; that leads to male infertility syndrome.

We also can understand in details with study of subs and their relations and dysfunctional organs. The star lord of ascendant is Venus that rules the male hormone secretion, is placed in fifth cusp and star lord of fifth cusp Moon occupied in ninth house afflicted by Mars and Ketu; again the lord of ninth house is Venus. The lord of fifth house is Saturn and placed in tenth house owned by Mercury placed in sixth house, so also the star lord of eighth house is Mars placed in ninth house conjoined with Moon and Ketu. It is noteworthy to understand here is that Moon also rules the secretion of NeuropeptideY and Beta adreno receptors which gives the signal for secretion of Testosterone, a male hormone; and production of sperms affected, either by deformed sperms or diseased and non motile count. Thus we can observe them making native totally infertile and causing hypogonadism. Further the sub lord of twelfth cusp is Saturn and that of sixth cusp also is Saturn placed in tenth house and lord of fifth and sixth house. The sub lord of Mercury is Sun and sub lord of Saturn is also Sun; the sub lord of eighth house is Saturn which is also Rahu occupied in third house, as such the disease is of chronic type and irrecoverable. The Saturn is also sub lord of twelfth house and is lord of sixth and fifth house; fifth house is here responsible for reproductive organs, further the Venus placed in fifth house is ninth house that rules the emotions and therefore the secretion of Alpha 2 adrenoreceptors which triggers the sperm count in semen, responsible for reproductive function.

Here the onset of the disease appears to be in puberty period only i.e. in adolescence when Rahu mahadasha was in progress and Saturn mahadasha was just started in 1988 at the age of 12th.

Planetary disposition

Sr.No	Zodiac	Degree: Min: Sec	Lord of zodiac	Star Lord	Sub Lord
01	Sun	194 : 59 : 25	Jupiter	Saturn	Jupiter
02	Moon	265 : 32 : 02	Venus	Mars	Rahu
03	Mars	263 : 39 : 47	Venus	Mars	Mars
04	Mercury	167 : 57 : 22	Saturn	Rahu	Sun
05	Jupiter	161 : 18 : 22	Saturn	Rahu	Saturn
06	Venus	148 : 42 : 23	Saturn	Mars	Saturn
07	Saturn	275 : 05 : 31	Mercury	Mars	Sun
08	Rahu	089 : 46 : 48	Mars	Mercury	Saturn
09	Ketu	269 : 46 : 48	Venus	Mars	Saturn
10	Uranis	032 : 59 : 09	Venus	Mars	Venus
11	Neptune	076 : 01 : 55	Mars	Saturn	Jupiter

Case No 018

Female born on 13th July 1975 at 1130 hrs. in Udgir Maharashtra Lat 018:24N Long 077:06E

This is a classic case generally found in tropical countries. The natal chart reveals Virgo ascendant and lord of ascendant placed in Gemini, own sign afflicted with Saturn; Saturn being lord of fifth and sixth house. The Venus responsible for the functioning of ovaries is placed in twelfth cusp conjoined with Moon which rules the hormonal balance in female; further Jupiter being responsible for the functioning of reproductive organs is placed in Pisces in seventh house, this house rules the female organs responsible for reproduction. The eighth cusp falls in Aries and Mars occupied in indicates the malfunctioning of the organ due to growth of poly cyst on ovaries causing functional problems in secretion of hormones required for ovulation cycle.

The star lord of ascendant is Moon which is responsible for secretion of hormones and ovulation is occupied in twelfth cusp Leo and under aspect of Saturn from tenth house, Moon is conjoined with Venus another planet related to the function of reproductive organs. The star lord of sixth cusp is Jupiter occupied in seventh cusp which falls in Pisces owned by Jupiter is under aspect of Saturn from tenth house; the star lord of eighth cusp is Venus which is also star lord of twelfth cusp is placed in twelfth house conjoined with Moon and under aspect of Saturn; further Venus is also sub lord of ascendant. The sub lord of sixth cusp is Saturn known to cause prolonged and chronic types of ailment is placed in tenth house; is also sub lord of eighth cusp and twelfth cusp indicating growth of tumors or fibroids in body as such the native had suffered from poly cystic ovarian syndrome since 28th March 2000 i.e. when Jupiter Mahadasha was in progress and in Saturn antardasha and Saturn prati antardasha was passing. In the year 2014 in Saturn Mahadasha Saturn antardasha and Saturn pratiantardasha was passing on 8th February 2014 the native was admitted to hospital for Pelvic Inflammation Disease caused severe pain in pelvic region and was required to undergo surgical operation and removal of both ovaries was carried leaving behind permanent infertility.

Planetary disposition

Sr. No.	Planet	Zodiac	Degrees: Min: Sec	Lord of zodiac	Star lord	Sub lord
01	Sun	Gemini	296 : 43 : 43	Mercury	Jupiter	Venus
02	Moon	Leo	352 : 25 : 21	Sun	Venus	Saturn
03	Mars	Aries	224 : 59 : 03	Mars	Venus	Venus
04	Mercury	Gemini	277 : 48 : 10	Mercury	Rahu	Rahu
06	Venus	Pisces	209 : 29 : 58	Jupiter	Mercury	Jupiter
07	Saturn	Leo	339 : 08 : 32	Sun	Ketu	Venus
08	Rahu	Gemini	298 : 40 : 29	Mercury	Jupiter	Saturn
09	Ketu	Scorpio	064 : 50 : 17	Mars	Saturn	Saturn
10	Uranus	Taurus	244 : 51 : 17	Venus	Mars	Venus
11	Neptune	Libra	075 : 33 : 38	Venus	Saturn	Jupiter

Case no 018

Female native born on 23rd February 1978   1930 hrs Mumbai, Mulund

Lat. 019:10N Long. 072:57E

The native is female had shown the severe fungal infection gone superficially treated for long period of more than almost four years, then all of sudden uterine bleeding occurred with severe pain in abdomen and therefore native was taken to hospital for further diagnosis. The diagnosis confirms the disease gonorrhea which was initially went untreated and came to notice after it had become severe; this creates further complications such as Pelvic Inflammatory Disease followed by blockages in fallopian tubes leading to chronic type of disease. This when was totally recovered relapsed after few years giving rise to Endometriosis and return of severe pain in abdomen caused due to bleeding into abdomen irritation and severe pain.

If we understand the planetary disposition with the help of Horoscope we see that Saturn being lord of sixth cusp Capricorn and seventh cusp is placed in ascendant house with moon lord of twelfth house; so also further the lord of ascendant Sun is placed in seventh house with Mercury and Venus and are under aspect of Saturn from first house which is a planet responsible for obstruction and inflammation making the disease chronic and prolonged. The Moon is lord of twelfth house is placed in ascendant afflicted with Saturn. The star lord of sixth cusp is Mars placed in Gemini with Jupiter which is also a sub lord of sixth house and star lord of eighth house. So also star lord of eighth house Mercury is also a star lord of twelfth house owns second house i.e. Virgo and eleventh cusp i.e. Gemini occupies seventh cusp with Sun and Venus; where Venus is sub lord of Saturn which owns sixth cusp and star lord of Moon owner of twelfth cusp is placed in seventh house conjoined with Mercury and Sun as explained above. Here noteworthy is that Venus is planet that governs diseases related to reproductive organs and Mercury rules the abdomen; so also the sixth house is cusp that denotes the disease and eighth cusp denotes the seriousness of the ailment with twelfth house being indicator of Hospitalization, Saturn being the cause of prolonged and chronic diseases occupies ascendant with Moon which governs the Hormonal disorder are conjoined indicating the chronic disease related to abdomen, reproductive organs, hormonal disorder with requiring hospitalization.

When after prolonged treatment the native was hospitalized when the disease was at its peak and with severe pain in abdomen and required to be surgically operated for Hysterectomy. To understand the onset and progress of disease we can confirm based on the connectivity of significators of sixth, eighth and twelfth cusps that as we see the onset of disease as indicated by sixth cusp and star lord, sub lord of sixth cusp are well connected with the lord of eighth house, star lord of eighth cusp and sub lord of eighth cusp. So we can see that sub lord of Saturn is Venus is conjoined with Saturn lord of sixth cusp and Sun lord of ascendant as also the star lord of eighth house Mercury. Thus further the lord of twelfth house Moon is placed with lord of sixth cusp Saturn; so also star lord of Saturn is Ketu occupying eighth cusp is also sub lord of Jupiter afflicted with Mars occupying Gemini, the lord of which is Mercury causative of diseases related to abdomen.

Here onset of disease if we look into can be understood with reference to the Mahadasha and antardasha of connected significators can be better understood by study of the respective periods. The disease occurred first and as reported to Doctor on 20th September 2003 when Moon mahadasha was in force and in Saturn antardasha with Moon prati antardasha continued. During this period the initial symptoms noticed were severe pain in abdomen causing continued unrest; this time it was well noted by Doctors and with great efforts the infection was suppressed leading to discharge of the native from hospital. Actually the disease must have existed even before that and went unnoticed. Further we can see there were consistent complains but native did not visit Doctor; during which period hormonal imbalance, frequent mood swing and cranky behavior was observed but remained unattended till the recurrence of severe pain followed by uterine bleeding occurred. On 20th February the native reported again to doctor when the level of infection was severe and serious, not only but also denoted the probability of growth of some tumor near cervix. Doctors when examined and diagnosed found that the native not only had Pelvic Inflammation Disease but is accompanied by growth of tumor near cervix inside the uterus; when doctor had to take native for surgical operation. As such the native was hospitalized and got operated for hysterectomy on 28th February 2011 when Mars mahadasha was due in which Saturn antardasha continued after completion of Mercury prati antardasha. This left behind the native infertile till life with great trauma and psychological troubles.   Planetary disposition is given as under.

Sr. No.	Planet name	Zodiac	Degree : Min : Sec	Lord of Zodiac	Star Lord	Sub Lord
01	Sun	Aquarius	191 : 02 : 52	Saturn	Rahu	Saturn
02	Moon	Leo	017 : 08 : 27	Sun	Venus	Moon
03	Mars	Gemini	329 : 01 : 00	Mercury	Jupiter	Sun
04	Mercury	Aquarius	188 : 05 : 22	Saturn	Rahu	Rahu
05	Jupiter	Gemini	302 : 32 : 20	Mercury	Mars	Ketu
06	Venus	Aquarius	198 : 51 : 05	Saturn	Rahu	Moon
07	Saturn	Leo	002 : 58 : 51	Sun	Ketu	Venus
08	Rahu	Virgo	044 : 09 : 49	Mercury	Moon	Ketu
09	Ketu	Pisces	224 : 09 : 49	Jupiter	Saturn	Rahu
10	Uranus	Libra	082 : 50 : 54	Venus	Jupiter	Saturn
11	Neptune	Scorpio	114 : 35 : 28	Mars	Mercury	Rahu

2)	Reproductive system Ailments in male native

In general the male reproductive system ailments are divided into two groups 1) Physiological type of ailments and diseases associated with pituitary gland and 2) Infectious type like Epididymis etc.

In male reproductive system major problems usually occur are

1) Prostate related either infection or cancerous growth. Prastatitis is normal in age group after 55 years of age. Where in normally no major symptoms are seen but eventually the bleeding occurs while urination.
2) Hypogonadism, In this syndrome normally testicular atrophy is observed sometimes because of bacterial or fungal infection.
3) Epididymis, In this normally inflammation associated with severe infection is noticed.

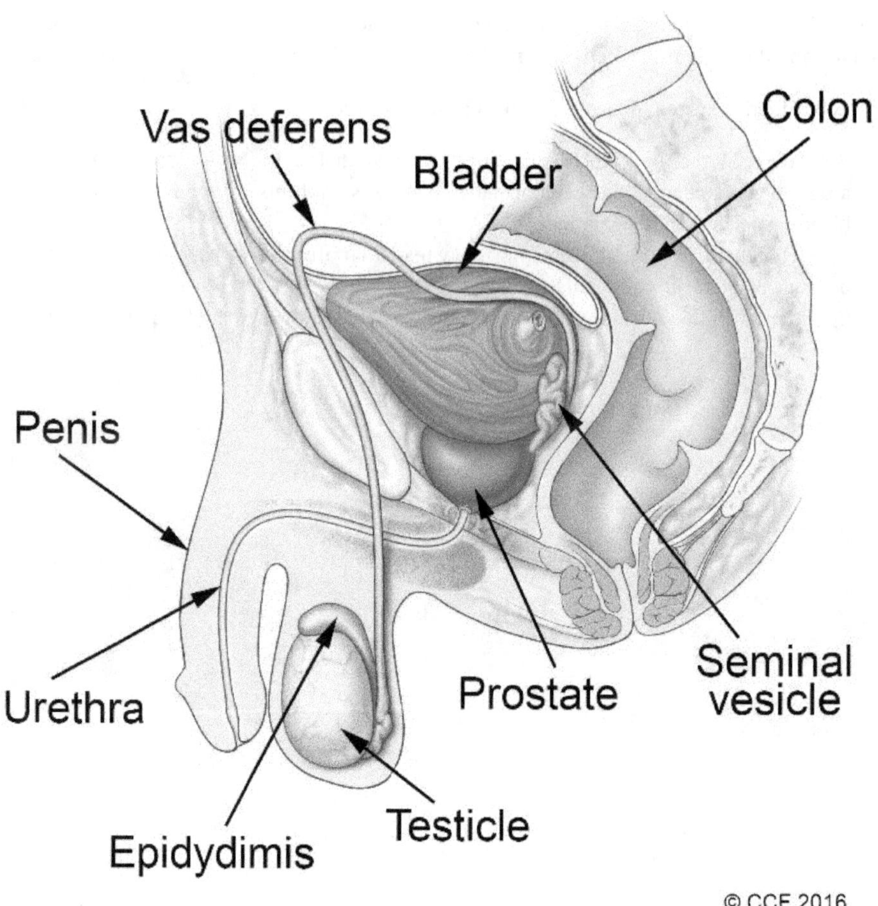

Case no 019

Female native born on 23rd February 1978   1930 hrs Mumbai, Mulund

Lat. 019:10N Long. 072:57E

The native is female had shown the severe fungal infection gone superficially treated for long period of more than almost four years, then all of sudden uterine bleeding occurred with severe pain in abdomen and therefore native was taken to hospital for further diagnosis. The diagnosis confirms the disease gonorrhea which was initially went untreated and came to notice after it had become severe; this creates further complications such as Pelvic Inflammatory Disease followed by blockages in fallopian tubes leading to chronic type of disease. This when was totally recovered relapsed after few years giving rise to Endometriosis and return of severe pain in abdomen caused due to bleeding into abdomen irritation and severe pain.

If we understand the planetary disposition with the help of Horoscope we see that Saturn being lord of sixth cusp Capricorn and seventh cusp is placed in ascendant house with moon lord of twelfth house; so also further the lord of ascendant Sun is placed in seventh house with Mercury and Venus and are under aspect of Saturn from first house which is a planet responsible for obstruction and inflammation making the disease chronic and prolonged. The Moon is lord of twelfth house is placed in ascendant afflicted with Saturn. The star lord of sixth cusp is Mars placed in Gemini with Jupiter which is also a sub lord of sixth house and star lord of eighth house. So also star lord of eighth house Mercury is also a star lord of twelfth house owns second house i.e. Virgo and eleventh cusp i.e. Gemini occupies seventh cusp with Sun and Venus; where Venus is sub lord of Saturn which owns sixth cusp and star lord of Moon owner of twelfth cusp is placed in seventh house conjoined with Mercury and Sun as explained above. Here noteworthy is that Venus is planet that governs diseases related to reproductive organs and Mercury rules the abdomen; so also the sixth house is cusp that denotes the disease and eighth cusp denotes the seriousness of the ailment with twelfth house being indicator of Hospitalization, Saturn being the cause of prolonged and chronic diseases occupies ascendant with Moon which governs the Hormonal disorder are conjoined indicating the chronic disease related to abdomen, reproductive organs, hormonal disorder with requiring hospitalization.

When after prolonged treatment the native was hospitalized when the disease was at its peak and with severe pain in abdomen and required to be surgically operated for Hysterectomy. To understand the onset and progress of disease we can confirm based on the connectivity of significators of sixth, eighth and twelfth cusps that as we see the onset of disease as indicated by sixth cusp and star lord, sub lord of sixth cusp are well connected with the lord of eighth house, star lord of eighth cusp and sub lord of eighth cusp. So we can see that sub lord of Saturn is Venus is conjoined with Saturn lord of sixth cusp and Sun lord of ascendant as also the star lord of eighth house Mercury. Thus further the lord of twelfth house Moon is placed with lord of sixth cusp Saturn; so also star lord of Saturn is Ketu occupying eighth cusp is also sub lord of Jupiter afflicted with Mars occupying Gemini, the lord of which is Mercury causative of diseases related to abdomen.

Here onset of disease if we look into can be understood with reference to the Mahadasha and antardasha of connected significators can be better understood by study of the respective periods. The disease occurred first and as reported to Doctor on 20th September 2003 when Moon mahadasha was in force and in Saturn antardasha with Moon prati antardasha continued. During this period the initial symptoms noticed were severe pain in abdomen causing continued unrest; this time it was well noted by Doctors and with great efforts the infection was suppressed leading to discharge of the native from hospital. Actually the disease must have existed even before that and went unnoticed. Further we can see there were consistent complains but native did not visit

Doctor; during which period hormonal imbalance, frequent mood swing and cranky behavior was observed but remained unattended till the recurrence of severe pain followed by uterine bleeding occurred. On 20th February the native reported again to doctor when the level of infection was severe and serious, not only but also denoted the probability of growth of some tumor near cervix. Doctors when examined and diagnosed found that the native not only had Pelvic Inflammation Disease but is accompanied by growth of tumor near cervix inside the uterus; when doctor had to take native for surgical operation. As such the native was hospitalized and got operated for hysterectomy on 28th February 2011 when Mars mahadasha was due in which Saturn antardasha continued after completion of Mercury prati antardasha. This left behind the native infertile till life with great trauma and psychological troubles.   Planetary disposition is given as under.

Sr. No.	Planet name	Zodiac	Degree : Min : Sec	Lord of Zodiac	Star Lord	Sub Lord
01	Sun	Aquarius	191 : 02 : 52	Saturn	Rahu	Saturn
02	Moon	Leo	017 : 08 : 27	Sun	Venus	Moon
03	Mars	Gemini	329 : 01 : 00	Mercury	Jupiter	Sun
04	Mercury	Aquarius	188 : 05 : 22	Saturn	Rahu	Rahu
05	Jupiter	Gemini	302 : 32 : 20	Mercury	Mars	Ketu
06	Venus	Aquarius	198 : 51 : 05	Saturn	Rahu	Moon
07	Saturn	Leo	002 : 58 : 51	Sun	Ketu	Venus
08	Rahu	Virgo	044 : 09 : 49	Mercury	Moon	Ketu
09	Ketu	Pisces	224 : 09 : 49	Jupiter	Saturn	Rahu
10	Uranus	Libra	082 : 50 : 54	Venus	Jupiter	Saturn
11	Neptune	Scorpio	114 : 35 : 28	Mars	Mercury	Rahu

In general the male reproductive system ailments are divided into two groups 1) Physiological type of ailments and diseases associated with pituitary gland and 2) Infectious type like Epididymis etc.

1) Physiological disorders --These are the diseases associated with functional disorders normally occurred in male reproductive system and can be further classified as Prostate related ailments ,Testicular diseases like Spermatorrhea etc. and hypogonadism related diseases.
2) Secondly diseases due to STD and infection are also occurred.

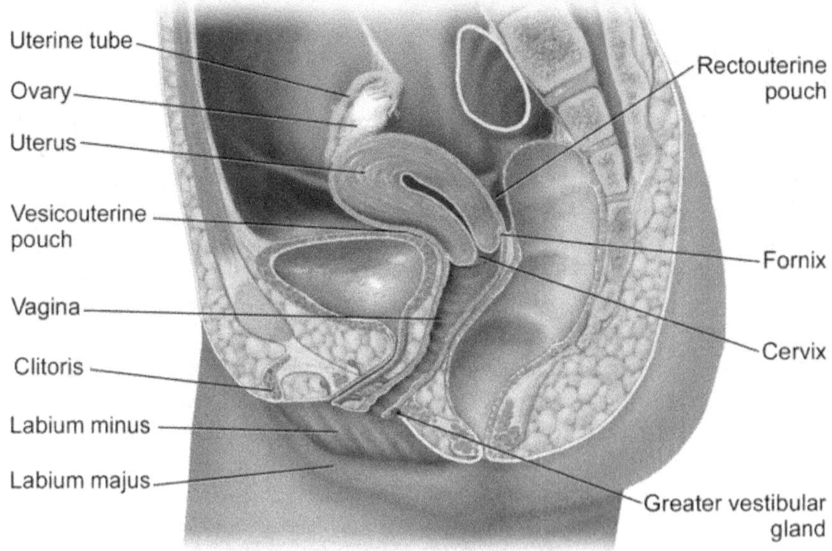

The Female Reproductive System

To understand in details we can see the natal chart and planetary disposition; this can be summarized as given under, it may be noted before that the seventh cusp rules the reproductive organs and eighth cusp represents the function. Malefic like Saturn and Rahu with Moon sign in ascendant indicate the probability of occurrence of these problems. Saturn and Ketu or Mars Saturn Ketu in eighth cusp give rise to functional disorders. Following points may be considered to find out the exact type of problem and subsequent solution to the ailment can be found out.

1) If the seventh cusp be occupied by Ketu or under aspect of Ketu the native may suffer from Hypogonadism.
2) If Venus and Mars occupy seventh cusp and are under aspect from Saturn native may have to suffer from pituitary dysfunction casing ED or spermatorrhea , oligospermia, azoospermia leading to infertility.
3) If Jupiter is placed in twelfth cusp and under aspect of Rahu diseases related to prostate are observed like prostate enlargement or prostate cancer occurs.
4) If Moon be hemmed in between malefic planets and eighth cusp is occupied by Ketu or Mercury the testicular torsion, testicular cancer or absence of testosterone occurs leading to infertility and lack of male signs are observed.
5) If Mercury is conjoined with Saturn in eighth cusp and Moon is afflicted anywhere in natal chart the Klinefelters syndrome is occurred where in abnormal testicles are formed.

6) If Rahu or Saturn in second cusp and Mercury occupies eighth with Moon being placed in twelfth cusp the native suffers from osteoporosis, epididymis, hot flashes, irritability with depression are noticed; which leads to infertility.

7) If Venus and Mars occupy the sign owned by Mars then also native suffers from either cancer of testicles or secretion of testosterone is affected.

8) If Mars, Saturn, Sun, and Moon are placed in second, sixth, eighth, twelfth cusp the native is likely to suffer from acute or chronic bacterial, fungal infection may lead to complication sometimes. Gonorrhea, Syphilis are also caused due to this type of planetary disposition.

9) Malefic planets in eighth house also indicate disorders related to sperm motility, azoospermia etc.

It is common as we know that seventh and cusps are responsible for the ailments associated with reproductive systems and Libra owned by Venus and Scorpio owned by Mars; causes the ailments and dysfunctions associated with the organs.

As such the diseases caused due to foreign molecule or microorganism can be studied well when we understand the role of Venus, Mars, and related zodiacs Libra and Scorpio; along with seventh and eighth cusp together. So also Rahu which if afflicts these planets or occupies these houses play important role in onset of the disease or making further complications in the progress of the disease. Also Neptune if afflicts ascendant or square aspect or seventh cusp, eighth cusp or Libra, Scorpio may be the native is likely to suffer from these infectious diseases; so also when we consider the combination of ascendant lord, the Moon, Rahu or Ketu.

The association of ascendant, Mars, Mercury, in fourth cusp or twelfth cusp or conjointly if the aspect sixth cusp; is certain to suffer from the infection in life. In addition to above it is also noticed that the nature of the disease or ailment depends on the sixth cusp sub lord, when connected to seventh, eighth cusp or signs Libra or Scorpio.

It is studied and noticed that following conditions either determine the occurrence of the disease or the intensity of the ailments.

1) If the sub lord of eighth cusp is Saturn and signifies eighth cusp the native will have acute or chronic bacterial infection of prostate.

2) If the sub lord of seventh cusp signifies seventh cusp the native suffers from STD.

3) If the sub lord of eighth cusp is Mars and signifies eighth cusp the native may suffer from frequent fungal infection and may be required to undergo circumcision surgery of penis.

4) If the sub lord of seventh cusp is Mars and signifies seventh cusp the native suffers from infections and may develop pituitary function disorder.

5) If the sub lord of eighth cusp is Jupiter and signifies eighth cusp the native is likely to suffer from frequent inflammation of the body part involved.

6) If the sub lord of eighth cusp is Sun and signifies eighth cusp then native will suffer from abnormal testicles and also likely to suffer from frequent infection.

7) If the sub lord of seventh house is Saturn and signifies the seventh house the native may suffer from cancerous growth in the reproductive organ.

8) If the sub lord of the eighth cusp is Venus and signifies eighth house the native will suffer from bacterial infection but the severity will be much less.

9) If the sub lord of the seventh house is Venus and signifies seventh house the native will be suffering from fungal infection due to unhygienic habits.
10) If the sub lord of seventh cusp is Rahu and signifies the seventh house the native will suffer from syphilis.
11) If the sub lord of seventh cusp is Sun and signifies seventh cusp the native will be suffering from repeated skin infections.
12) If the sub lord of eighth cusp is Mercury and signifies eighth house the native will suffer from depression and irritability towards the act.
13) If the sub lord of seventh cusp is Mercury and signifies the seventh house the native is likely to suffer from severe infection due to Gonorrhea.
14) If the sub lord of eighth cusp be Moon and signifies the eighth cusp the native is likely to suffer from ED (erectile dysfunction).
15) If the sub lord of seventh house is Ketu and signifies seventh cusp the native will suffer from some or the other infection frequently.
16) If the sub lord of seventh cusp is Jupiter and signifies the seventh house native is likely to suffer from repeated infections and may develop further cancerous growth.

This can further be studied with the following case

Case no 019

The native born on 02^(ND) November 1926 at 2038 hrs in Mumbai/Mulund

Lat. 019:10 N   Long. 072:57E

Ascendant of this native being Taurus owned by Venus which is also a lord of sixth cusp indicates malefic house related to diseases. The Venus occupies Libra the seventh sign in natures chart indicating diseases related to reproductive organs and is placed in sixth cusp; the Venus is also under aspect from Mars placed in twelfth house again ruler of diseases related to reproductive organs. The star lord of ascendant is Mars and is also lord of seventh cusp Scorpio which in its turn is eighth sign in natures chart indicating diseases related to reproductive organs. The star lord of Mars is Venus which is lord of ascendant and sixth cusp occupying seventh house and afflicted by Saturn in Scorpio. The sub lord of ascendant is Jupiter which is also lord of eighth cusp causative of prostate related disorders. Mercury is the lord of fifth cusp and rules the reproductive system and emotions is placed in seventh cusp afflicted with Saturn in the zodiac owned by Mars paced in twelfth house, Mars also governs the lower abdomen and abdominal cavity. Another important cusp is sixth cusp that rules the nature of the ailment and lord of the sixth cusp is placed in Libra i.e. seventh cusp of natures chart ruled by Venus and as we know the Venus is significator of first, sixth and seventh and sign Libra and Scorpio.   The star lord of sixth cusp is Jupiter; which is lord of eighth house and placed in ninth house under

aspect of Saturn, Saturn occupies seventh house that indicates diseases of reproductive organ. The other important planet is sub lord of sixth house that is Mercury; a lord of fifth cusp related to emotions and abdomen occupies seventh house, i.e. Scorpio, important sign for infection and inflammation. Sub lord of Mercury is Venus and occupant of Libra i.e. sixth cusp is an important planet related to reproductive organs. Hence considering all the significators of ascendant, sixth house, are well connected to the ascendant, sixth cusp, eighth cusp, and twelfth cusp; so also the sign Libra, Scorpio it can be concluded that native will suffer from chronic bacterial prostatic inflammation along with epididymis ; an infectious disease commonly referred to as Gonorrhea. One more important house to be examined here is eighth with seventh together; the sub lord of seventh house is Jupiter and the sub lord of eighth cusp is Saturn, where Saturn is placed in seventh cusp aspect ninth cusp where Jupiter is occupied. Star lord of Jupiter is Mars and is also lord of cusp occupied by Saturn, thereby confirming the occurrence of the disease.

The occurrence of the disease was reported when Saturn mahadasha started and Saturn antardasha was on its way in prati antardasha of Mercury i.e. 29th January 1976 when the dasha lord was in its own star. The native died due to septicemia leading to multiple organ failure.

Planetary disposition is as given under.

Sr. no	Planet	Zodiac	Degree: Min :Sec	Lord of zodiac	Star Lord	Sub Lord
01	Sun	Libra	166 : 36 : 39	Venus	Rahu	Venus
02	Moon	Virgo	133 : 52 : 02	Mercury	Moon	Rahu
03	Mars	Aries	349 : 00 : 10	Mars	Venus	Rahu
04	Mercury	Scorpio	189 : 40 : 31	Mars	Saturn	Venus
05	Jupiter	Capricorn	265 : 06 : 04	Saturn	Mars	Rahu
06	Venus	Libra	161 : 53 : 24	Venus	Rahu	Saturn
07	Saturn	Scorpio	183 : 35 : 10	Mars	Saturn	Saturn
08	Rahu	Gemini	047 : 17 : 30	Mercury	Rahu	Venus
09	Ketu	Sagittarius	227 : 17 : 30	Jupiter	Venus	Moon
10	Uranus	Pisces	303 : 07 : 58	Jupiter	Jupiter	Rahu
11	Neptunr	Leo	093 : 57 : 34	Sun	Ketu	Moon

Case no 020

Male native born on 26th June 1964 at 0345hrs in Akole/Ahmed nagar
Lat- 019:32N Long- 074:03E

The native whose chart is mentioned here is classic example of the relation between planetary disposition and the occurrence of ailment. The natal chart denotes Taurus Ascendant occupied by Mars, the sixth house lord is Venus occupies second house and afflicted with Rahu the lord of eighth cusp is Jupiter placed in twelfth house in Aries. Here first thing we can note from the birth chart is that the lord of sixth house is also sub lord of seventh house and star lord of ascendant occupies the second house with lord of sixth cusp Venus; which is also a star lord of Jupiter placed in eighth cusp and lord of ascendant is afflicted conjoined with Rahu a malefic that is responsible for tumor and any malignant growth in body.

The sub lord of sixth cusp Venus is lord of sixth cusp and occupies second house under aspect from Ketu placed in eighth cusp afflicting Moon , lord of third house and star lord of Mars occupying ascendant owned by Venus; and Mars aspects seventh house owned by itself causing the onset of disease, Mars is also lord of twelfth cusp where lord of eighth cusp Jupiter is placed; whereas the Jupiter is star lord of Neptune occupying sixth house, this indicates the occurrence of disease related to prostate enlargement so also the sub lord of Neptune is Saturn and Saturn is also sub lord of Jupiter placed in twelfth cusp, which indicates the disease related to Reproductive system as well indicates hospitalization. Further we can see the sub lord of Ascendant is Sun which is also sub lord of fifth house is placed in second house and conjoined with Mercury, lord of fifth cusp and both are afflicted by Rahu. Also Sun is sub lord of eighth cusp which denotes the severity and intensity of the ailment apart from diseases related to the reproductive organs, Ketu which occupied eighth house is also sub lord of eighth cusp directly aspect the Venus, Sun and Mercury placed in second house. Here important is to that the Mercury is responsible for diseases related to abdominal cavity and kidney and Venus denotes the ailments related to the reproductive system conjoined with rahu. Rahu being sub lord of Mars which is lord of seventh and twelfth house and occupies ascendant is also causative of inflammatory and infectious diseases of reproductive system and the lord of ascendant is Venus which is also lord of sixth cusp. Considering all the above points it is observed that all the significators of sixth, Fifth, Eighth and twelfth cusp are well connected with that of ascendant and the sign Venus Scorpio indicating the occurrence of the prostate infection with prolonged chronic ailment which subsequently gave rise to prostate cancer.

As well the onset of disease i.e. first appearance of the disease occurred on 30th October 1994 when Mahadasha of Mars was in progress with antar dasha of Venus and prati antardasha of Mars. The medical and hospital treatment the native availed was of excellent grade and the disease apparently disappeared temporarily.

The diagnosis was the benign prostate hyperplasia associated with acute bacterial infection leading to dribbling urine, frequent urination, and stiffness in back along with burning sensation. There was also severe pain occurred frequently with urinary incontinence. After almost twenty years the same symptoms were noticed and native complained of frequent passing of blood along with urine. The native was advised to get hospitalized again on 20th July 2014 when Rahu mahadasha was in progress with antar dasha and prati antar dasha of Mars. Again when diagnosed the doctor reported that native may have developed prostate cancer which was confirmed after few weeks of diagnosis.

As it is clear from the chart that the Sun, and Jupiter along with Venus in favorable condition the native got totally recovered and was discharged on eve of new year on 28th December 2014.

Planetary disposition as in birth chart

Sr. No.	Name of planet	Name of Zodiac	Degrees: Min :Sec	Lord of Zodiac	Star Lord	Sub Lord
01	Sun	Gemini	040 : 59 : 09	Mercury	Rahu	Saturn
02	Moon	Sagittarius	230 : 36 : 02	Jupiter	Venus	Jupiter
03	Mars	Taurus	012 : 38 : 24	Venus	Moon	Rahu
04	Mercury	Gemini	039 : 16 : 57	Mercury	Rahu	Jupiter
05	Jupiter	Aries	353 : 37 : 41	Mars	Venus	Saturn
06	Venus	Gemini	031 : 39 : 56	Mercury	Mars	Mercury

07	Saturn	Aquarius	281 : 35 : 22	Saturn	Rahu	Saturn
08	Rahu	Gemini	038 : 38 : 04	Mercury	Rahu	Rahu
09	Ketu	Sagittarius	218 : 38 : 04	Jupiter	Ketu	Jupiter
10	Uranus	Leo	103 : 22 : 38	Sun	Venus	Venus
11	Neptune	Libra	171 : 57 : 21	Venus	Jupitr	Saturn

Chapter No 18

Diabetes scanned under Horoscope

The term diabetes indicates the malfunctioning of Pancreas which secrets insulin that controls the free glucose in blood and level of glycogen in human body; and it is disorder of metabolism. In almost all cases of diabetes there is insufficiency of insulin due to malfunction in pancreas. And if insulin is not produced due to the malfunctioning of pancreas the very process of converting excess glucose in blood to form glycogen and stored in pancreatic cells. This leads mainly into glycosurea resulting because of excess glucose in blood. This also leads to excessive fatigue as sufficient glucose is not available when required so also polyurea may occur which causes elimination of extra fluid from body and increase in thirst; also marked by loss in weight. Jupiter rules over pancreas, liver, and carbohydrates and in birth chart if found badly afflicted.   Diabetic natives also suffer from cardiovascular and renal dysfunction or ailments related and it becomes necessary to take in to account all these factors to understand the physiology of native. As such the planetary disposition in natal chart of diabetics must be studied through different perspectives; whether planes and significators denotes the atherosclerosis, hypertension, cerebral hemorrhage, renal dysfunction, sores on feet etc., along with the metabolism of the native. In many chronic cases nephritis is also occurred, so also thrombotic non bacterial endocarditic. Pancreas is governed by the sign Cancer and any affliction of Cancer by malefic may make native suffer from diabetes; the function of pancreatic cells is disturbed because of faulty food habits or because of genetic factors, or stress related is denoted by second cusp in natal chart so also indicated by disposition of Venus in chart. As the Jupiter governs the liver, is responsible for secretion of bile that aids the very process of digestion; and if Jupiter if afflicted leads to malfunctioning of liver and pancreas. When planet Jupiter is afflicted in Libra or Scorpio the very secretion of insulin is affected or cellular storage sugar in form of glycogen is hampered; Jupiter if conjoined with Saturn also leads to the condition called diabetic. The seventh house in natures chart is Libra which rules the function of kidney also causes insulin secretion; as zodiac Libra is owned by Venus and if Venus is afflicted in Libra or Scorpio the native suffers from diabetes. Venus and Moon are watery planets and if afflicted by Mars or other malefic in Cancer, Scorpio or Pisces the native is likely to suffer from type 2 diabetes and may become chronic. So also if ascendant, sixth cusp, and their lord conjoin with Venus, Moon in ascendant or sixth cusp the native suffers from diabetes and is likely to suffer from complications related to renal function disorder. In case Mercury placed in the sign of Jupiter or Libra and under aspect from Mars the functional disorder of pancreas associated with kidney failure.

If Jupiter is placed in sign of Libra which rules the kidneys; Saturn in the sign of Cancer which indicates diseases related to metabolism and endocrine glands and in conjunction or in aspect of Uranus the diabetes and complications are certain to appear. Pancreas is ruled by sixth cusp while endocrine dysfunction by Venus and as such if both are afflicted by Rahu or by Mars the diabetic disorder is occurred. Jupiter governs the function of glycogen cycle in body; Venus and Moon denotes the metabolism while Mercury denotes the imbalanced blood sugar levels if both are afflicted diabetes is indicated.

Saturn denotes the chronic ailments or prolonged and chronic diseases even sometimes disease goes unnoticed for long period and occurs all of sudden when it is difficult to control. And as such Saturn, Venus, Moon, Jupiter and Mercury play vital role in onset of the disease and also in further complications. To summarize we find that if sub lord of sixth cusp is either Venus, Jupiter, or Moon, and watery sign Cancer, Scorpio, and Pisces the native is certain to suffer from incurable diseases like diabetes.

Anatomical correlation of diabetes with Zodiac and organs affected are as

1) Cancer—Stomach, Esophagus, pancreas, blood serum, upper lobe of liver.
2) Libra ---- Kidney, Adrenal glands, Lumbar region, vasomotor nerves, skin.
3) Scorpio—Bladder, Urethra, Genitals, Prostate, Pubic area.
4) Pisces --- Feet, Toes, Fibrinogen; in blood that causes the blood to clot.

Physiological afflictions to the sign

1) Cancer--- Indigestion, Gastric upsurge, Flatulence, dropsy.
2) Libra----- Nephritis, urine incontinence, glycos urea, Uremia.
3) Scorpio—Skin infection, gangrene, constipation.
4) Pisces ---- Gout, tumors, infection and wounds of heals.

Venus, the main planet denotes the diabetes type 2 and resistance to insulin which causes sugars builds up in blood; secondly Jupiter which rules the obesity, spleen, liver, and function of pancreatic cells to convert free glucose in to glycogen thereby maintaining the blood sugar level under control, and nerves. The hormone insulin that moves free sugar from blood into cells to be stored as glycogen or to be freed for generating energy for body movements; in case native suffers from diabetes the either body doesn't make sufficient insulin or can't use it efficiently. Untreated high blood sugar from diabetes can damage nerves, eyes, kidneys, and even skin at certain body parts. That is all the planets those rule these parts of the body are also required to be scanned under horoscope. In pre diabetic stage; when blood sugar level is high but still not exceed enough to cause diabetes type2. So also in gestational diabetes the temporary escalation of blood sugar indicating diabetes is observed in many cases of pregnancy where Venus occupies either sixth cusp or occupies eighth house as lord of sixth house. This is being of temporary type doesn't need to be considered but needs treatment.

To study further we may consider few cases and analyze under horoscope as given bellow.

Case no 21

This is classic case for study of diabetic native and its planetary disposition.

The native is female with Birth date 16th June 1975 at 1820 hrs in Krishna giri

with Lat- 015:34 N and Long- 077: 49 E

The chart shows Scorpio ascendant with Mars as lord of ascendant which occupies fifth cusp i.e. Pisces conjoined with Jupiter; the Mars is also a lord of sixth house indicating the occurrence of disease. The lord of eighth cusp is Mercury a planet responsible for the function of endocrine glands and thus controls the secretion of insulin, occupies seventh house owned by Venus. The Star lord of sixth cusp is Sun and occupies eighth house afflicted by Saturn; Saturn also star lord Rahu placed in ascendant. Saturn is under aspect of Mars from fifth cusp is also lord of sixth cusp and ascendant thus denotes the disease related to blood disorders. Further we can note that Mars is star lord of Sun and Uranus occupied in twelfth house which denotes a disease of chronic type and associated with hyper thyroid type of disease. So also Lord of eighth cusp Mercury is placed in seventh cusp afflicted with Ketu, again lord of seventh house is Venus a planet rules the blood sugar or diabetes; is placed in ninth house Cancer owned by Moon. Venus being the major planet to be considered as planet causative of diabetes; the star lord of Venus is Saturn and placed in eighth cusp conjoined with Sun, which is star lord Moon; another major planet to be considered for Diabetes is placed in fifth house is connected with sixth cusp as it is lord and star lord of sixth house. Venus being also lord of twelfth house and placed in Cancer

clearly indicate the complications of the disease diabetes. But as Saturn lord of third another malefic cusp and Star lord of Rahu and Moon indicates the disease giving rise to diabetes and gets complicated due to presence of Uranus in twelfth cusp and Neptune being placed in ascendant. Saturn also star lord of Neptune and Sun being star lord of sixth cusp confirms the onset of the disease in natives chart. Now sub lord of sixth cusp is Rahu placed in ascendant and conjoined with Neptune; sub lord of eighth cusp Mercury is placed in seventh house afflicted with ketu and under direct aspect of Rahu and Neptune. Also the sub lord of eighth cusp Mercury is also sub lord of Saturn placed in eighth cusp. Saturn from eighth house aspect Mars in fifth cusp a lord of sixth cusp and causative of serious blood disorder, and Jupiter which rules the secretion of insulin in body; as such the sub lord of sixth house, eighth cusp and twelfth cusp are well connected with each other and ascendant to cause the disease diabetes. Here further we can note that the causative of mysterious disease Uranus is placed in twelfth cusp and sub lord of which is Jupiter afflicted with Mars and under direct aspect by Saturn occupied in eighth cusp causes onset of hyperthyroidism along with diabetes which creates further obesity leading to severing diabetes.

The planetary disposition of the chart is as tabled bellow.

Sr. No.	Name of planet	Name of zodiac	Degree: Min: Sec.	Lord of Zodiac	Star Lord	Sub lord
01	Sun	Gemini	211 : 14 : 54	Mercury	Mercury	Mercury
02	Moon	Virgo	300 : 04 : 03	Mercury	Mars	Rahu
03	Mars	Pisces	145 : 57 : 26	Jupiter	Sun	Rahu
04	Mercury	Taurus	202 : 48 : 37	Venus	Moon	Sun
05	Jupiter	Pisces	145 : 57 : 26	Jupiter	Mercury	Rahu
06	Venus	Cancer	256 : 35 : 43	Moon	Saturn	Jupiter
07	Saturn	Gemini	235 : 16 : 47	Mercury	Jupiter	Mercury

08	Rahu	Scorpio	006 : 15 : 15	Mars	Saturn	Mercury
09	Ketu	Taurus	186 : 15 : 15	Venus	Sun	Mercury
10	Uranus	Libra	335 : 01 : 19	Venus	Mars	Sun
11	Neptune	Scorpio	016 : 30 : 22	Mars	Saturn	Jupiter
12	Pluto	Virgo	312 : 57 : 57	Mercury	Moon	Rahu

The disease was noticed when the native visited doctor for severe fatigue followed by vertigo, sometimes frequent urination specifically during night leading to sleep disturbances with continuous increase in body weight was reported. After initial diagnosis doctor advised hospitalization as blood sugar was found to have crossed 450 mark. This was occurred during dasha period of ascendant i.e. when maha dasha of Rahu was about to finish and in Mars antardasha and Moon prati antar dasha on 1st December 2014. Now even the native has resumed daily work she is consistently under treatment and periodic tests she has to undergo; It is clearly revealed that the diabetes associated with complications and added disorder called hyperthyroidism, which actually is result of the planet Moon; lord of ninth cusp and known causative of thyroid function disorder placed in Virgo under direct aspect of Mars and star lord of Moon being Sun which is placed in eighth house afflicted with Saturn. This indicates the disease that causes hyperthyroidism was occurred at the same time when diabetes is detected. The entire study indicates that the disease Diabetes and Hyperthyroidism are of chronic type and will stay till life. The native was also advised to take care of feet as Jupiter placed in fifth house afflicted with Mars in Pisces which may cause wounds to feet or heals leading and may also lead to gangrene requiring amputation in future.

Case no 22

Native is a male born on 03rd October 1982 at 2257 hrs in Mumbai/Goregaon

Lat – 019:10 N   Long – 072:51 E

The chart is of male native having Gemini ascendant and Rahu occupied the ascendant; the lord of ascendant Mercury is placed in fourth house in own house Virgo conjoined with Sun, Venus afflicted with Saturn. The Venus being lord of fifth cusp Libra indicating diseases related to stomach and pancreas; is also afflicted with Saturn, and Sun lord of third house afflicted with Saturn lord of eighth cusp and ninth cusp. Here the lord of sixth cusp and eleventh cusp is Mars which is malefic planet and rules the body metabolism along with blood; so also the lord of seventh house Jupiter is conjoined with Mars; Jupiter rules the stomach related, liver related diseases. The Moon that denotes diseases related to endocrine glands is placed in tenth cusp and under aspect of Saturn. The lord tenth cusp occupying sixth house conjoined with Mars, which is also a lord of seventh cusp. Now Lord of eighth house is placed in fourth cusp that indicates the diseases related to pancreas; Saturn conjoined with Venus, indicator the disease diabetes, and Mercury causative of nerve system and Sun, lord of third house i.e. malefic house; in Virgo , a sixth zodiac in natures chart responsible for diseases related to liver, pancreas. Star lord of sixth cusp is Jupiter placed in Scorpio i.e. eighth cusp conjoined with Mars which owns the cusp; here Scorpio is sign denotes the disease related to blood so also Mars. Further star lord of eighth cusp is Sun, which is again star lord of twelfth cusp;

afflicted with Saturn, which aspect the sixth cusp and is star lord of Mars and Uranus significator of the chronic disease related to blood. Star lord of Jupiter is Rahu placed in ascendant in Gemini, a zodiac owned by Mercury which is already afflicted by Saturn in fourth house and the sub lord is Moon placed in Pisces in tenth house under aspect of Saturn, the lord of house is Jupiter occupying sixth house is also sub lord of Mars. Venus is sub lord of Uranus and Ketu malefic planets which aspect Rahu in ascendant causing the diabetes and complicating the disease. Moon being the planet responsible for mood swing and psychosomatic disorders is also known to rule endocrine gland function thus causing diabetes as result of stress developed; Moon is also sub lord of third house and star lord of Mercury is thus major planet that makes native suffer. Here wecan clearly see that sub lord of ascendant is Ketu occupying seventh house and placed in square of Moon that is sub lord of sixth cusp and under direct aspect of Sun which is sub lord of eighth cusp are well connected so also sub lord of twelfth cusp is Rahu placed in ascendant is sub lord of Moon and sub lord of Mercury placed in fourth cusp also a lord of ascendant indicating the ascendant sub lord and star lord are well connected to the disease causing planets Moon and Mercury; so also further the sub lord of seventh cusp is Venus is also sub lord of Rahu, Ketu and Uranus leading to the prolonged and chronic type of disease.

The seventh cusp which is responsible for kidney and urinary tract function and ailments is afflicted by presence of Ketu and Uranus of which Uranus is planet of mysterious diseases denotes the kidney related and also blood related disease of unknown origin; here the sub lord of Uranus is Venus and sub lord of Ketu is also Venus which is related to diseases like diabetes, is placed such the result is diagnosis was diabetes indicating high blood sugar levels but after sometime it was found that native was also suffering from auto immune disease called "type1 diabetes. So also the native was victim of renal function disorder due to nephritis. This gives us the connectivity of above mentioned combinations of sub lord, star lords and causative planets and the disorders occurred.

The occurrence of the disease was noticed on 20th April 2015 when Venus mahadasha and Ketu antardasha and Mars prati antardasha was in progress. The native was hospitalized on 20th April 2015 and after 12rd May 2015 the native was discharged but with life time gift of irrecoverable diabetes and disturbed kidney function.

Planetary disposition chart as given here with,

Sr. No.	Planet	Zodiac	Degrees: Min : Sec	Lord of Zodiac	Star Lord	Sub Lord
01	Sun	Virgo	106 : 33 : 31	Mercury	Moon	Saturn
02	Moon	Pisces	295 : 06 : 37	Jupiter	Mercury	Rahu
03	Mars	Scorpio	165 : 52 : 37	Mars	Saturn	Jupiter
04	Mercury	Virgo	103 : 24 : 59	Mercury	Moon	Rahu
05	Jupiter	Libra	138 : 30 : 10	Venus	Rahu	Moon
06	Venus	Virgo	098 : 27 : 47	Mercury	Sun	Venus
07	Saturn	Virgo	119 : 43 : 20	Mercury	Mars	Saturn
08	Rahu	Gemini	014 : 58 : 34	Mercury	Rahu	Ketu
09	Ketu	Sagittarius	194 : 58 : 34	Jupiter	Venus	Venus
10	Uranus	Scorpio	158 : 14 : 34	Mars	Saturn	Venus
11	Neptune	Sagittarius	180 : 52 : 22	Jupiter	Ketu	Venus
12	Pluto	Libra	122 : 34 : 35	Venus	Mars	Ketu

Chapter 19

Rheumatism and planetary disposition

This is group of diseases related to those conditions when immune system gets awry and attacks own tissues. Commonly occurred diseases are Osteoarthritis, Rheumatoid arthritis, Lupus, Spondylo arthropathys, Psoriatic arthritis, Sjoren syndrome, gout, Scleroderma, Infectious arthritis, Juvenile idiopathic arthritis, Poly mialgia, Rheumatic a. The causes for these diseases are often considered to be genetic or result of environment around and mostly the victims are women than men.

Osteoarthritis is not connected to immunity related disorders but only damage to cartilage in joints is found, indicating pain, swelling, stiffness, and muscle weakness is observed. Rheumatoid arthritis is related to immune system and immune system attacks own tissues, giving rise to joint pain, swelling, stiffness, even eye and lungs get affected. Sometimes severe fatigue and lumps which are called rheumatoid nodules are observed; this may be due to antinuclear antibodies, anti cyclic citrullinated peptides are the responsible factors, found by testing. C reactive protein and Erythrocyte sedimentation rate can lead to exact intensity and cause of the disease in diagnostic tools.

Lupus is another rheumatoid related disorder normally found in women; which is auto immune disease and can affect many organs in body, this can be confirmed by testing for antinuclear antibobdy and anti double stranded DNA antibody test or Anti smith antibody test. The one more of this group commonly reported is ankylosing spondylitis where in severe lower back pain and pelvic region, sacroiliac joints pain observed sometimes shoulder blades, buttocks are also painful. Rarely found is Sjorens syndrome which attacks normally eyes, mouth are the body parts affected; is also a auto immune disease where immune system creates dryness in eyes, mouth etc.

Psoriatic arthritis is auto immune arthritis linked with skin and gives distal affects the end of the fingers, toes, spine, neck, and small joints.

In all these types of disease if we study together few common things are found those are

1) Immune system
2) Bones and Joints,
3) Tissues, and muscles
4) Organs like eyes, Lungs, Kidneys
5) Blood cells

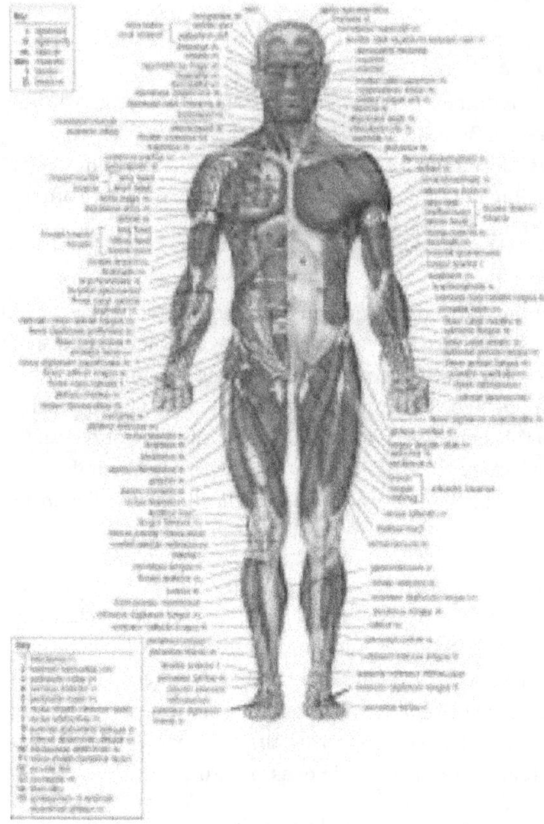

And accordingly we can correlate the syndromes to different combinations of constellations and sub lord associated with the respective planet responsible for the body part; further we can certainly predict with most accuracy the type of the disease which further can be confirmed by actual diagnostic tools. As we have already seen the significators of sixth cusp and sub lord of the sixth cusp either falls in Capricorn or Saturn occupies the sixth house along with other malefic in first , eighth or twelfth cusp clearly indicates the rheumatic types of disorders. The sub lord of Jupiter if placed in eighth cusp with Pisces like watery sign gives the information about relation between immune system and affected joints in body; so also if Jupiter be the sub lord of sixth cusp and placed in fiery sign Leo then also the symptoms related to Rheumatoid arthritis, osteo arthritis, and spondylitis are observed. Further if Jupiter is in the star lord of Ketu in Aquarius the also we find the native will be suffering from Lupus, and if Jupiter being sub lord of sixth cusp and well connected to signs Leo, Aquarius, and Pisces then Psoriatic arthritis or infectious arthritis is observed. In addition to all these we also can correlate the Rheumatic Arthritis and other immunity related diseases like Sjors syndrome , Lupus, Poly mailgia rheumatica, and Schleroderma with that of Saturn being sub lord of sixth cusp and in Jupiter's sign or if star lord of sixth house is Sun and Jupiter is sub lord and placed in ascendant then we notice these types of diseases in native. Further if Sun in the star of Venus, and Venus occupies ascendant then also we observe the diseases like Juvenile idiopathic arthritis, and if the ascendant is afflicted by Mars or Ketu then we see the native is suffering from gout, or osteo arthritis. In all these cases the fatal effect of the disease can be predicted by eighth cusp; if malefic occupies and sub lord is either Jupiter or Saturn and if well connected with sub lord of twelfth cusp. If ascendant sub lord is Saturn and is lord of sixth cusp; be placed anywhere in chart produces auto immune disease, so also if Uranus ne placed in ascendant and if the star lord is either Rahu or Ketu and if ascendant is under aspect of Saturn or Mars the native is certain to suffer from Rheumatism related disorders.

In many cases of Rheumatoid Arthritis we prominently see that Saturn in sixth cup with lord of house Mars and sub lord be Jupiter the disease occurs during the dasha period of the planets; so also if Mars be occupying ascendant and owns the house then if at same time star lord of eighth cusp and twelfth cusp is also Mars the native is certain to suffer from Osteo arthritis. Also Saturn Mars conjunction in ninth, tenth, and eleventh house also causes Rheumatoid Arthritis or related disorder; because ninth house rules pelvic joints, hips joints; tenth house governs joints in legs like knee whilst eleventh house governs the feet and toes, and if are afflicted by malefic leads to auto immune diseases.

Summarizing all the above observations we can further correlate with actual natives who suffered these diseases we clearly see the planets responsible for the disease are Saturn, Jupiter, Mars and if they are well connected with ascendant sixth house, eighth house, ninth house, tenth house, eleventh house and twelve house as star lord, sub lord or as lord of house the rheumatic Arthritis related ailments are occurred; which we can confirm with few examples. The planetary disposition for Rheumatism and associated diseases is as given bellow based on study of few Native who suffered it.

1) Malefic in Scorpio, Capricorn, Aquarius, or Pisces with special reference to Saturn.
2) Saturn in ascendant and Mars in ninth may give rise to Rheumatoid Arthritis.
3) Saturn and Moon in twelfth cusp is certain to cause Schleroderma.
4) Mars in Sagittarius denotes Spondyloarthrtis.
5) The sign Sagittarius or Pisces if under aspect from Saturn causes Psoriatic Arthritis.
6) IF in seventh house Sturn and Mars conjoin and are under aspect from Rahu causes Sjoren syndrome.
7) Mars in tenth cusp, if afflicted by Saturn causes poly myalgia Rheumatica.
8) Mars in Capricorn gives Rheumatoid Arthritis.
9) Rahu in Sagittarius gives infectious arthritis, and in Capricorn gives juvenile idiopathic Arthritis.
10) Saturn and Moon in twelfth cusp gives Gout.

Here we can confirm that major causative planet is Saturn because it rules Bones and joints; whilst Mars gives infectious arthritis, and inflamed joints.

We further study these collective data by referring few cases as described here with.

Case no. 023

Female native born on 13th July 1982 at 0741hrs. in Buldhana Nandur Lat 020:42N and Long 076:12E

In this chart ascendant is Cancer and Lord of house is Moon placed in ninth house under direct aspect of Saturn conjoined with Mars in first instance it is clear that the native is suffering from Rheumatoid arthritis. In this case sixth house is occupied by Ketu, a planet known to complicate the disease; and Neptune which denotes auto immune types of diseases and the cusp lord is placed in fourth house owned by Venus. Jupiter being the main supposedly signifying the disease rheumatism is hemmed in between two malefic Saturn and Uranus thus debilitating the Jupiter; and also lord of ninth house that is responsible for Arthritis. Saturn is also conjoined with Mars lord of tenth house which further confirms the disease, The Mars is placed in Virgo a sign known for muscular atrophy is also confirmed as the palm fingers were found affected severely. The lord of second house and which is responsible for the body metabolism is placed in twelfth house and is under aspect of Saturn thus indicating disease related to immunity; the Sun also is causative of disorders related to brain and face as indicated by the butterfly marks indicative of syndrome known as Lupus. This disease is earmarked by specific sign of this butterfly marks on face. The Moon which denotes the blood disorder is placed in ninth house as it is observed that in Lupus Erythromatosus the blood plays vital role in this disease. Now the sub lord of fifth house is Venus occupying eleventh house, an important house as we have noted earlier for the disease. So also the sub lord of sixth house is also Venus and that of eighth house is also Venus confirming the disease. Sub lord of ninth house is Jupiter and that of eleventh house is Ketu, Ketu is placed in Sixth house owned by Jupiter and Star lord of Neptune. Further we can clarify that the Saturn placed in conjunction with Mars is star lord of Moon which occupies ninth cusp and Mars is sub lord of Venus placed in eleventh cusp thus ninth and eleventh cusp are well connected and are indicative of chronic arthritis. As well as we can see further that Saturn is lord of seventh and eighth house; also aspect fifth cusp and denotes the auto immunity type of disease. Here it is also observed that the cause of damage to skin i.e. Mercury, a lord of third and twelfth cusp is placed in twelfth house conjoined with Sun indicating serious skin flares called as butterfly marks on face and making native allergic to Sun light. As we also observe here that the Venus is sub lord of twelfth cusp, eighth cusp and fifth cusp confirms the occurrence of the disease; and being star lord of tenth and sixth house further ascertains the dreaded disease. We also can see here that the lord of ascendant Moon is placed in tenth cusp under aspect from Saturn and Mars which leads the damage to cartilage types of bones in between joints making movements of joints difficult. Here it is also important to be noted that the firth cusp falls Scorpio owned by Mars which is afflicted by Saturn is occupied by Uranus that is responsible for rheumatoid arthritis types of diseases causing skin flares; is also under aspect of Saturn clarifies the occurrence of the disease. Here debilitated Moon being also ruler of psychology of the native indicates the stress level the native had to pass through which in its course made appearance of the disease. Noteworthy is that Venus is sub lord of Saturn is also placed in twelfth cusp under aspect of Saturn; and sub lord of Jupiter a causative of the joint disorders and is also sub lord of Mars placed in twelfth cusp under aspect from Ketu, this gives us the confirmation of the type and occurrence of the disease along with parts of body affected.

The onset of the disease in the period can be assessed with reference to the Ketu occupied sixth cusp leads the confirmation and as such the disease made its appearance on 20th December 2009 first time by appearance of flares on face and may be the disease had started its root in earlier period which is not afflicted with Saturn. As exactly recorded, the antardasha commenced was Mercury and prati anterdahsa was also of Mercury.

The planetary disposition in birth chart,

Sr. No.	Name of Planet	Name of the zodiac	Degrees : Min : Sec.	Lord of Zodiac	Star Lord	Sub Lord
0	Sun	Gemini	356 : 45 : 52	Mercury	Jupiter	Venus
02	Moon	Pisces	253 : 37 : 40	Jupiter	Saturn	Rahu
03	Mars	Virgo	084 : 58 : 56	Mercury	Mars	Rahu
04	Mercury	Gemini	343 : 01 : 00	Mercury	Rahu	Mercury
05	Jupiter	Libra	097 : 10 : 32	Venus	Rahu	Rahu
06	Venus	Taurus	327 : 17 : 37	Venus	Jupiter	Mars
07	Saturn	Virgo	082 : 23 : 23	Mercury	Moon	Venus
08	Rahu	Gemini	349 : 21 : 17	Mercury	Rahu	Mars
09	Ketu	Sagittarius	169 : 21 : 17	Jupiter	Venus	Rahu
10	Uranus	Scorpio	127 : 16 : 33	Mars	Saturn	Mercury
11	Neptune	Sagittarius	151 : 23 : 22	Jupiter	Ketu	Venus

Case No 24

A   classic case of Stefan Jorens Syndrome

Female native born on 23rd February 1970 at 0532 hrs in Mumbai/Girgaum
With Lat. 018: 57 N Long. 072: 49 E

This is classic case to understand the rare but dreaded disease under the family of Rheumatism occurred. Here we can see the most affected organ in body is eyes specifically the glands those produce water to keep eye watery and as such causing damage to eyes. In this particular case we also find some ailments related to Arthritis as well as Rheumatism. In the chart under consideration it is clear that the ruler of eyes Moon and Sun both are afflicted seriously so also the lord of sixth house occupies ascendant and under aspect of Saturn; the Saturn is also lord of ascendant and placed in fourth cusp with Mars as lord of fourth house which occupied third cusp, a known malefic cusp. So also the lord of eighth house is Sun occupied in second cusp indicating diseases of eyes, is afflicted with Rahu and the lord of third cusp being Saturn which occupies fourth cusp. Another planet responsible for function of eyes is Moon, placed in eighth cusp and afflicted conjoined with Ketu. Lord of twelfth house which also denotes malfunctioning of eyes is Jupiter, placed in tenth house; as we know this cusp is responsible for rheumatism, so also the lord of ninth cusp is Mercury placed in ascendant and under aspect of Saturn. Further the lord of Fifth cusp is Venus, placed in second house conjoined with Sun as lord of eighth house and Rahu indicating the disease arthritis. So also the star lord of sixth cusp is Rahu and is placed in second house indicating disease related to eyes and Sun and star lord of Jupiter denoting ailments connected with arthritis; here sub lord of sixth cusp Venus is also placed along with Rahu in second cusp conjoined with lord of eighth cusp Sun. Note worthy is that the planet related with water secreting glands in eyes is placed in eighth house conjoined and afflicted by Ketu is under aspect of Sun as such the disease denoted by Jupiter and Saturn is also associated with eyes leading eyes dry; so the name Sjorens Syndrome.

The major joints are ruled by Saturn and Jupiter and as Saturn and Jupiter both are under aspect of each other and Mars that governs the function of cartilage are debilitated causing the complex related to Rheumatoid Arthritis, and further Mars being the ruler of blood cells and its function placed in third house owned by Jupiter gives the disease related to immunity. Here in this case the native first was diagnosed for only Arthritis and after passage of time RA factor was found increased with higher value antinuclear antibody, Anti cyclic citrullinated peptides, and C - reactive protein value. This also was diagnosed as Rheumatoid nodules were observed; casing drying out of eyes, because of affected lachrymal layer in eyes.

The first reported occurrence was noted on 18th February 2010 when the native reported causing swelling in small joints and stiffness observed in carpel muscles. Doctor after thorough diagnosed the native as Rheumatic Arthritis associated with rheumatic nodules, after few days the burning sensation in eyes leading dryness of eyes was noticed. That is in progression of Rahu mahadasha and Mars antar dasha period when Rahu prati antar dasha was passing the disease was occurred or was noticed.

Case no 025

Another classic case of Rheumatoid arthritis with immunity function disorder is mentioned below.

The native is again female born on 26th July 1967 at 1413hrs in Ratnagiri/Khed

With   Lat 017:44 N Long 073:25 E

The another classic case related to complications associated with Rheumatoid arthritis, the chart shows at first instance the lord of sixth cusp Mars is placed in ascendant and afflicted with Neptune in Scorpio indicating the type of disease was associated with immune system; so also the planet related to i.e. bones and joints is Saturn which occupies sixth cusp in Aries owned by Mars denoting this combination the occurrence of disease Rheumatism, which further also is important to note here that the ninth house occupied by Mercury a planet rules the skin and nerve system with Sun responsible for blood disorder in Cancer, a sign that is related with the metabolism in body gives an indication of disease associated with Skin, Blood, and joints.

Further if we note the star lord of fifth house that denotes the pelvic bone diseases is Saturn, placed in sixth cusps also the lord of fifth house is Jupiter which is also star lord of fifth house denotes diseases of joints. The star lord of Saturn is Venus, placed in seventh house in Taurus; is lord and sub lord of twelfth cusp Libra again related to small joints under aspect from Mars and Neptune gives disease related to immune system. Thus lord of eighth cusp is Mercury and also lord of eleventh cusp where Uranus Ketu; are conjoined with Jupiter indicates the disorder that gives swellings to joints due to debilitated Mercury. The sub lord of eighth house is Mars and star lord of twelfth cusp so also the sub lord of twelfth cusp is Venus is also sub lord of Saturn and Jupiter and lord of twelfth cusp as such well connecting the houses sixth eighth and twelfth confirms the rheumatism associated with Jupiter and Saturn, further the sub lord of sixth cusp Moon placed in second house Sagittarius responsible for joints disorder and sub lord of ninth house also responsible for bones and joints. The Rahu a malefic planet placed in Pisces in fifth cusp is also a sub lord of Mercury confirming the complications are connected with connective tissue i.e. Skin; which is observed by occurrence of Psoriasis associated with Rheumatoid arthritis. Here the ends of fingers, toes, nails and spine are observed to have been affected and small joints were constantly showing swelling associated with stiffness.

Here if we notice the occurrence of disease we find that even though the disease supposedly existed the native had not reported till it becomes difficult for her to move in daily routine. The first time reported on 15th December 2015 but it is presumed that must have started its root long back in initial period of Mars mahadasha though the period reported falls on 15th December 2015 which was Mars Mahadasha with mercury antardasha and Ketu prati antar dahsa. Doctor after diagnosis reported that the native is suffering from Psoriatic Arthritis which also involves the skin due to reduced immunity. The normal other signs like involvement of small and larger joints with swelling was also noticed along with distal effects on fingertips, toes, and nail occurred.

The native was hospitalized for short period and had resumed her daily routine with effect from June 2016 but the complaints though reduced persists and native is likely to consume medicines till life for survival.

Planetary disposition in case no 024

Sr. No.	Name of planet	Name of zodiac	Degrees : Min : Sec	Lord of zodiac	Star Lord	Sub Lord
01	Sun	Cancer	249 : 44 : 47	Moon	Saturn	Venus

02	Moon	Sagittarius	030 : 40 : 38	Jupiter	Ketu	Ketu
03	Mars	Scorpio	010 : 26 : 53	Mars	Saturn	Sun
04	Mercury	Cancer	254 : 00 : 50	Moon	Saturn	Rahu
05	Jupiter	Virgo	308 : 08 : 43	Mercury	Sun	Venus
06	Venus	Taurus	207 : 43 : 17	Venus	Mars	Jupiter
07	Saturn	Aries	164 : 56 : 07	Mars	Venus	Venus
08	Rahu	Pisces	120 : 15 : 09	Jupiter	Jupiter	Moon
09	Ketu	Virgo	300 : 15 : 09	Mercury	Sun	Rahu
10	Uranus	Virgo	307 : 28 : 07	Mercury	Sun	Ketu
11	Neptune	Scorpio	002 : 32 : 45	Mars	Jupiter	Rahu

Case no 0256

Female native born on 11th June 1981 at Ahmed nagar Maharashtra

Lat. 019:05 N Long. 074:44 E

This chart if looked at will reveal three major things first being the ascendant is occupied by Uranus in Scorpio; secondly Mars occupies the seventh house conjoined with Sun lord of tenth house, and thirdly Mercury a causative planet of skin diseases is placed in eighth cusp under aspect of Saturn from eleventh house. This can be further explained as the lord of sixth house is Mars placed in seventh cusp conjoined with Sun in Taurus indicates the diseases Rheumatism, also as Saturn placed in eleventh house causes arthritis; which further aspect the fifth house where Zodiac Pisces falls indicating immunity related diseases, so also Saturn aspects the Mercury placed in eighth house denoting Rheumatic Arthritis relating to effect on skin due to decreased immunity. Also the ninth house occupied by Rahu indicates the arthritis associated with immunity disorder and the lord of ninth house is Moon, placed in eleventh cusp afflicted with Saturn and Jupiter; the sign lord Mercury being placed in eighth cusp rules the skin and nerves. This has led the native suffer from Lupus a type of Rheumatoid Arthritis in which skin becomes sun rays sensitive and causes flares, called as Butterfly marks. Here fifth, ninth, and eleventh cusps are connected to cause the disease, Lord of tenth house is Sun and is placed in seventh cusp afflicted by Mars and under direct aspect of Uranus; which itself is planet known to cause mysterious diseases. Another important planet Rahu is placed in ninth house and the cusp is undr Aspect of Ketu from third house denoting the frequent ups and downs in the symptoms of the disease. As it was discussed earlier the Saturn in eleventh house, Rahu in Ninth house and tenth house being hemmed in between two malefic planets Rahu and Saturn causes the Rheumatic Arthritis Here Saturn also indicates prolonged and chronic type of disease sometimes produces inflamed joints. The ninth cusp rules the pelvic joints and tenth house legs it is noticed that because of malefic present in ninth house, and tenth house being hemmed in between two malefic planets the effect of the pain in joints will occur more in legs and pelvic joints. The signs Taurus, Virgo, and Capricorn are earthy signs and if afflicted due to malefic or under aspect of malefic mainly give rise to arthritis that produces pain in flesh.

Further we can note that star lord of ascendant is Mars placed in seventh house in Taurus conjoined with Sun, that rules the face causing skin flares on face and head. Also star lord of ascendant is Saturn along with star lord of ninth house is placed in eleventh house with star lord of third cusp Moon and sub lord of eighth house causing immunity dysfunction; where Moon is the ruler of Blood. Sub lord of twelfth cusp is Venus which is also sub lord of Saturn that causes chronic type prolonged diseases related to Rheumatism. Further sub lord of sixth cusp is Sun placed in seventh house with Mars in Taurus, the lord of Taurus being Venus placed in eighth house is sub lord of Saturn and placed in eighth cusp associated with Mercury which further is sub lord of Venus; and is also lord of twelfth cusp Libra thus connected well with sixth eighth and twelfth house. Sub lord of Mercury is Saturn so also sub lord of eighth cusp and is star lord of ascendant connecting the sixth, eighth, twelfth, and ascendant confirms the occurrence of the disease. Saturn also directly aspect the second house which falls in Sagittarius, with fifth cusp both owned by Jupiter that rules the disease rheumatic Arthritis with debilitated Mercury giving rise further to immunity complications and causes Lupus.

Planetary disposition for case no025

Sr. No.	Name of Planet	Name of Zodiac	Degrees :Min :Sec	Lord of Zodiac	Star Lord	Sub Lord
01	Sun	Taurus	206 : 53 : 09	Venus	Mars	Jupiter
02	Moon	Virgo	319 : 44 : 19	Mercury	Moon	Ketu
03	Mars	Taurus	190 : 53 : 04	Venus	Moon	Moon
04	Mercury	Gemini	221 : 27 : 52	Mercury	Rahu	Saturn
05	Jupiter	Virgo	307 : 10 : 31	Mercury	Sun	Ketu
06	Venus	Gemini	224 : 02 : 50	Mercury	Rahu	Mercury

Case No 027

A   classic case of Stephan jorens Syndrome

Female native born on 23rd February 1970 at 0532 hrs in Mumbai/Girgaum

With Lat. 018: 57 N Long. 072: 49 E

This is classic case to understand the rare but dreaded disease under the family of Rheumatism occurred. Here we can see the most affected organ in body is eyes specifically the glands those produce water to keep eye watery and as such causing damage to eyes. In this particular case we also find some ailments related to Arthritis as well as Rheumatism. In the chart under consideration it is clear that the ruler of eyes Moon and Sun both are afflicted seriously so also the lord of sixth house occupies ascendant and under aspect of Saturn; the Saturn is also lord of ascendant and placed in fourth cusp with Mars as lord of fourth house which occupied third cusp, a known malefic cusp. So also the lord of eighth house is Sun occupied in second cusp indicating diseases of eyes, is afflicted with Rahu and the lord of third cusp being Saturn which occupies fourth cusp. Another planet responsible for function of eyes is Moon, placed in eighth cusp and afflicted conjoined with Ketu. Lord of twelfth house which also denotes malfunctioning of eyes is Jupiter, placed in tenth house; as we know this cusp is responsible for rheumatism, so also the lord of ninth cusp is Mercury placed in ascendant and under aspect of Saturn. Further the lord of Fifth cusp is Venus, placed in second house conjoined with Sun as lord of eighth house and Rahu indicating the disease arthritis. So also the star lord of sixth cusp is Rahu and is placed in second house indicating disease related to eyes and Sun and star lord of Jupiter denoting ailments connected with arthritis; here sub lord of sixth cusp Venus is also placed along with Rahu in second cusp conjoined with lord of eighth cusp Sun. Note worthy is that the planet related with water secreting glands in eyes is placed in eighth house conjoined and afflicted by Ketu is under aspect of Sun as such the disease denoted by Jupiter and Saturn is also associated with eyes leading eyes dry; so the name Sjorens Syndrome.

The major joints are ruled by Saturn and Jupiter and as Saturn and Jupiter both are under aspect of each other and Mars that governs the function of cartilage are debilitated causing the complex related to Rheumatoid Arthritis, and further Mars being the ruler of blood cells and its function placed in third house owned by Jupiter gives the disease related to immunity. Here in this case the native first was diagnosed for only Arthritis and after passage of time RA factor was found increased with higher value antinuclear antibody, Anti cyclic citrullinated peptides, and C- Reactive protein value. This also was diagnosed as Rheumatoid nodules were observed; casing drying out of eyes, because of affected lachrymal layer in eyes.

The first reported occurrence was noted on 18th February 2010 when the native reported causing swelling in small joints and stiffness observed in carpel muscles. Doctor after thorough diagnosed the native as Rheumatic Arthritis associated with rheumatic nodules, after few days the burning sensation in eyes leading dryness of eyes was noticed. That is in progression of Rahu mahadasha and Mars antar dasha period when Rahu prati antar dasha was passing the disease was occurred or was noticed.

Planetary disposition for this natal chart is given here with.

Sr. NO.	Planet	Zodiac	Degrees: Min : Sec	Lord Zodiac	Star Lord	Sub Lord
01	Sun	Aquarius	040 : 31 : 01	Saturn	Rahu	Saturn
02	Moon	Leo	238 : 43 : 40	Sun	Sun	Mars
03	Mars	Pisces	087 : 52 : 23	Jupiter	Mercury	Jupiter
04	Mercury	Capricorn	019 : 34 : 36	Saturn	Moon	Mercury
05	Jupiter	Libra	287 : 30 : 44	Venus	Rahu	Saturn
06	Venus	Aquarius	047 : 33 : 36	Saturn	Rahu	Sun
07	Saturn	Aries	100 : 50 : 33	Mars	Ketu	Saturn
08	Rahu	Aquarius	049 : 02 : 11	Saturn	Rahu	Moon
09	Ketu	Leo	229 : 02 : 11	Sun	Venus	Rahu
10	Uranus	Virgo	254 : 37 : 38	Mercury	Moon	Jupiter
11	Neptune	Scorpio	307 : 25 : 44	Mars	Saturn	Ketu

Case no 028-- Another classic case of Rheumatoid arthritis with immunity function disorder.

The native is again female born on 26th July 1967 at 1413hrs in Ratnagiri/Khed

With   Lat 017:44 N Long 073:25 E

The another classic case related to complications associated with Rheumatoid arthritis, the chart shows at first instance the lord of sixth cusp Mars is placed in ascendant and afflicted with Neptune in Scorpio indicating the type of disease was associated with immune system; so also the planet related to i.e. bones and joints is Saturn which occupies sixth cusp in Aries owned by Mars denoting this combination the occurrence of disease Rheumatism, which further also is important to note here that the ninth house occupied by Mercury a planet rules the skin and nerve system with Sun responsible for blood disorder in Cancer, a sign that is related with the metabolism in body gives an indication of disease associated with Skin, Blood, and joints.

Further if we note the star lord of fifth house that denotes the pelvic bone diseases is Saturn, placed in sixth cusps also the lord of fifth house is Jupiter which is also star lord of fifth house denotes diseases of joints. The star lord of Saturn is Venus, placed in seventh house in Taurus; is lord and sub lord of twelfth cusp Libra again related to small joints under aspect from Mars and Neptune gives disease related to immune system. Thus lord of eighth cusp is Mercury and also lord of eleventh cusp where Uranus Ketu; are conjoined with Jupiter indicates the disorder that gives swellings to joints due to debilitated Mercury. The sub lord of eighth house is Mars and star lord of twelfth cusp so also the sub lord of twelfth cusp is Venus is also sub lord of Saturn and Jupiter and lord of twelfth cusp as such well connecting the houses sixth eighth and twelfth confirms the rheumatism associated with Jupiter and Saturn, further the sub lord of sixth cusp Moon placed in second house Sagittarius responsible for joints disorder and sub lord of ninth house also responsible for bones and joints. The Rahu a malefic planet placed in Pisces in fifth cusp is also a sub lord of Mercury confirming the complications are connected with connective tissue i.e. Skin; which is observed by occurrence of Psoriasis associated with Rheumatoid arthritis. Here the ends of fingers, toes, nails and spine are observed to have been affected and small joints were constantly showing swelling associated with stiffness.

Here if we notice the occurrence of disease we find that even though the disease supposedly existed the native had not reported till it becomes difficult for her to move in daily routine. The first time reported on 15th December 2015 but it is presumed that must have started its root long back in initial period of Mars mahadasha though the period reported falls on 15th December 2015 which was Mars Mahadasha with mercury antardasha and Ketu prati antar dahsa. Doctor after diagnosis reported that the native is suffering from Psoriatic Arthritis which also involves the skin due to reduced immunity. The normal other signs like involvement of small and larger joints with swelling was also noticed along with distal effects on fingertips, toes, and nail occurred.

The native was hospitalized for short period and had resumed her daily routine with effect from June 2016 but the complaints though reduced persists and native is likely to consume medicines till life for survival.

Planetary disposition in case no 028

Sr. No.	Name of planet	Name of zodiac	Degrees : Min : Sec	Lord of zodiac	Star Lord	Sub Lord
01	Sun	Cancer	249 : 44 : 47	Moon	Saturn	Venus
02	Moon	Sagittarius	030 : 40 : 38	Jupiter	Ketu	Ketu
03	Mars	Scorpio	010 : 26 : 53	Mars	Saturn	Sun
04	Mercury	Cancer	254 : 00 : 50	Moon	Saturn	Rahu
05	Jupiter	Virgo	308 : 08 : 43	Mercury	Sun	Venus
06	Venus	Taurus	207 : 43 : 17	Venus	Mars	Jupiter
07	Saturn	Aries	164 : 56 : 07	Mars	Venus	Venus
08	Rahu	Pisces	120 : 15 : 09	Jupiter	Jupiter	Moon
09	Ketu	Virgo	300 : 15 : 09	Mercury	Sun	Rahu
10	Uranus	Virgo	007 : 28 : 07	Mercury	Sun	Ketu
11	Neptune	Scorpio	002 : 32 : 45	Mars	Jupiter	Rahu

Case no 029

Female native born on 11th June 1981 at Ahmed nagar Maharashtra

Lat. 019:05 N Long. 074:44 E

This chart if looked at will reveal three major things first being the ascendant is occupied by Uranus in Scorpio; secondly Mars occupies the seventh house conjoined with Sun lord of tenth house, and thirdly Mercury a causative planet of skin diseases is placed in eighth cusp under aspect of Saturn from eleventh house. This can be further explained as the lord of sixth house is Mars placed in seventh cusp conjoined with Sun in Taurus indicates the diseases Rheumatism, also as Saturn placed in eleventh house causes arthritis; which further aspect the fifth house where Zodiac Pisces falls indicating immunity related diseases, so also Saturn aspects the Mercury placed in eighth house denoting Rheumatic Arthritis relating to effect on skin due to decreased immunity. Also the ninth house occupied by Rahu indicates the arthritis associated with immunity disorder and the lord of ninth house is Moon, placed in eleventh cusp afflicted with Saturn and Jupiter; the sign lord Mercury being placed in eighth cusp rules the skin and nerves. This has led the native suffer from Lupus a type of Rheumatoid Arthritis in which skin becomes sun rays sensitive and causes flares, called as Butterfly marks. Here fifth, ninth, and eleventh cusps are connected to cause the disease, Lord of tenth house is Sun and is placed in seventh cusp afflicted by Mars and under direct aspect of Uranus; which itself is planet known to cause mysterious diseases. Another important planet Rahu is placed in ninth house and the cusp is undr Aspect of Ketu from third house denoting the frequent ups and downs in the symptoms of the disease. As it was discussed earlier the Saturn in eleventh house, Rahu in Ninth house and tenth house being hemmed in between two malefic planets Rahu and Saturn causes the

Rheumatic Arthritis Here Saturn also indicates prolonged and chronic type of disease sometimes produces inflamed joints. The ninth cusp rules the pelvic joints and tenth house legs it is noticed that because of malefic present in ninth house, and tenth house being hemmed in between two malefic planets the effect of the pain in joints will occur more in legs and pelvic joints. The signs Taurus, Virgo, and Capricorn are earthy signs and if afflicted due to malefic or under aspect of malefic mainly give rise to arthritis that produces pain in flesh.

Further we can note that star lord of ascendant is Mars placed in seventh house in Taurus conjoined with Sun, that rules the face causing skin flares on face and head. Also star lord of ascendant is Saturn along with star lord of ninth house is placed in eleventh house with star lord of third cusp Moon and sub lord of eighth house causing immunity dysfunction; where Moon is the ruler of Blood. Sub lord of twelfth cusp is Venus which is also sub lord of Saturn that causes chronic type prolonged diseases related to Rheumatism. Further sub lord of sixth cusp is Sun placed in seventh house with Mars in Taurus, the lord of Taurus being Venus placed in eighth house is sub lord of Saturn and placed in eighth cusp associated with Mercury which further is sub lord of Venus; and is also lord of twelfth cusp Libra thus connected well with sixth eighth and twelfth house. Sub lord of Mercury is Saturn so also sub lord of eighth cusp and is star lord of ascendant connecting the sixth, eighth, twelfth, and ascendant confirms the occurrence of the disease. Saturn also directly aspect the second house which falls in Sagittarius, with fifth cusp both owned by Jupiter that rules the disease rheumatic Arthritis with debilitated Mercury giving rise further to immunity complications and causes Lupus.

Planetary disposition for case no 027

Sr. No.	Name of Planet	Name of Zodiac	Degrees :Min :Sec	Lord of Zodiac	Star Lord	Sub Lord
01	Sun	Taurus	206 : 53 : 09	Venus	Mars	Jupiter
02	Moon	Virgo	319 : 44 : 19	Mercury	Moon	Ketu
03	Mars	Taurus	190 : 53 : 04	Venus	Moon	Moon
04	Mercury	Gemini	221 : 27 : 52	Mercury	Rahu	Saturn
05	Jupiter	Virgo	307 : 10 : 31	Mercury	Sun	Ketu
06	Venus	Gemini	224 : 02 : 50	Mercury	Rahu	Mercury
07	Saturn	Virgo	309 : 26 : 06	Mercury	Sun	Venus
08	Rahu	Cancer	250 : 22 : 11	Moon	Saturn	Sun
09	Ketu	Capricorn	070 : 22 : 11	Saturn	Moon	Moon
10	Uranus	Scorpio	003 : 34 : 24	Mars	Saturn	Saturn
11	Neptune	Scorpio	029 : 58 : 28	Mars	Mercury	Saturn

The occurrence of the disease if observed falls in the dasha period of Jupiter and antar dasha of Mercury with prati antar dasha also of Jupiter was in progress. That is the occurrence of disease was noticed first on 5th August 2015 with frequent ups and downs tending to reduce the suffering when Jupiter transited in to Capricorn in 2020 January.

Chapter no 20

Human nervous system is a complicated and mainly divided into two sub parts; one being Central nervous system and second is peripheral nervous system. The principal organs of the nervous system also include eyes, ears, sensory organs of taste, sensory organs of smell and sensory receptors located in skin, joints, muscles, and other parts of body. The nervous system is vulnerable to various disorders and can be affected or damaged by Trauma, Infection, Degeneration, Structural defects, Tumors, Blood flow disruption, and Auto immune disorders.

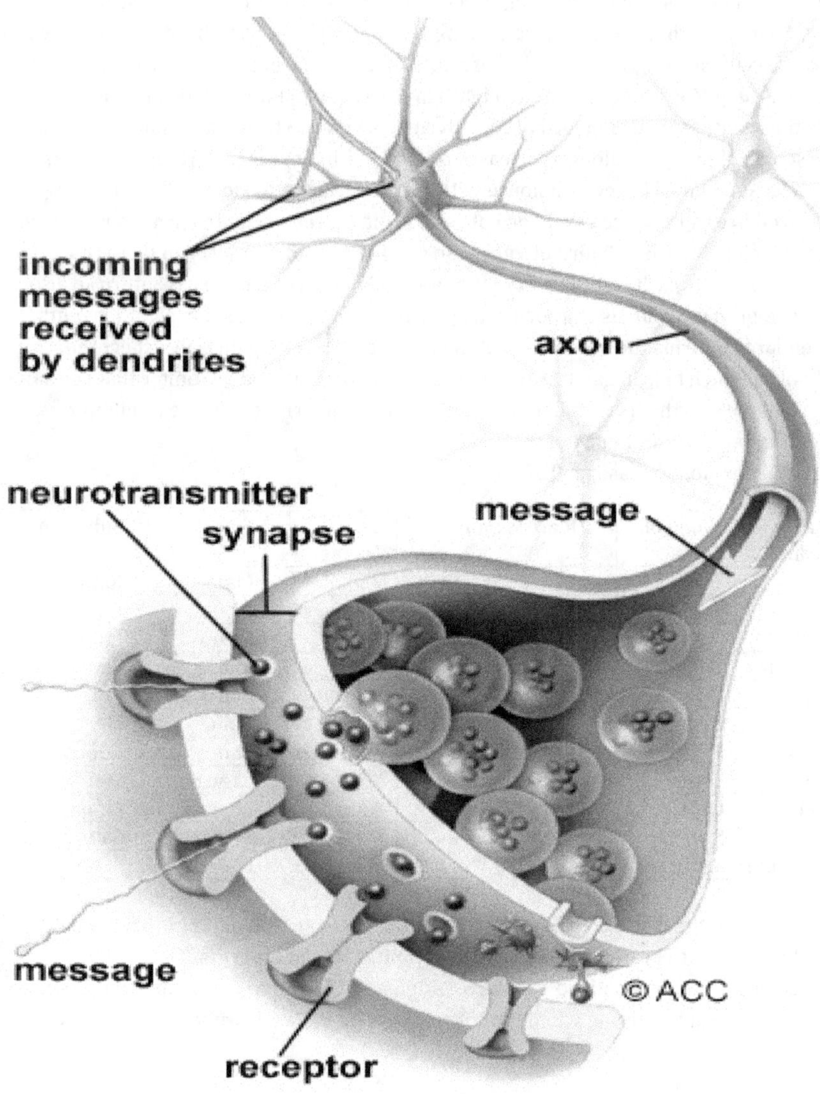

And As such may include.

1) Vascular disorders such as strokes, transient ischemic and hematoma, extra Dural hemorrhage.
2) Infection such as meningitis, encephalitis, polio, epidural abscess.
3) Structural disorder such as brain or spine cord injury, Belly's palsy, cervical spondylosis, carpal tunnel, brain or spinal cord tumors, peripheral neuropathy, and guillian barre syndrome.
4) Functional disorders such as headache, epilepsy, dizziness, neuralgia.
5) Degenerative disorders which include Parkinson's disease, Multiple sclerosis, amyotrophic, lateral sclerosis, Hutingtone chorea, Alzheimer's disease.

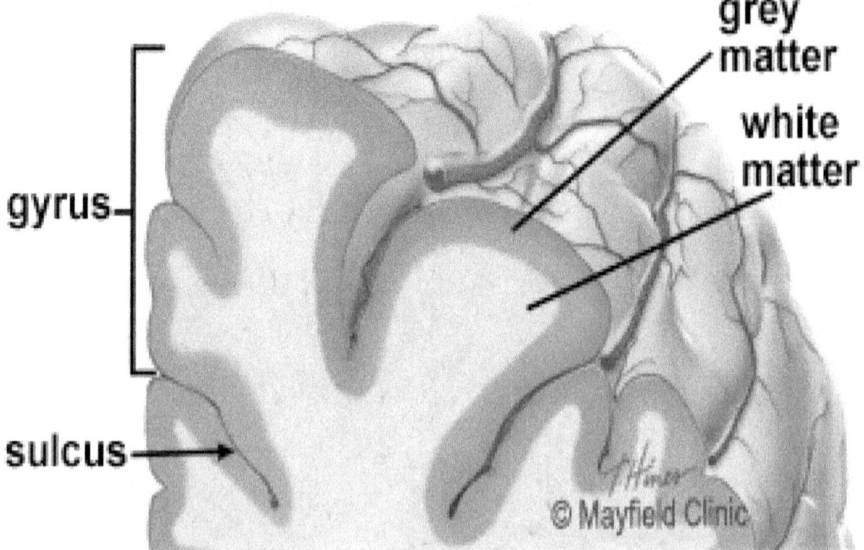

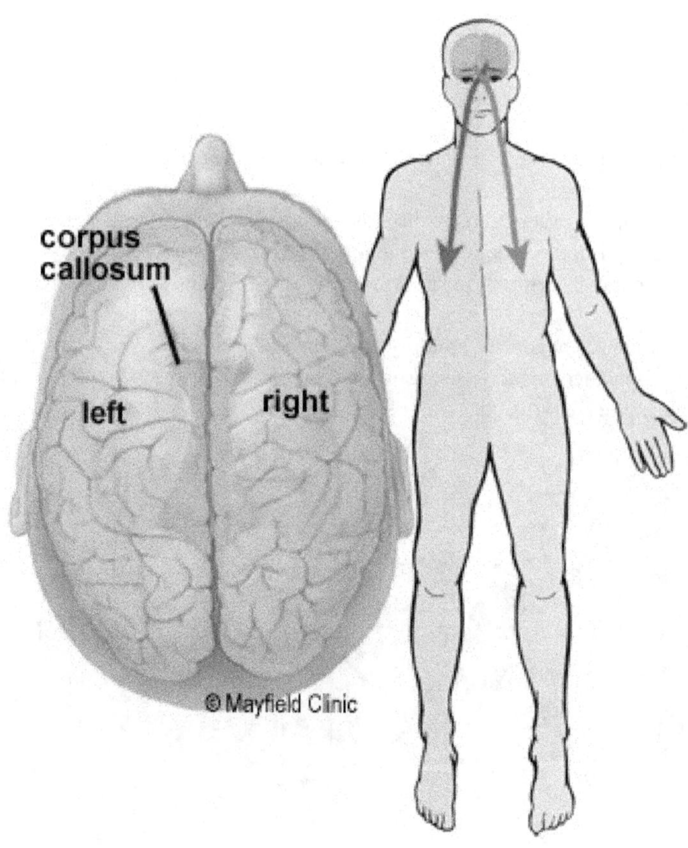

Following are the few signs normally observed

1) Persistent or sudden onset of headache
2) Headache that changes with time and or is different
3) Loss of feeling and tingling
4) Weakness or loss of muscle strength
5) Loss of sight or double vision
6) Memory loss
7) Impaired mental ability
8) Muscle rigidity
9) Tremors and seizers
10) Back pain which radiates to the feet, toes, or other parts of body
11) New language impairment i.e. expression or comprehension.

To diagnose and understand the exact nature of disease lot of time is required to be spend with patient before making a probable diagnosis of specific condition. And exactly it is achieved just by spending few minutes at the natal chart of patient.

Major branches of health care those provides the cure for disease include

1) Neurology that treat acute strokes and cerebral aneurysms using endovascular techniques.
2) Neurosurgery i.e. surgical intervention of nervous system.
3) Neuroradiologists and interventional radiologists mainly for cerebral aneurysms, vertebral fractures, certain tumors.
4) Rehabilitation for neurological disorders called psychiatrists.

Nervous system is complex collection of highly sophisticated specialized cells and nerves that transmit signals between different parts of body; essentially an electric wiring. Functionally the nervous system has two main sub divisions; the somatic or voluntary component and Autonomic or involuntary component. The autonomic nervous system regulates certain body processes such as blood pressure and breathing that works with conscious efforts.

The Somatic nervous component is ruled by Mercury and the Autonomic or involuntary component is ruled by Saturn. So also Mars and affliction of these planets in Aries may give rise to neurological diseases. In addition the influence of Ketu in evil aspect to Moon, and Mercury in Aries also cause these disorders as Ketu is responsible for mysterious diseases. At the same time Aries and Ascendant represents the function of nervous system and if any malefic present in these cusps and if sixth cusp, eighth cusp, and twelfth cusp are well connected or sub lords of these houses are well connected the disorders associated with nervous systems are occurred. The trauma leading to damage of nervous system is occurred due to presence of Mars with Uranus in eighth or third cusp and the sixth, twelfth cusp are either afflicted by malefic planets or under aspect of Ketu, Saturn, and Neptune. Also the infection to nerve system is caused when Sub lord of sixth cusp is in twelfth cusp and becomes strong significator of sixth cusp then inefectious disease like Meningitis, encephalitis is observed. If Mercury occupies eighth or sixth cusp and is afflicted with Rahu, so also if at the same time Sun is under aspect from any malefic and occupies eighth house the degeneration in nerve cells occurs causing degenerative type of nervous disease. Further if Aries be placed in eighth cusp and occupied by Sun which is under aspect from Mars and the ascendant is occupied by Saturn at the same time if lord of sixth cusp Saturn also aspects the Mercury in seventh cusp then structural disorders or even tumors are found. It is also noticed that in case if ninth, tenth, eleventh, and fifth cusps are either afflicted or under aspect from Saturn or malefic and occupied by Jupiter, Mars or Moon then blood flow obstruction or autoimmune type of disorders are observed.

Moon rules the complex collection of nerves and neurons (specialized cells) which transmits the signal between different parts of the body. As such if Moon is afflicted or adversely placed or under aspect of malefic, then native is certain to suffer from strokes or cerebral aneurism; also if along with Mercury, Moon is afflicted or Mercury is placed in eighth house and under aspect from Ketu the native is likely to suffer from neurological disorders such as Parkinson's disease. Further the beneficial conjunction of Moon and Mercury makes native highly intelligent; Saturn if aspect the conjoined planet native suffers from neurological disorders like depression, anxiety, schizophrenia, sleep apnea and sometimes leads to violent type of personality. If only Moon is placed in eighth cusp and Mercury be in sixth cusp and both are under aspect from Neptune and Saturn respectively the tumor is likely to develop either in brain or vertebral fracture may occur. In case Mercury is placed in sixth cusp and Saturn aspect it from twelfth house and Moon be placed in second hose then native may develop disorders requiring Surgical intervention.

As such to summarize we can conclude in short following combination of Planet indicate the neurological disease.

1) The fifth house is related to intelligence and any affliction to this and Moon or Mercury certain to cause neurological disorders specifically Structural defect, and blood flow disruption.
2) Jupiter in fifth house if afflicted or placed in third house and under aspect from Ketu cause degenerative type of neurological disorder.
3) The Moon and Rahu are placed in ascendant and malefic in fifth cusp or ninth cusp then blood flow disruption or subarachnoid hemorrhage, hematoma may occur, in these cases if extra Dural hemorrhage occurs the serious and chronic neurological disorders are certain to take place.
4) Moon and Mercury if are afflicted by Saturn or Rahu in Saturn's cusp like Capricorn or Aquarius the native suffers from hysteria or Belly's palsy or cervical spondylosis, carpal tunnel syndrome are certain to occur.
5) Moon, Mars, Saturn if all three conjoined in eighth cusp also gives spinal cord tumors or peripheral neuropathy and Guillian syndrome may occur.
6) If Moon and Rahu or Mercury and Saturn in Gemini or Virgo give functional disorder such as headache, epilepsy, dizziness, neuralgia is observed.
7) If Jupiter and Saturn in twelfth house are under aspect from Mercury or Saturn and Mercury placed in twelfth house are under aspect from Jupiter from sixth house then the native is certain to suffer from degenerative types of diseases like Parkinson's disease, Multiple sclerosis, Amyotrophic lateral sclerosis, Huttingtons chorea and Alzheimer disease are likely to occur.
8) Sun in ascendant and Mars or Saturn in seventh house causes persistent sudden head ache, loss of feeling, tingling, and weakness of sight or double vision, memory loss may be observed which is related to some or other neurological disorders.
9) Saturn in Ascendant and Mars in fifth, seventh or ninth house the impaired mental ability, Lac of coordination, Muscle rigidity may occur.
10) Jupiter in Ascendant while Mars or Saturn in seventh cusp causes tremors, seizers, or weakness in muscle may occuer.
11) Conjunction of Moon, Mars, Saturn, in eighth cusp give rise to back pain which radiates to feet or other parts of body is noticed along with slurred speech or muscle wasting or impairment in expression, or comprehension is noticed.
    In all of these cases to diagnose and understand lot of time is required to be spend with patient before making probable diagnosis of specific condition and exact can be noticed in this study of Birth chart.

This further can be explained well by understanding few examples given herewith.

Case no 030

This case is of female child born on 13th January 2007 at 1630 hrs in Pune/Nigdi

Lat 018:30 N Long 073:48 E

The birth chart is Gemini ascendant and lord of ascendant Mercury is placed in Eighth cusp in Capricorn with lord of twelfth cusp Venus and Neptune, also the Mars is placed in seventh cusp in Sagittarius conjoined with Sun, lord of third house. The Moon is placed in fifth house in Libra owned by Venus, so also Mars is lord of sixth house which is occupied by Jupiter. The lord of ninth cusp is Saturn which occupies Cancer in second house; Saturn directly aspect the Mercury and Venus in eighth house. So also Uranus conjoined with Rahu are placed in ninth house owned by Saturn i.e. Aquarius aspects Moon in fifth cusp indicating disease related to nervous system. Further Aries falls in eleventh cusp is also under aspect of Saturn which confirms the disease related to cerebral aneurysm causing inability to control movement of right hand and facial palsy. So also we can see the Mercury placed in eighth cusp is lord pf ascendant and seriously afflicted by Neptune denoting structural defects; further Aries is major sign which rules the brain and spinal cord; is under aspect of Saturn from second house indicates either injury to spinal cord or Belly's palsy. The Cancer is sign owned by Moon and this governs the nerve motor function i.e. entire peripheral nervous system is afflicted by Saturn occupying in it also confirms the peripheral neuropathy with Belly's palsy. Moon which is significator of diseases related to nervous system is occupied in fifth house again that fifth cusp is related to somatic or voluntary nervous system. Another house related to neurons, that transmit signals between different body parts is afflicted severely by Rahu conjoined with Uranus indicating the disease related to neurons; the lord of ninth house is Saturn that directly aspect the eighth house occupied by Mercury and Venus as discussed earlier, is also afflicted by Neptune, that confirms the occurrence of disease. Further the other planet that rules the complex collection of nerves and neurons causing the spastic syndrome observed; the lord of sixth cusp is Mars is placed in seventh house conjoined with Sun in Sagittarius owned by Jupiter thus making interchange between Mars and Jupiter leading to complex irrecoverable nervous system disorder.

Now we can also note here that star lord and sub lord of sixth house is Saturn placed in second cusp aspect eighth house, the star lord of eighth house is Sun placed in seventh cusp conjoined with Mars, sub lord of Neptune. Sub lord of twelfth house is Saturn which is also sub lord of Venus, lord of twelfth cusp thus indicating the severity of the disease. The sub lord of eighth cusp is Rahu placed in Aquarius in ninth cusp owned by Saturn and Rahu aspects Moon in Libra, the fifth cusp; also the lord of ascendant is Mercury placed in eighth cusp under aspect of Saturn, the sub lord of Mercury is Jupiter placed in sixth house owned by Mars which is sub lord of Sun and star lord of ninth house and fifth house is also star lord of ascendant. Thus we can confirm here that all the significators of sixth, eighth, and twelfth cusp are well connected so also the significators of fifth, ninth cusp are also well connected confirming the occurrence, growth and complications of the disease.

The onset of disease can be observed with respect to the dasha lord being Jupiter and in Jupiter mahadasha and Mercury antar dasha was in progress on 20th October 2013 while Saturn pratiantar dasha was passing. The disease being chronic and as such the life expectancy appears to be short.

Sr. No	Name of Planet	Name of Zodiac	Degree: Min : Sec	Lord of Zodiac	Star Lord	Sub Lord
01	Sun	Sagittarius	208 : 54 : 44	Jupiter	Sun	Mars
02	Moon	Libra	140 : 00 : 57	Venus	Jupiter	Jupiter
03	Mars	Sagittarius	183 : 32 : 31	Jupiter	Ketu	Sun
04	Mercury	Capricorn	212 : 48 : 19	Saturn	Sun	Jupiter
05	Jupiter	Scorpio	166 : 43 : 14	Mars	Mercury	Mercury
06	Venus	Capricorn	227 : 42 : 06	Saturn	Moon	Saturn
07	Saturn	Cancer	059 : 48 : 54	Moon	Mercury	Saturn
08	Rahu	Aquarius	265 : 03 : 03	Saturn	Jupiter	Mercury
09	Ketu	Leo	085 : 03 : 03	Sun	Venus	Mercury
10	Uranus	Aquarius	258 : 03 : 28	Saturn	Rahu	Sun
11	Neptune	Capricorn	234 : 34 : 26	Saturn	Mars	Rahu

Case no 031

Native is male and born on 21st August 1954 at 1240 hrs in Mumbai/ Sion

Lat- 019: 03N Long 072: 52E

In this chart it is observed that the ascendant Mars is placed in Sagittarius second house and afflicted with Rahu; also lord of second house ij Jupiter occupies eighth house in Gemini and under aspect fro Mars. The lord of ascendant is also under aspect fro Saturn occupied in twelfth cusp. Here noteworthy

is that the Mars is also lord of sixth house Aries which is under direct aspect from Saturn denoting the disease related to neurological disorder; further it can be seen that the lord of second house Sagittarius Jupiter is placed in eighth cusp afflicted with Ketu in Gemini, Jupiter being the planet causative of major diseases related to nervous system. So also further the Jupiter is also lord of fifth house that is known to rule the intelligence indicating diseases related to peripheral nervous system; the malefic present along with is Ketu which gives mysterious diseases of unknown origin and difficult to diagnose. The Mars being lord of ascendant and afflicted by Rahu in Sagittarius denotes the serous disorder related to nervous system and as under aspect from Saturn the Sagittarius and Mars together produces the disease known as peripheral neuropathy causing carpal syndrome first which then progresses into legs giving loss of sensitivity that leads to the disease gangrene leading to amputation of one leg. Further the Venus that is responsible for diseases related to metabolism like diabetes also occur making the native vulnerable further for neurological complications. Venus being lord of twelfth house is placed in Virgo in eleventh cusp is hemmed in between two malefic Saturn and Sun indicating the delayed onset of diabetes which worsens the peripheral neuropathy syndrome, The ninth cusp Cancer is afflicted by Uranus again a planet denoting mysterious diseases related to nervous system, the lord of ninth cusp is Moon placed in seventh house owned by Venus; the lord of seventh house also making Moon debilitated and leads to diseases related to degenerative type of nervous disorsers clearly indicates the loss of sensitivity. Here long before onset of the disease the native complained about weakness in muscles and loss of strength, which further progressed with occurrence of carpal tunnel syndrome and then within few months sudden rise in random blood sugar indicating occurrence of diabetes observed. The major point in this case is that the native has developed continuous depression much before the disease was diagnosed; that tells us about the how loss of feeling and depression are well connected with this disease. The native unfortunately had undergone several surgical interventions for either amputation of limb or for other types of neuro surgeries as indicated by lord of sixth house placed in Sagittarius and afflicted by Rahu.

It is interesting here to note that the star lord of ascendant is Jupiter placed in eighth cusp which conjoined with star lord of sixth cusp Ketu indicating repeated hospitalization also further the star lord of twelfth cusp is Mars which occupied in Sagittarius is also star lord of twelfth house and lord of ascendant and sixth house, Mars is again star lord of eighth cusp confirms the progressive complications in disease that is related to peripheral neuropathy. Sub lord of twelfth cusp is Moon placed in seventh house with Venus as lord of house, Moon sub lord of Mercury another major planet that denotes the disease related to nervous system and sub lord of Ketu placed in eighth cusp which had afflicted Jupiter. The Sub lord of ascendant is Rahu which is also sub lord of sixth house and ninth house, placed in Sagittarius in second house; Rahu is also sub lord of Uranus placed in ninth house, and conjoined with Mars   lord of ascendant. The sub lord of eighth house and fifth house is Mercury which is placed in tenth house conjoined with Sun; is also Sub lord of Moon, and Neptune thus indicates the worsening of case over passage of time requiring repeated hospitalization and surgical operations. So also it is clear that all the significators of ascendant, sixth house, eighth house and twelfth house are well connected denoting and confirming the disease.

The occurrence of the disease can be confirmed by the dassha period of the causative planets was admitted to hospital on 15th August 2009 for the first time before which no information is available, i.e. in Mahadasha of Saturn and antardasha of Saturn was in progress with prati antar daha of Mars and was advised to undergo first surgery on 20th October 2009 i.e. in Rahu prati antar dasha period. The native had undergone four major surgeries including one leg amputation.

Sr. No.	Name of planet	Name of zodiac	Degrees: Min : Sec	Lord of zodiac	Star Lord	Sub Lord
01	Sun	Leo	274 : 27 : 56	Sun	Ketu	Moon
02	Moon	Taurus	185 : 44 : 06	Venus	Sun	Mercury
03	Mars	Sagittarius	035 : 46 : 56	Jupiter	Ketu	Rahu
04	Mercury	Leo	273 : 54 : 54	Sun	Ketu	Moon
05	Jupiter	Gemini	236 : 23 : 04	Mercury	Jupiter	Ketu
06	Venus	Virgo	319 : 56 : 13	Mercury	Moon	Ketu
07	Saturn	Libra	341 : 03 : 34	Venus	Rahu	Saturn
08	Rahu	Sagittarius	049 : 13 : 03	Jupiter	Venus	Rahu
09	Ketu	Gemini	229 : 13 : 03	Mercury	Rahu	Moon
10	Uranus	Cancer	242 : 14 : 03	Moon	Jupiter	Rahu
11	Neptune	Libra	300 : 38 : 04	Venus	Mars	Mercury

Case No032

Male native born on 06th June 1990 at 0550 hrs Bhalvani / Solapur Lat 017: 42N and Long 075: 55 E

The native born in solapur was taken to psychiatrist for behavioral problems and frequent episodes of suicide attempt. If we observe the natal chart the reason behind the disease will be clear. The chart shows Taurus ascendant with Sun , the lord of fourth house is placed; the causative planet of behavioral disturbance is placed in twelfth cusp Aries responsible for nervous disorder and is conjoined with lord of ascendant Venus, so also the lord of twelfth cusp and seventh cusp Mars is placed in eleventh house owned by Jupiter which is placed in second house Gemini owned by Mercury. The lord of third cusp which is occupied by Ketu is placed in sixth house owned by Venus and under aspect of Saturn occupied in ninth house; Saturn is afflicted with Rahu in ninth cusp also under aspect of Ketu. The lord of eighth cusp Jupiter is placed in third house and under direct aspect of Uranus known to cause mysterious disease, Mars the lord of twelfth house is placed in eleventh house and aspect Jupiter in Gemini is also lord of seventh cusp. Here few noteworthy points to be considered are The main zodiac Aries responsible for the Psychological diseases falls in twelfth house whilst the major planet that denotes the occurrence Moon is placed in sixth cusp, further the lord of sixth cusp is placed in twelfth house. In addition the eighth house is occupied by Uranus so called planet that causes mysterious diseases and aspect the lord of eighth cusp Jupiter in second cusp; the Ketu occupied in third cusp directly aspect the ninth house that is further responsible for the severe depression, anxiety, and frequent suicidal tendency. This further can be confirmed by correlating the significators of ascendant, sixth, eighth and twelfth cusp and ninth house.   The star lord of ascendant is Moon placed in sixth cusp is also star lord of fifth, ninth cusp; the star lord of sixth cusp is Rahu placed in ninth cusp conjoined with Saturn which aspects the third cusp Cancer denoting the blood supply to nerve system or organs; again lord of Cancer is Moon placed in sixth cusp which is main planet that is responsible for severe mood swing condition. Also star lord of eighth cusp is Venus placed in twelfth cusp, is also star lord of twelfth cusp and sub lord of sixth cusp indicating severity of the disease. Sub lord of ascendant is Moon which is also star lord of ninth house and sub lord of third house and twelfth cusp is placed in sixth house. In addition star lord of Moon is Jupiter, is also sub lord of Neptune and Ketu which are malefic planets. The sub lord of Sun in ascendant , Venus is also sub lord of Uranus in eighth cusp and sub lord of Venus in twelfth house; is lord of sixth cusp and ascendant thus indicating the well connected houses ascendant, sixth, eighth, and twelfth houses confirming the disease. The Moon occupied in sixth house under aspect from Venus placed in twelfth cusp is the major responsible planet for the disease.

The Moon, Mars, Jupiter and signs Aries, Cancer, and Sagittarius shows the type of disease being Memory loss, impaired mental ability, lack of coordination, and mainly severe depression that led the native frequently trying to commit suicide or harming self. The onset of disease may have occurred prior also but was first noticed on 8th December 2012 when native was required to be admitted to hospital for serious injury occurred while native was trying to commit suicide, when mahadasha of Saturn, antardasha of Moon was in progress and Mercury prati antardasha was just started.

Sr. No.	Planet	Zodiac	Degrees: Min : sec	Lord of zodiac	Star Lord	Sub Lord

01	Sun	Taurus	020 : 17 : 52	Venus	Moon	Venus
02	Moon	Libra	021 : 20 : 07	Venus	Jupiter	Mercury
03	Mars	Pisces	174 : 34 : 07	Jupiter	Saturn	Sun
04	Mercury	Aries	310 : 26 : 56	Mars	Sun	Moon
05	Jupiter	Gemini	050 : 08 : 06	Mercury	Jupiter	Jupiter
06	Venus	Aries	343 : 56 : 21	Mars	Venus	Venus
07	Saturn	Capricorn	240 : 48 : 44	Saturn	Sun	Rahu
08	Rahu	Capricorn	256 : 28 07	Saturn	Moon	Saturn
09	Ketu	Cancer	076 : 28 : 07	Moon	Saturn	Jupiter
10	Uranus	Sagittarius	224 : 47 : 42	Jupiter	Venus	Venus
11	Neptune	Sagittarius	230 : 13 : 04	Jupiter	Venus	Jupiter

Case no 033

Native is male born on 27th April 1979 at 1334 hrs in Pimpri/ Pune with Lat- 018:30 N, Long - 073:52E.   This is classic case of Cognitive Behavioral defects and ascendant falls in Cancer a causative zodiac of neurological disorders. The lord of ascendant is Moon occupied in tenth cusp in Aries; as we have seen before also Moon in Aries denotes the learning deficiency disorder or inability/ impaired mental ability. The lord of fifth cusp is Mars which also rules the brain function is placed in ninth house in Pisces and fifth cusp is occupied by Neptune, another malefic planet denoting the disturbed function of expression

Or comprehension; and ninth house occupied by Mars denotes the ability of cognitive functions are affected. The owner of ninth house and sixth house is Jupiter which is placed in ascendant in Cancer, indicating confused state of native at all the times. The lord of ascendant Moon is placed in tenth house conjoined with Sun in Aries are under aspect of Uranus a known malefic planet that causes mysterious diseases. Mercury, the lord of twelfth cusp is placed in ninth house afflicted by Mars indicates the nervous system related disorder. So also the second house known to rule the function of speech is occupied by Saturn conjoined with Rahu and thus leaving an impact on speech; Saturn and Rahu also aspect the eighth house Aquarius and Ketu placed in. The Mercury is causative of fluent or disturbed speech is lord of twelfth and third cusp and placed in ninth house afflicted with Mars, also shows the onset of the disease related to peripheral nervous system in addition to impaired mental ability. As Moon placed in Aries and under aspect from fourth house by Uranus indicates the frequent mood swing and cranky nature of the native; lord of sixth cusp Jupiter placed in ascendant also leads to the disorders related to peripheral nervous system.

To understand further we can see that the star lord of ascendant is Mercury which is also star lord of fifth house and ninth house confirming the lack of coordination and impaired mental ability. Further the star lord of sixth cusp is Sun conjoined with Mercury lord of twelfth cusp; and star lord of eighth cusp Jupiter is occupied in ascendant is also star lord of twelfth house. In addition to above the sub lord of sixth cusp is Rahu placed in second house aspect the sub lord of eighth cusp Ketu and Saturn, sub lord of ascendant is also sub lord of twelfth cusp denotes the cognitive behavioral dysfunction.

The same can also be explained in case of planetary disposition. The sub lord of Moon is Saturn, is also sub lord of ascendant and star lord of Mercury, Jupiter indicates the nervous system disorder.

All these observations certainly indicate the irrecoverable impairment of mental ability and diseased speech.

Sr. No	Planet	Zodiac	Degrees: Min : Sec	Lord of zodiac	Star Lord	Sub Lord
01	Sun	Aries	282 : 54 : 37	Mars	Ketu	Mercury
02	Moon	Aries	293 : 00 : 20	Mars	Venus	Saturn
03	Mars	Pisces	262 : 07 : 03	Jupiter	Mercury	Sun
04	Mercury	Pisces	256 : 24 : 51	Jupiter	Saturn	Jupiter
05	Jupiter	Cancer	007 : 01 : 46	Moon	Saturn	Mercury
06	Venus	Pisces	251 : 27 : 20	Jupiter	Saturn	Moon
07	Saturn	Leo	043 : 38 : 17	Sun	Venus	Venus
08	Rahu	Leo	051 : 29 : 55	Sun	Venus	Jupiter
09	Ketu	Aquarius	231 : 29 : 55	Saturn	Jupiter	Jupiter

Chapter 21

Diseases in reference with Drekkan

In natal chart there are twelve cusps as there are twelve Zodiacs and as entire universe of 360 degrees if divided into twelve cusps or houses each house occupies 30 degrees, this each house if further divided into three divisions and each division such obtained is called as drekkan. Each drekkan rules specific organ of the body and can clearly be understood by following Drekkan chart. Each Drekkan will be of 10 degrees. This what we study according to KP in 249 sub lords.

Cusp No.	First Drekkan	Secodn Drekkan	Third Drekka
Ascendant	Head, Face, Lumbar Region.	Brain, Neck, Throat, Kidney, Epigastria Region.	Facial bones, Bladder, Urethra, Feet, Pelvic, Legs.
Second and twelfth	Neck, Thyroid, Right eye, Left eye, Feet, Toes,	Lateral ventricles of brain, Choroid plexus, Central canal, Prefrontal cortex, Larynx, Lymphatic system, Shoulder blades. Rt. and Left shoulder.	First vertebra, Anterior sub mandibular, Sub mental, carotid triangles, posterior occipital and omoclavicular triangle, 9 cartilages of Larynx, Hyoid bones, hyoid muscles.
Third and eleventh	Cochlea, Epiglottises,Right and Left eye.	Lymphatic system, Lungs, Blood, Rt. Hand, Left hand, Arms, Circulation.	Collar bone, Shoulder joints, Right and Left testicles.
Fourth and Tenth	Breast, Thoracic bones, Epigastria region, Nostrils, Right Knee.	Stomach, Intestine, Right and Left armpit.	Breast bones, Ribs, Right and Left thigh, Knee cap, petal.

Fifth and ninth	Spine, Hips, Back muscles, Peripheral nervous system, C14 TO L6 Vertebra, Lamen.	Right and left ventricle, Inferior vena cava and Superior vena cava, Aorta, Nerves of thoracic region.	T1 to C13 Vertebra, Gluteus muscles, Left knee.
Sixth and Eighth	Umbilical region, Abdomen, Right chin, Jaws, Anorectal region, Urinary tract, Reproductive organs.	Bowels, Large Intestine, Liver, Spleen, Pancreas, Uterus, Ovaries, Pelvic region.	Nerve of spine, lower limbs, Calf muscles, Kidneys, Prvic girdle, Hip joints.
Seventh	Skin, Coccygeal bone, Tibia, Fibular bones, Femur bone, Sciatic nerve.	Calcaneous Talus, Navicular Cuboids, Cunieform bones, Metatarsals.	Quadriceps, Femoris, Hamstrings, Rectus femoris, Soleus, Medial and lateral condoyle.

If any particular drekkan is conjoined with or aspected by any benefic planet there will be a mole or an attractive mark on limb signified while in case malefic planet there will be some form of deformity or that part is likely to get affected by some disease. We can locate which decanate a planet is placed and in which cusp or the concerned lord of house is placed to know the type of disease and organ affected. If a planet is in fourth cusp and first decanet then there will be some defect in Breast or Thoracic bones or epigastric area or nostrils or right knee then if planet is Moon and afflicted by malefic the thoracic disease can be considered and diagnosed with tools; if it is Saturn then right knee may have problem if Mercury then it is epigastirca region and if Mars then breast or nostrils may have disease. Even though the diagnosis appears to be easy the accuracy is suspected but we can get approximate clue regarding the disease. Thus we can use this table to find out pathogenic effect of twelve zodiac signs.

1) Aries: Head, Neurological disorders, Diseases of brain, Cerebral hemorrhage, Insomnia, Epileptic disease, Psychological disorders, Acute strokes, Alzheimer, Transient ischemic attack, Hematoma, Meningitis, Encephalitis, Subarachnoid hemorrhage.
2) Taurus: Diphtheria, Apoplexy, Goiter, Thyroxin related disorder, Cervical vertebrae Piles, Fistula, Amenorrhea, Ovulation disorders, Endometriosis, Pelvic Inflammation Disease, Polycystic ovarian disorder, Ear and nose related diseases, sinus tachycardia.
3) Gemini: Pulmonary diseases, Eosinophillia, Asthma, Tuberculosis, Pneumonia, Bronchitis, Pleurisy, Inflammation of pericardium, Peripheral nervous system related disorders.
4) Cancer: Digestive system related disorders, Liver disorders, Gall bladder stones, Dropsy, Jaundice, Melancholia, Irritable bowel syndrome, Appendicitis, Hysteria, Hypochondria.
5) Leo: Blood related disorders, Aneurism, Cardiac system disorders, Spinal meningitis, Arteriosclerosis, Angina pectoris, Anemia, Spinal cord related disorders, Spondylosis.
6) Virgo: Worms in intestine, Peritonitis, digestive disorders related to small and large intestine. Vitamin B deficiency disorders, Colic pains.
7) Libra: Poly urea, Urine incontinence, Renal function disorders, Hormonal disorders, Bright's disease, Lumbar region diseases, Rheumatoid Arthritis, Skin diseases, Hernia, Prolapsed uterus.

8) Scorpio: Bladder related diseases, Coli form infection, and Uric acid stones, and Uremia, prostate related diseases, and infertility related disorders in females, Fibroid growth in uterus, Kidney stones.

9) Sagittarius: Hips bone disorders, Ilium locomotors, ataxia, Fracture of femur bones, Varicose veins.

10) Capricorn: Psoriasis, Fracture of knee bones, Patella degenerative changes, Knee cap related diseases, Leprosy, Leucoderma, Vitiligo, Blood cancer, Cancer of colon, Piles.

11) Aquarius: Ankles related disorders, Lower limb disorders, Cardiac function disorders related to blockages in vessels, Cholesterolmia, Eye related diseases like cataract, Attention deficiency disorder.

12) Pisces: Diseases of feet and toes, Deformities in feet, Delirium, Drug addiction, Tremors, Parkinson's disease, Auto immune diseases, Degenerative disorders in brain, Structural defects in brain.

Further we also can find the relation between diseases and planets as detailed bellow,

1) Sun: Right eye related diseases, Fever, Jaundice, Cardiac functioning, Stomach related diseases, Sin disorders, Bones related diseases, Diseases of brain, Baldness, Typhoid, Polyps, Epilepsy, Bile related problems, Sunstroke, speech disorders.

2) Moon: Cardiac function disorders, Pulmonary diseases, Uterus related disorders, Tuberculosis, Hormonal disorders, Mental aberrations, Anemia, Pleurisy, Nervous system diseases, Psychological disorders, Left eye problems, Sleep disorders, Diarrhea, Poisoning, Gastric diseases, Appendicitis, Breast cancer, Mammary gland disorders, Colic pains, Tumors, Hyper and hypothyroidism, Bronchitis, Dyspepsia, Typhoid.

3) Mars: Blood disorders, Tissue torture, Burns, Mental aberrations, Epilepsy, Tumors, Sjoren disorder leading to dryness of eyes, Itches, Cuts, Wounds, Hypertension, Fatigue, Hormonal disorders, Fracture of bones, Urinary diseases, Cancers, Ulcers, Anorectal diseases, Mumps, Encephalitis, Fistula, Muscular rheumatism, Septic poisoning, Herniated disorders, Abortions, Tetanus.

4) Mercury: Diseases of chest, Trauma, Blood flow disruption in brain, Auto immune diseases, Vascular disorders, Stroke, Structural disorders, Brain spinal cord injuries, Belly's palsy, Cervical spondylosis,   Spinal cord tumors, Peripheral neuropathy, Parkinson's syndrome, Multiple sclerosis, Paralysis, Ulcers, Impaired mental function, Lack of coordination, Muscle rigidity, Tremors and seizers, Slurred speech, New language impairments, Huntington's disease, Vertigo, Skin diseases, Deafness and dumbness.

5) Jupiter: Liver, Kidney, Pulmonary function disorders, Dropsy, Obesity, Tumors, Morbid growth, enlargements of organs, Diabetes, Nephritis, Dyspepsia, Abscess, Kidney function disorders.

6) Venus: Eye diseases, Reproductive organ diseases, Maxillofacial diseases, Digestive system diseases, Thyroid function dis orders, Diabetes, Carbuncle, Urethra inflammation, Cataract, Tonsillitis, Ovary function disorders, Venereal diseases, Goiter, Gout, Cyst anywhere in body.

7) Saturn: Paralysis, Insanity, Cancers, Elephantiasis, Endocrine gland disorders, Loss of limbs, Teeth related disorders, Fracture of bones, Connective tissue diseases, Rheumatoid

Arthritis, Depression and anxiety related diseases, Obstruction causing diseases, Atrophy of muscles.

8) Rahu: Pulmonary function disorders, Pulmonary artery blockages, Spleen enlargement, Ulcers in intestine, Bone tuberculosis, Cataract, frequent ailments, Edison's disease, Varicose veins.

9)   Ketu: Intestinal infection, Epidemics, Low blood pressure, Deafness, Non diagnosable diseases of eye, Boils, Stammering,.

10) Uranus:
   a)   Uranus in Aries gives accidents; that causes injuries to brain, skull, Migraine.
   b)   Uranus in Taurus gives infectious diseases to throat, Swelling, Mumps, Dumbness.
   c)   Uranus in Gemini gives Pneumonia, Bronchial infection, Cough.
   d)   Uranus in Cancer causes Dyspepsia, Fracture of ribs, Ulcers in breast.
   e)   Uranus in Leo causes degenerative diseases of vertebral column, Cardiac diseases.
   f)   Uranus in Virgo causes Digestive system chronic diseases, accident due to electric shock.
   g)   Uranus in Libra gives Inflammation in kidneys, Uric acid stones, pain in hips, Bladder cancer.
   h)   Uranus in Scorpio gives herniated growth in abdomen, Reproductive system disorders.
   i)   Uranus in Sagittarius gives Tetanus, dog bite, Fractures of hips and thighs.
   j)   Uranus in Capricorn gives Rheumatoid arthritis, Sjoren disease, Psoriatic arthritis.
   k)   Uranus in Aquarius causes sudden Cardiac arrest, Death due to poisoning.
   l)   Uranus in Pisces causes Accidents leading to amputation or disease leading to amputation.

We also can refer the constellation that are related to defects in specific organs and is listed as given in chapter 5.

Chapter 22

Miscellaneous cases that explains the Horoscope

There are many instances where the diagnosis itself misleads the doctors and the patient suffers for long time due to undiagnosed disease. To understand the exact cause we can study few cases as detailed bellow. The nature of disease is indicated by the sixth cusp and its significators, the sub lord of sixth cusp if falls in Capricorn which indicates skin diseases, Stomach ailments, and Rheumatism. And many times the diagnosis is misled if this house is occupied by Ketu and Uranus then the symptomatic indications lead doctors to go for exactly the diagnosis is different and doctors are misled; even complaints that patient registers also give wrong directions to the doctors.

Case No 033

Native born on 01st April 1978 at Pimpri/Pune with Lat 018:30N and Long. 073:52 E

The native visited doctor for frequent vertigo associated with severe headaches; initially doctor considered the case as usual related to either Anemia or Hypertension and may have some vitamin deficiency disorder and was treated accordingly, but even after almost one year the complaints remained and therefore patient was referred to neurologists for further diagnosis and treatment. Still the efforts were in vein and then to find out any spiritual remedy the patient approached some Astrologer for finding out the culprit planet and to perform some PENANCE for the evil planet according to Hindu. When the natal chart was referred following observations were noted.

The sub lord of sixth cusp is Jupiter and is also the lord of eighth house, as Jupiter is causative of diseases related to Kidney Function i.e. filtration of blood but the diagnostic reports were indicting that there is no ailment of any type related to kidney; further the Jupiter was occupied in constellation Mrugasira, i.e. indicative of Arteries that supply blood to Kidney. Further it is important to note that the sixth house is occupied by Uranus which is also a planet of mysterious diseases and as such again indicates the renal function disorder. In fact after several pathological tests it was confirmed that there was dysfunction at kidney which was not indicated by routine tests like Serum Creatine level and others. The native was then referred to Urologist and then it was diagnosed the growth of cancer cells in glomeruls of left kidney. The patient was then hospitalized and then operated surgically. If we study the natal chart in detail we find that Lord of ascendant is Venus, occupied in twelfth house in Aries conjoined with Mercury and both are under aspect from Uranus from sixth cusp; so also the star lord of sixth cusp is Jupiter which is also the lord of eighth house and occupied in Gemini and in third cusp. The Star lord of eighth cusp is Venus occupied in twelfth house, is also star lord of twelfth cusp as such connecting sixth, eighth and twelfth houses. Further sub lord of ascendant Mars directly aspect the Moon in eighth house, the Uranus Saturn placed in fourth cusp aspect ascendant, the sub lord of eighth cusp is Rahu which is occupied in fifth cusp indicating abnormal growth in kidney and as also Moon in eighth cusp indicates problems related to nervous system along with the kidney function further the Saturn occupied in fourth cusp directly aspect the sixth cusp indicating obstructive type of chronic disease. As also the planet Mercury lord of fifth cup is placed in twelfth house indicates problems related to nerves; the lord of ascendant and sixth house Venus is conjoined with Mercury indicating surgical procedure but as Jupiter aspect the eighth house from second cusp and Moon as well indicate total recovery. The native was required to get operated and the tumor type growth removed successfully. Indicating the confusion in diagnosis and suffering of native for long period was caused due to 1) Uranus, 2) Mercury 3) Moon and constellation Mrigasira.

Kidneys filter blood in three stages, firstly Nephrons filter blood that runs through the capillary network in Glomerular network by a process called glomerular filtration, secondly the filtrate is collected in renal tubules where most of the solutes get re absorbed in PCT, by process called tubular re absorption; thirdly in loop of Henle's loop filtrate continues to exchange solute and water with renal medulla and the peri tubular capillary network. Water is also reabsorbed in this stage and then additional solutes and wastes are secreted into kidney tubules during tubular secretion which in essence the opposite process to tubular re absorption. The collecting duct called filtrate commeasure from the nephron and fuse in medullar papillae deliver the filtrate and now it is called Urine. Here the cancerous growth doctor found was in medulla and that disturbed the process of filtration in Nephron stage that is in first stage leading to uremia that caused vertigo and nervous disorder. In first stage the diagnosis misled the doctors and delayed the exact required treatment.

Planetary disposition in natal chart

Sr. No	Planet	Zodiac	Degree: Min : Sec	Lord of Zodiac	Star Lord	Sub Lord
01	Sun	Pisces	317 : 33 : 28	Jupiter	Mercury	Mercury
02	Moon	Sagittarius	235 : 10 : 19	Jupiter	Venus	Mercury
03	Mars	Cancer	063 : 24 : 34	Moon	Saturn	Saturn
04	Mercury	Aries	332 : 33 : 42	Mars	Ketu	Venus
05	Jupiter	Gemini	035 : 01 : 48	Mercury	Mars	Sun
06	Venus	Aries	334 : 22 : 41	Mars	Ketu	Moon
07	Saturn	Leo	090 : 36 : 54	Sun	Ketu	Ketu
08	Rahu	Virgo	132 : 13 : 24	Mercury	Moon	Rahu
09	Ketu	Pisces	312 : 13 : 24	Jupiter	Saturn	Mars
10	Uranus	Libra	172 : 09 : 29	Venus	Jupiter	Saturn
11	Neptune	Scorpio	204 : 43 : 57	Mars	Mercury	Rahu

Case no 34

Male native born on 21st August 1980 at 2215 hrs in Pune Lat. 018:30N Long. 073:48

This classical chart shows the irrecoverable insanity leading to alcoholics, Repetition several times of the same thing gives the truest conceivable clinical picture of incurable cretinism. This is mental defect that may lead to insane obsession; nervous exhaustion of the person by over work. The nervous system is complex collection of nerves and specialized cells called neurons that transmit signals between different parts of body; which is essential electrical wiring. Functionality of nervous system has two main sub divisions, the somatic or voluntary component and autonomic or involuntary component. The native in initial stages complained of insomnia i.e. loss of control over sleep leading to loss of feeling and tingling. Further the native started feeling weakness in muscles and sometimes double vision. The native could not get relief even after medical treatment for long time; and started consuming alcohol and got addicted. After few months native had complained about impaired mental ability and lack of coordination. If we analyze the natal chart it is seen that, the lord of second house, Venus is placed in third house Gemini and under aspect from Saturn occupied in Sixth cusp; also the lord of ascendant Mars is placed in seventh cusp conjoined with Mercury in Virgo. The ascendant falls in Aries which is sign governing the nervous system, Mercury again rules the somatic or voluntary component of nervous system is placed in fifth cusp conjoined with Sun and Jupiter both the planet that rule the mental ability and hemmed in between Rahu and Saturn as malefic planets. The Moon that rules the mood and emotions occupied in ninth house i.e. Sagittarius indicating the behavioral disorder r and again hemmed in between two malefic planets Ketu and Neptune. Further the lord of ascendant Mars placed in Seventh cusp afflicted with Uranus giving rise to the aggressive and hot constitution that led the native suffer from impaired mental ability and muscle rigidity. The exact cause of the disease was not diagnosed and the native was under treatment for long time; when native lost control over sleep and suffered from insomnia. To overcome the insomnia native turned alcoholics which crossed the limit. This is indicated by the debilitated Venus which is lord of second cusp, here the lord of second cusp is responsible for addiction and afflicted Mars is responsible for insanity that went irrecoverable.

The star lord of ascendant is Jupiter is placed in fifth cusp hemmed in between Rahu and Saturn; the Jupiter is also star lord of twelfth house indicating the nervous disorder. The star lord of sixth house is Sun which is also lord of fifth cusp is occupied in fifth house hemmed in between two malefic, and conjoined with lord of twelfth cusp and lord of sixth cusp and thereby aggravating the disease. The sub lord of sixth house is Rahu occupied in fourth cusp Cancer owned by Moon, squared with Mars the lord of ascendant and eighth cusp. The Mars is also sub lord of twelfth house, also Venus the lord of second cusp is sub lord of eighth house and sub lord of third cusp indicating insomnia associated with addiction. It again noteworthy that in such cases even though the doctor advises the patient doesn't abide by the instructions falling prey to the addiction, also the close relatives play important role in such cases. Here the lord of second house is primarily responsible for the addiction and the cusp Aries, Leo, Sagittarius and planets Moon, Venus and Jupiter are the important factors are responsible and need to be accounted.

The planetary disposition is as given here with,

Sr. NO.	Planet	Zodiac	Degrees: Min : Sec.	Lord zodiac	Star Lord	Sub Lord
01	Sun	Leo	125 : 10 : 28	Sun	Ketu	Mars
02	Moon	Sagittarius	247 : 15 : 56	Jupiter	Ketu	Rahu
03	Mars	Libra	181 : 33 : 53	Venus	Mars	Mercury
04	Mercury	Leo	120 : 14 : 15	Sun	Ketu	Ketu
05	Jupiter	Leo	142 : 17 : 36	Sun	Venus	Saturn
06	Venus	Gemini	079 : 26 : 18	Mercury	Rahu	Mars
07	Saturn	Virgo	152 : 41 : 47	Mercury	Sun	Jupiter
08	Rahu	Cancer	115 : 56 : 18	Moon	Mercury	Rahu
09	Ketu	Capricorn	295 : 56 : 18	Saturn	Mars	Rahu
10	Uranus	Libra	208 : 07 : 46	Venus	Jupiter	Venus
11	Neptune	Scorpio	236 : 20 : 53	Mars	Mercury	Jupiter

Case no 35

Male native born on 13th September 1975 at 1200 hrs in Pune Lat: 018: 30N Long. 073: 48 E

In this case chart shows the ascendant is occupied with Rahu and Neptune and lord of ascendant Mars is placed in seventh cusp afflicted with Ketu; so also the lord of sixth cusp is again Mars which aspect in Moon occupied in second house, Moon is responsible for nervous disorders, and is lord of ninth cusp which is occupied by Saturn. The lord of eighth cusp is Mercury placed in Virgo under aspect of Saturn. As such we get clear indication that Moon, which rules nervous system, Mars which causes functional disorder and ascendant all are debilitated showing the degenerative type of disorder in nervous system. The native suddenly starts complaining about the severe headaches and was treated accordingly, the disease suppresses for short time and again relapse occurs after few days. When the patient was thoroughly examined by team of doctors was observed to be suffering from some ailment related to brain function disorder and then after prolonged period the treatment for cause started. The native being auto rickshaw driver could not understand the severity of the disease and resumed the work after short relief ignoring the medication. This has led to the complications and was required again to be hospitalized where he underwent treatment under specialized neurologists.   The native complained about continuous headaches, dizziness, and over sleep, had also complained of intermittent vertigo and tremors and seizures associated with back pain and slurred speech; all these complaints indicate the serious brain function disorder. In birth chart we can see that the ruler of peripheral nervous system Mars is seriously afflicted and the planet that governs the function of involuntary nervous system is also debilitated; further the ascendant is occupied with Neptune in Scorpio indicative of acute stroke and cerebral aneurism. So also the Mercury which rules the nerve function is also under aspect from Saturn, the Sun causative of cranial nervous network is also under aspect from Mars and thus shows the problem related to cranial nerves. Further the twelfth cusp is occupied by Uranus, planet of mysterious diseases indicating the frequent hospitalization. It is important to note here that the onset of the disease was very slow and native had ignored the initial symptoms that led doctors to diagnose the disease late after it has become serious.   The planetary disposition if we study we find that the star lord of ascendant is Saturn placed in Cancer owned by Moon, the star lord of sixth cusp is Venus placed in tenth house under aspect of Mars, which is also lord of sixth house and ascendant; the star lord of eight cusp is Rahu occupied in ascendant thus indicating the disease and Rahu is also sub lord of sixth cusp and star lord of twelfth cusp thus confirming the ailment. Secondly the sub lord of twelfth cusp is Moon placed in second cusp aspect the eighth house, in addition sub lord of eighth cusp is Mercury which is under aspect from Saturn, and Mercury is also sub lord Saturn. Sub lord of Sun which is causative of cranial nerve system is Ketu placed in seventh house afflicting the Mars which is lord of ascendant. Sub lord of Moon is Rahu which is also sub lord of Uranus thus establishes the connection with twelfth cusp, the sub lord of Mars is Sun and is also sub lord of Mercury is placed in tenth house under aspect of Mars conjoined with Venus which is lord of twelfth house. All these planetary dispositions shows that the native is suffering from functional nervous system disorder.

Here onset of the disease can easily be confirmed with reference to the sixth house significators. The occurrence of the disease noticed on 18th November 1989. The Venus Mahadasha was in progress and in antar dasha of Rahu with prati antardasha of Mars. The suffering was continued till the 10th December 2004 i.e. till the end of Sun Mahadasha. The native is discharged on 10th December 2004 in Antar dasha of Venus.

Planetary disposition is tabled bellow.

Sr. No	Planet	Zodiac	Degrees : Min: Sec	Lord of Zodiac	Star Lord	Sub Lord
01	Sun	Leo	296 : 20 : 14	Sun	Venus	Ketu
02	Moon	Sagittarius	035 : 34 : 53	Jupiter	Ketu	Rahu
03	Mars	Taurus	203 : 07 : 23	Venus	Moon	Sun
04	Mercury	Virgo	322 : 59 : 42	Mercury	Moon	Sun
05	Jupiter	Pisces	149 : 46 : 53	Jupiter	Mercury	Saturn
06	Venus	Leo	272 : 22 : 20	Sun	Ketu	Venus
07	Saturn	Cancer	246 : 05 : 24	Moon	Saturn	Mercury
08	Rahu	Scorpio	001 : 33 : 06	Mars	Jupiter	Rahu
09	Ketu	Taurus	181 : 33 : 06	Venus	Sun	Jupiter
10	Uranus	Libra	336 : 43 : 53	Venus	Rahu	Rahu
11	Neptune	Scorpio	015 : 38 : 26	Mars Saturn		Jupiter

Case No 36

Female native born on 09th March 1990 at 1030 hrs in Siliguri/Assam Lat 023:18N Long 085:48E

The native complained initially of bleeding through nostrils very frequently and after repeated occurrence the doctor's advice was sought which diagnosed as infectious sputum leading to ischemic condition and bleeding. After almost a month's time she was taken to hospital for finding out the cause behind frequent bleeding through nose; and was diagnosed for bilateral maxillary poly poidal sinusitis with mild DNS towards left side that also indicated the growth of tumor. The observations noted were mucoplypoidal thickening involving bilateral maxillary and posterior ethmoidal sinuses, whilst frontal and sphenoidal sinuses were clear; so also it was noted that the nasal septum appears mildly deviated with convexity towards left side. Now when her natal chart was observed that shows following indications,

1) Lord of ascendant Venus was placed in ninth cusp afflicted with Mars and Rahu, further the the planet that rules the olfactory lobes and olfactory ganglions Moon is occupied in third house afflicted with Ketu in own sign Cancer,
2) The Saturn, planet that is known for obstructions and inflammations is placed in eighth house in Sagittarius and afflicted with Uranus, the planet known for mysterious diseases.
3) The lord of sixth cusp Venus placed in ninth cusp is under aspect from Ketu.
4) The planet that denotes diseases related to nasal bones Mars is placed in ninth cusp afflicted with Rahu and under aspect of Ketu.
5) The lord of second house that rules the nasal cavity is Mercury occupied in tenth house conjoined with Sun and under aspect from Saturn from eighth cusp.
6) The ascendant falls in sign Taurus which governs the function of nasal cavity is owned by Venus and Venus which is also lord of sixth cusp indicating disease occurrence.
7) Lord of eighth cusp that denotes the seriousness of the disease Jupiter is occupied in second cusp indicating the acute abnormal growth in nasal cavity, and the Saturn placed in eighth cusp indicates the inflammation with infection that necrotizes the fleshy part in nasal cavity.

After analyzing the natal chart native went to another Hospital and the diagnosed that there is acute necrotizing inflammation with fungal organism which is morphologically consistent with Aspergllosis, no granuloma or malignancy was occurred. We can find out the correlativity of the disease causing cusps and planets so also their significators.

The star lord of ascendant is Moon and occupied in third cusp afflicted with Ketu, where Ketu is also star lord of eighth cusp; the star lord of sixth cusp is Rahu and it is placed in ninth cusp under aspect from Ketu. The star lord of twelfth cusp is Saturn occupied and conjoined with Uranus and Neptune; Saturn is also sub lord of Moon and Mars. The sub lord of Sixth cusp is Jupiter occupied in second cusp sub lord of Neptune placed in eighth house. Further sub lord of eighth cusp is Saturn and placed in eighth house; is also sub lord of twelfth house. This shows that ascendant, sixth cusp and eighth cups and its significators are well connected gives the clear indication of infective inflammation of septum in nostrils which was confirmed by clinical diagnosis.

Planetary disposition of the natal chart is tabled as under.

Sr. no.	Planet	Zodiac	Degrees: Min : Sec	Lord of zodiac	Star Lord	Sub Lord
01	Sun	Aquarius	294 : 38 : 20	Saturn	Jupiter	Mercury
02	Moon	Cancer	088 : 22 : 14	Moon	Mercury	Saturn
03	Mars	Capricorn	244 : 27 : 46	Saturn	Sun	Saturn
04	Mercury	Aquarius	285 : 50 : 31	Saturn	Rahu	Venus
05	Jupiter	Gemini	037 : 20 : 17	Mercury	Rahu	Rahu
06	Venus	Capricorn	250 : 16 : 30	Saturn	Moon	Moon
07	Saturn	Sagittarius	239 : 06 : 45	Jupiter	Sun	Mars
08	Rahu	Capricorn	261 : 10 : 29	Saturn	Moon	Venus
09	Ketu	Cancer	081 : 10 : 29	Moon	Mercury	Venus
10	Uranus	Sagittarius	225 : 19 : 28	Jupiter	Venus	Venus
11	Neptune	Sagittarius	230 : 27 : 05	Jupiter	Venus	Jupiter

Occurrence of the disease as rule of sixth cusp was appeared on 6TH January 2019 when Venus mahadasha was in progress and in Ketu antar dasha with Saturn prati antar dasha. The native was hospitalized on 07th January 2019 and after diagnosis was discharged on 20th January 2019

The native got totally recovered without operative surgery, and was declared by doctors was on

14th April 2019.

Case no 37

The female native born on 16th December 1969 at 0937 hrs in Nagaon /Assam

 Lat.027: 01 N and Long. 094: 10 E

The native reported to doctor regarding some skin type of infection of breast caused specific red coloration and was initially treated for fungal type of infection but the red coloration and swelling persisted rather increased. After thorough clinical diagnosis doctor confirmed that it was type of breast cancer having swelling in left side of breast. In initial period the swelling and red coloration appeared to be fungal infection and rate of proliferation was also slow and there was no any sign of cancer being of malignant nature. After almost two months the doctor advised the biopsy after assuring the patient that no threat of further proliferation, doctor found that the cancer was malignant and was of Inflammatory Breast cancer that gives characteristic red colorization and swelling. It normally is confused with breast infection which is more common cause of breast redness and swelling. This is being locally advanced cancer that spread from its point of origin to nearby lymph nodes.

Lord of ascendant and lord of sixth cusp in tenth house and under aspect from Saturn or Mars denote the breast cancer. In the present natal chart lord of ascendant is Saturn is placed in fourth cusp which falls in Aries and lord of sixth cusp occupied in twelfth cusp which falls in Sagittarius; further the lord of fourth cusp, Mars is placed in second house afflicted with Rahu and aspect the eighth cusp. Lord of twelfth cusp Jupiter is placed in tenth house under aspect of Saturn. Further the ninth cusp is occupied by Uranus, a planet known to cause mysterious diseases. The owner of the ninth cusp Mercury is placed in twelfth house conjoined with Sun, so also the Sun is lord of eighth cusp and aspect sixth house owned by Mercury. Thus lord of sixth house and eighth house are conjoined and placed in twelfth cusp; whereas the lord of twelfth cusp is Jupiter placed in tenth house and under aspect of Saturn which is lord of ascendant and second house. Thus sixth cusp and eighth cusp ascertain the presence of cancer; whilst the twelfth cusp throws light on convalescence. If we correlate the primary characteristics of the disease with symbolic attribute of planet we find the growth is in lymphatic duct in breast, here we can correlate growth of cancerous cells with planetary parlance; Jupiter signifies the growth of cancerous cells and is lord of twelfth cusp clarifies the breast cancer. Further shadow planet Rahu is astrologically associated with morbid and erratic growth in addition to swelling; pain and discomfort is also despised. And as such Rahu is key symbol in our interpretation of natal chart to signify Breast cancer. The Moon rules the breasts and is placed in third cusp hemmed in between Rahu and Saturn; indicating chronic prolonged disease. Moon in third cusp Pisces is under aspect from Uranus, Uranus is responsible for abnormal cells growth and severe inflammation with pain. The breast cancer of this type that is inflammatory type and always mislead with simple fungal infection which is the characteristic of Uranus is known to be the mysterious effect of Uranus when it aspect the Moon.

Saturn occupied in fourth house which is indicative of breast related obstructive diseases, is star lord of Neptune and thus indicative of lymphatic obstruction is observed. Star lord of ascendant is Mars afflicted with Rahu denotes the inflammatory and chronic type of disease related to breast. The sub lord of ascendant Mars which is also star lord of sixth cusp and sub lord of Cancer that occupies seventh cusp indicating difficulty and delay in diagnosis leading to complication of disease. The sub lord Mercury is also sub lord of twelfth house and placed with lord of eighth cusp Sun and lord of sixth cusp, thus well connected with ascendant, sixth cusp, eighth cusp, and twelfth cusp, so also their significators. This confirms the type and intensity of the disease.

The onset of disease was noticed on 10th February 2014 when Ketu mahadasha and Mercury atardasha was in progress and in Jupiter prati antardasha. And was recovered in mahadasha of Venus was in progress i.e. in May 2017 in Mercury prati antardasha.

Planetary disposition of the natal chart is tabled bellow.

Sr. No.	Planet	Zodiac	Degrees: Min : Sec	Lord of Zodiac	Star Lord	Sub Lord
01	Sun	Sagittarius	300 : 35 : 53	Jupiter	Ketu	Ketu
02	Moon	Pisces	062 : 09 : 15	Jupiter	Jupiter	Rahu
03	Mars	Aquarius	036 : 59 : 20	Saturn	Rahu	Rahu
04	Mercury	Sagittarius	346 : 36 : 35	Jupiter	Venus	Moon
05	Jupiter	Libra	276 : 28 : 46	Venus	Mars	Moon
06	Venus	Scorpio	321 : 06 : 06	Mars	Mercury	Venus
07	Saturn	Aries	099 : 56 : 25	Mars	Ketu	Jupiter
08	Rahu	Aquarius	052 : 41 : 04	Saturn	Jupiter	Saturn
09	Ketu	Leo	232 : 41 : 04	Sun	Venus	Saturn
10	Uranus	Virgo	254 : 58 : 58	Mercury	Moon	Jupiter
11	Neptune	Scorpio	305 : 55 : 35	Mars	Saturn	Mercury

Case no 38

Male native born on 22nd May 1963 at 0026 hrs in Satara Lat. 017: 40 N Long. 073: 58 E
This is also one of the classic case to understand the relation planet establishes and the
body organ response to that and fall sick over passage of time.

The chart denotes Capricorn falls in ascendant and lord of the house occupies it i.e. Saturn. The
fourth cusp that rules the cardiac function is occupied by Moon conjoined with Venus where Venus
is lord of fifth and tenth cusps and Moon is lord of seventh house and is planet that controls the
mood and emotions along with blood function. The Mars which rules the composition of blood and
and lord of fourth cusp is placed in eighth cusp afflicted with Uranus. The lord of eighth cusp is Sun
which is placed in fifth house conjoined with Mercury which is lord of sixth and ninth cusp. Sixth
cusp is occupied by Rahu and twelfth cusp by Ketu aspect each other. Jupiter which is lord of
twelfth house and third house is occupied in third house Pisces, and under aspect of Saturn. Further
the Moon is under aspect from Ketu and Neptune as such debilitated giving cranky mood and
causes severe depression. So also the Jupiter lord of twelfth cusp placed in third house rules the
arteries and superior and inferior vena cava, indicating the trouble associated with arteries and
Moon indicates troubles associated with blood flow. Saturn which occupied ascendant gives
depression and stress level linked cortisol in blood. Saturn also reduces the secretion of endorphins
causing nervous syndrome that leads to insomnia. So also the Mercury rules nerve supply to heart
and malefic present in Leo indicates the disease related to arteries and blood vessels connected to
heart, Saturn that governs the breath also indicates the ailments associated with heart. In this chart
fourth cusp is occupied by sign Aries denotes the malfunctioning of blood circulation, and the sign
which rules the cardiac diseases i.e. Cancer is placed in seventh and under aspect from Saturn. Mars
that denotes the blood circulation is placed in eighth house indicating some problems associated
with blood circulation.

1) The Moon that rules blood function and if afflicted or under aspect of malefic gives an
   indication of diseases and as such the Moon in this chart signifies the defect in either
   composition of blood or deformed cells in blood.

2) The other planet Mars that controls the blood circulation is placed in eighth house is afflicted with Uranus, which indicates mysterious diseases also denotes something that increases the heart problems.
3) The Saturn which is causative of obstructive and inflammatory type of diseases is occupied in ascendant also indicates obstruction in blood flow leading to cardiac disease.
4) The cancer which also indicates the heart related disorder is under aspect from Saturn denotes the cardiac problems.
5) The Leo sign that rules the function of heart falls in eighth cusp and occupied by Mars and Uranus give the indication of circulation related disease.
6) The Sun that is responsible for cardiac function i.e. the diastolic and systolic pressure is placed in fifth house conjoined with lord of sixth house; also the Sun is lord of eighth cusp indicates the obstruction in pulmonary artery and is required to be examined.
7) The Jupiter which is responsible for growth is under aspect from Saturn and as such indicates the accumulation or growth of some kind in arteries.

All these signs indicate the problems related to heart, but when examined thoroughly it was diagnosed that there is enlargement of heart and also the sudden rise in blood pressure was observed, also the ventricular tachycardia was noted which is indicative of obstruction in pulmonary artery. The native was advised bypass surgery and accordingly the native underwent the surgery and now after almost two months resumed normal routine life.
The star lord of ascendant is Mars occupied in eighth cusp is also lord of fourth house; the star lord of sixth house Jupiter placed in third house is also star lord of Rahu occupied in sixth cusp that aspect twelfth cusp. The star lord of twelfth cusp is sun placed in fifth house conjoined with Mercury lord of sixth cusp and Sun is also star lord of eighth cusp. Further the sub lord of ascendant is Rahu placed in sixth cusp and Ketu is sub lord of Mars placed in eighth cusp and occupied in twelfth cusp aspect directly the sixth cusp indicating occurrence of the disease, hospitalization followed by surgery and also recovery. The occurrence of the disease was reported on 20th August 2017 and was diagnosed for ventricular tachycardia related to pulmonary artery as it was found blocked almost 92 %. Doctor advised immediate surgery and as such was required to get operated on 15th November 2017. He got successfully operated and recovered.

Planetary disposition in natal chart is tabled as given under.

Sr. No	Planet	Zodiac	Degrees: Min : Sec	Lord of Zodiac	Star Lord	Sub Lord
01	Sun	Taurus	126 : 39 : 25	Venus	Sun	Mercury
02	Moon	Aries	107 : 06 : 54	Mars	Venus	Moon
03	Mars	Leo	210 : 38 : 42	Sun	Ketu	Ketu
04	Mercury	Taurus	121 : 03 : 40	Venus	Sun	Rahu
05	Jupiter	Pisces	077 : 13 : 11	Jupiter	Mercury	Mercury
06	Venus	Aries	099 : 57 : 44	Mars	Ketu	Saturn
07	Saturn	Capricorn	029 : 38 : 27	Saturn	Mars	Saturn
08	Rahu	Gemini	179 : 53 : 29	Mercury	Jupiter	Moon
09	Ketu	Sagittarius	359 : 53 : 29	Jupiter	Sun	Rahu

| 10 | Uranus | Leo | 217 : 52 : 30 | Sun | Ketu | Jupiter |
| 11 | Neptune | Libra | 290 : 31 : 17 | Venus | Jupiter | Jupiter |

Case No. 39

A female native born on 27th December 1987 at 1559 hrs in Sangli Lat. 016:55N Long. 074:37E

This is typical case that denotes organ affected and planetary disposition and their transit. It is known fact that normally the problems associated with women in India are concerned with mostly female organs and as such the natal chart when denotes malefic occupied in fifth, seventh, eighth cusp or Mars placed in sixth oreighth and Moon placed in eighth cusp the disease associated with female reproductive system exists.

In the chart under discussion we find that Ketu occupied sixth cusp and Mars is placed in sixth cusp which indicates the disease associated with Uterus. Further Mercury is placed in eighth cusp afflicted with Saturn, that gives obstructive disorders and Uranus that causes mysterious and difficult to diagnose diseases. Mercury it self governs the function ovaries in body and denotes diseases related to reproductive system. Secondly the planet that rules the secretion of homones in body Moon is occupied in Pisces in twelfth cusp afflicted with Rahu indicates the hormonal imbalance, so also the Sub lord of seventh house is Mars and it also signifies the seventh cusp indicates growth of tissues in ovary which referred to as Polycystic ovarian disorder. Further the Sun occupied in eighth cusp afflicted with Saturn, Uranus and Neptune indicates the obstruction in ovulation and denotes the incapacitance for conception. The lord of eighth cusp Jupiter is placed in eleventh cusp under aspect from Ketu denotes the delayed or absence of menstrual cycle and as such the disease associated with ovaries.

The lorde of fifth cusp which governs the menstrual cycle in female Mercury is placed in eighth cusp afflicted with Saturn, Uranus and Neptune denotes the ailment related to ovulation cycle. Further we can see that the lord of seventh house Mars which signifies blood is occupied in sixth cusp indicating the hormonal imbalance along with cyst formation in ovaries. The lord of ascendant Venus is palced in ninth cusp owned by Saturn and under aspect from Mars indicates the disease also related to reproductive system and so also the relation with emotional imbalance. The star lord of ascendant is Moon occupied in eleventh cusp conjoined with Rahu and Jupiter and under aspect from Ketu from fifth cuspwhere Rahu is star lord of sixth cusp and Ketu is star lord of eighth cusp and twelfth cusp. The Sub lord of ascendant is Rahu which is also sub lord of sixth cusp is placed with Jupiter which is sub lord of eighth and twelfth cusp, thus ascendant, sixth house, eighth and twelfth cusp are well connected indicating the disease diagnosed as Poly Cystic Ovarian Disorder. Occurrence noted in the the dasha period of Ketu and Antardasha of Rahu on 08th July 2015when Mercury prati antardasha was in progress. Planetary disposition is as bellow given.

Sr. No.	Planet	Zodiac	Degree: Min: Sec	Lord of Zodiac	Star Lord	Sub Lord
01	Sun	Sagittarius	221 : 26 : 08	Jupiter	Ketu	Saturn
02	Moon	Pisces	311 : 41 : 00	Jupiter	Saturn	Moon

03	Mars	Libra	178 : 12 : 46	Venus	Jupiter	Venus
04	Mercury	Sagittarius	223 : 48 : 02	Jupiter	Venus	Venus
05	Jupiter	Pisces	326 : 19 : 11	Jupiter	Mercury	Jupiter
06	Venus	Capricorn	252 : 41 : 44	Saturn	Moon	Rahu
07	Saturn	Sagittarius	201 : 14 : 41	Jupiter	Ketu	Venus
08	Rahu	Pisces	303 : 43 : 06	Jupiter	Saturn	Saturn
09	Ketu	Virgo	123 : 43 : 06	Mercury	Sun	Saturn
10	Uranus	Sagittarius	213 : 41 : 58	Jupiter	Ketu	Moon
11	Neptune	Sagittarius	223 : 55 : 26	Jupiter	Venus	Venus

Chapter no 23

Digestive system scaned under horoscope

Human digestive system is principal system in body that makes body available the essential Vitamins, Minerals, Proteins, Fats, and carbohydrates and as such serves as major system of human body.   Non functioning or poorly functioning of Gastro Intestianl tract can be the source of many chronic health problems, that can interfere with the quality of life and in many instances the death of person begins in the intestine. Gastro Intestine system is responsible for the break down and absorption of various foods, liquids needed to sustain life. Many different organs have essential roles in the digestion of food from the mechanical disrupting by teeth to the creation of bile by liver used for emulsification of fats. Bile production of the liver plays an important role in digestion from being uring this two main stored and concentrated in gall bladderduring fasting stages for being discharged to small intestine. In order to understand the interaction of the different components and their relation ship with planets and zodiacs we have to study the journey of food through human body and during these two main processes occur at the same time.

1. Mechanical Digestion; In this larger pieces of food are trituarated into micro particles; naturally the Teeth are the most important organ and falls under the sign Taurus and plnet Jupiter and Saturn rules the teeth, any malefic if occupied in Taurus or Jupiter be under aspect of malefic planet or Saturn falls in Leo may cause malfunctioning of teeth and thereby digestion of food.

2. Chemical Digestion this starts in mouth and continues into intestines, Several different enzymes break down macro molecules into micro moleculesthat can be absorbed by the body.

GI tract starts with mouth and proceeds to the esophagus, stomach, small intestine, Jejunum, Ilium, and then into large intestine, colon, and rectumthen terminates in anus. Also Pancreas, Liver contributes materials to small intestine. G.I. tract is composed of four layers or tunics and each has different tissuesand functions. There are specialized goblet cells that secrets mucos through out G. I. tract located within.

1) Mucosa layer on this mucosa layer there are villis and microvillis.
2) Submucosa layer which is relatively thick and serves as mucosa that allows absorbed element pass through the mucosa are picked up from blood vesselsof submucosa. It has glands and nerve plexuses.
3) Muscularis, This layer is responsible for segmental contraction and peristaltic wave's movment in G.I.tract. The muscularis is composed of two layers of muscles, an inner circular and outer longitudinal layer. These cause food to move further and churn with digestive enzymes down the G.I. tract.
4) Serosa, this is last layer is protective layer composed of avascular connective tissue and simple epithelium. It secrets lubricating serous fluid. This is visible layer on outside of the organ.
Now in above system the deuodenum, small intestine, Jejunum, is ruled by sign Gemini and any malefic in this sign or aspect of any malefic planet causes the malfunctioning of these parts of digestive system. Futher the later part of small intestine, Ilium, Liver, Pncreas, are ruled by sign Virgo and if under aspect of any malefic or present of any malefic gives the diseases related to these organs. The transverse colon, ascending colon, descending colon are controlled by Virgo and any malefic or Jupiter in this sign dnotes the disease related to these organs. Sigmoid colon rectum and anus are ruled by Sagittarius and planet Saturn. Further the liver, spleen, gall bladder, and secretion of enzymes is conroled by Scorpio and Sagittarius and planet Jupiter, Mars and Mercury. The artery that supply blood to G.I. tract and absorb the neutrients and fluid containing urea is ruled by Mars.
Accesory organs are detailed as bellow.
1. Salivary glands, parotid glands, submandibular glansds, are exocrine glands that produce saliva which begins the process of digestion with amylase.
2. Tongue this manipulates food for swallowing with taste bud placed in the tongue also senses the taste of food.
3. Teeth these are used to disintegrate the food into micro particles and churn that with amaylaze to get digested. Here the ascendant and Jupiter rules the process and if afflicted with Saturn gives major problems related to teeth or above secretary gland.
4. Liver this is most vital organ of the body that produces and excrets bile required for emulsifying fat, some part of it is drained directly into deuodenum and some part is stored in gall bladder. Bile helps in metabolizing protein, lipids, carbohydrates and urea a chief end product of human metabolism is formed in liver from amino acid and compound of ammonia. The function of liver is governed by Jupiter and Saturn and sign Virgo and Leo.
5. Gall bladder this is bile storage pouch stors the excess bile and releases when protei and fat enter the G.I.tract. It is ruled by the sign Leo with planet Mercury.

6. Pancreas the exocrine functions of pancreas is to produce digestive enzymes and stores zymogen that will be activated by the brush border membrane in small intestine when person eats proteins, Trpsinogen, Chymotypsinogen, carboxy peptidase, lipase, Amylase, etc. The endocrine function of pancreas include somatstatins in bile that inhibits the function of insulin, Glucagon that stimulates the stored glycogen in liver to convert into glucose incase required. Insulin made in beta cells of islets of langerhans of pancreas; thus insulin regulates the glucose. This endocrine function ruled by sign Cancer and any affliction of Cancer indicates malfunctioning of pancreas leading to diabetes.

7. Vermiform Appendix this part vestigal organ that takes part in producing immunoglobulines and maintains gut flora that produces vitamin B called neurovitamins in human body. This is ruled by sign Gemini and Scorpio with sixth cusp and Uranus, Mercury planets.

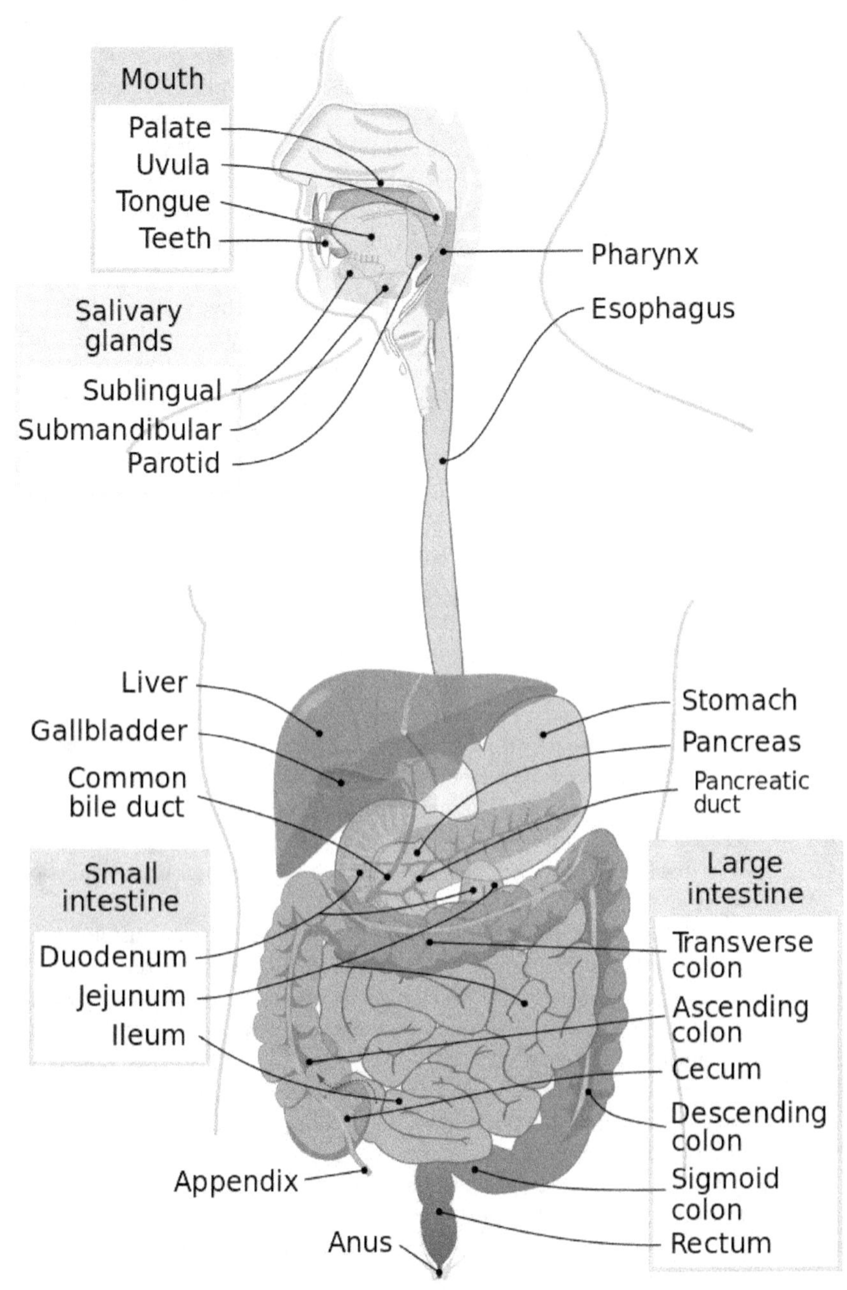

Mouth
Palate
Uvula
Tongue
Teeth
Salivary glands
Sublingual
Submandibular
Parotid
Pharynx
Esophagus
Liver
Gallbladder
Common bile duct
Small intestine
Duodenum
Jejunum
Ileum
Appendix
Anus
Stomach
Pancreas
Pancreatic duct
Large intestine
Transverse colon
Ascending colon
Cecum
Descending colon
Sigmoid colon
Rectum

In large intestine there is re absorption of some minerals and water and then feces are formed. Further there is sphincter in descending colon that acts as valves; the digested food is not allowed to return its way by these sphincters. The Uranus causes malfunctioning of these sphincters; if Saturn and Uranus conjoin in Virgo or Libra with constellation Hstha and Chitra produce malfunctioning of sphincters lading to diseases piles, Fistulla etc. If Mars be the planet conjoined with Uranus in Virgo the iiretable bowel syndrome occurs and may also lead to surgical operation of anorectal reagion. If Saturn and Mars occupy the eighth cusp and are afflicted by Rahu or Ketu produces colon cancer. So also if Sun occupies the eighth cusp and is afflicted with Rahu or Ketu and under aspect of Mars produces pile and gives hot constitution.

Mars is the major causative planet for the ailments of digestive system specifically the intestine and if offlicted by Saturn or Rahu in Virgo or Scorpio may give rise to ailments related to the function of deuodenum and Jejunum which is responsible for digestion of protein and fat from the food leading to specific malneutrition disorder. Mars is responsible for function of Anorectal part of large intestine that causes elimination of feces and also Mercury is responsible for function of rectum which finally eliminates feces through anus, where the fuction of sphincters and the specific movement of descending colon are important; thus Mars and Mercury if occupies the eighth cusp and sixth cusp and are under aspect from Saturn or Rahu causes poor function of rectum causing repeated constipation and gives rise to associated diseases. Further if Jupiter be placed in sixth or eighth cusp and at the same time Mars or Mercury is afflcted leads to irritable bowel syndrome; if Jupiter be placed in sixth cusp and Uranus occupies twelfth cusp also indicated poor elimination of feces from body which causes many more ailments. Neptune deals with exocrine function that; the glands that secrets the enzymes and called zymogen which further gets activated by brush border membrane of small intestine into Trypsinigen, chymotypsinogen, carboxypeptidase, Lypase Amylase etc which take part in digestion as catalyst.

1. The sign Gemini Virgo, Scorpio, and Pisces are prominent signs if falls in sixth cusp causes poor digestion or poor absorption of digested food.
2. The sixth eighth and twelfth cusp are relevant to the diseases related function of large intestine.
3. Uranus, Mercury, Mars, and Neptune are the major planets responsible for function of exocrine and endocrine functions of Pancreas that takes part in digestion.
4. Jupiter, Mars, Mercury if afflicted by Rahu or Ketu either by aspect, Semisquare, Square, Quincunx and Opposition may cause the malfunctioning of liver, pancreas, Spleen, and function of large intestine.
5. Saturn in fifth house makes a person voracious eater with consequent disease of over eating and diseases like constipation, indigestion, and associated effects like headaches, hypertention are caused.

    As the cecum a part of large intestine and bowels movment falls under theses planetary disposition any ailment if appears must be studied accordingly and appropriate diagnosis may arrived at and be treated. Mars is the causative for all ruptures, inflammation, tumors, abscesss, boils, etc and causes it is essential to understand the status of Mars first. Uranus causes inflammation and ischemia of colon. Uranus in Virgo,

Libra and in the constellation Hasta and Chitra leades to the diseases of colon and anorectal part of large intestine. This can well be explained with practical observations listed below.

Case No 40

The female native born on 14th September 1983 at 1922 hrs in Thane

Lat. 019:12 N Long. 072: 05 E

The natal chart shows Pisces ascendant and lord of ascendant is placed in ninth house owned by Mars i.e. Scorpio afflicted with Uranus and Ketu. The lord of fifth cusp is Moon placed in Sagittarius in tenth cusp afflicted with Neptune and under aspect from Saturn. Fifth cusp is occupied by Venus conjoined with Mars is also under aspect of Saturn, The Mercury is placed in sixth cusp conjoined with Sun in Leo. Saturn occupied in eighth cusp in Libra and in quincunx with Rahu from third house in Taurus. Thus we can observe here that, the Mars that is causative of function of large intestine; and is indicativeof the disease irritable bowel syndrome is under aspect from Saturn from eighth cusp and the Moon that rules the secretion of endocrine glands in pancreas is afflicted with Neptune in tenth cusp. Further the Neptune also afflicts the zodiac Sagittarius denoting the problem with bowel movement. It is note worthy in this case that eighth cusp is occupied by Saturn placed in Libra indicates the obstructive type of ailment causing constipation repeatedly. S also we can note here is the Uranus which is responsible for exocrine function of pancreas leads to improper and incomplete digestion of food causing formation of toxic compounds in colon.

The Mars which is responsible for the formation of feces and elimination through anus causes the problems associated with bowel movment, another planet Neptune whis is known to cause the malfunctioning of sphincters in descending colon and anorectal region.

The Jupiter that is responsible for smooth functioning of large intestine is afflicted with Uranus and Ketu in ninth cusp so also is under aspect of Rahu denoting the persistent and chronic problem of absorption in small intestine and removal of feces from body. Further sign Libra is afflicted with presence of Saturn which is known to cause obstructive and inflmatory diseases denotes the existence of ailment in intestines. When the native was reffered by doctor to undergo Colonoscopy it was revealed that the descending colon was found to have inflamed and also affected due to some microbial infection.

If we take account of significators it is revealed that the star lord of ascendant Saturn is placed in eighth cusp in Libra and is also star lord of fifth cusp and ninth cusp confirming the above findings. Fuerter star lord of sixth cusp is Ketu placed conjoined with Jupiter in ninth cusp under aspect of Rahu which is star lord of eighth cusp, the star lord of twelfth cusp is Mars occupied in fifth cusp conjoined with Venus the sub lord of twelfth house. Sub lord of Ascendant is Sun placed in sixth house with Mercury which is star lord of Ketu. Sub lord of sixth cusp is Moon occupied in tenth house under aspect of Saturn in eighth cusp and star lord of twelfth cusp in fifth cusp under aspect of Saturn thus well connecting the ascendant, sixth cusp, eighth cusp and twelfth cusp.

Planetary disposition of this natal chart is given in this table.

Sr. No.	Planets	Zodiac	Degrees: Min:Sec	Lord of Zodiac	Star Lord	Sub Lord
01	Sun	Leo	177 : 33 : 23	Sun	Sun	Moon
02	Moon	Sagittarius	272 : 58 : 20	Jupiter	Ketu	Venus
03	Mars	Cancer	146 : 43 : 12	Moon	Mercury	Jupiter
04	Mercury	Leo	179 : 43 : 59	Sun	Sun	Rahu
05	Jupiter	Scorpio	250 : 39 : 23	Mars	Saturn	Sun
06	Venus	Cancer	149 : 36 : 10	Moon	Mercury	Saturn
07	Saturn	Libra	218 : 17 : 29	Venus	Rahu	Rahu
08	Rahu	Taurus	086 : 38 : 54	Venus	Mars	Jupitewr
09	Ketu	Scorpio	266 : 38 : 54	Mars	Mercury	Jupiter
10	Uranus	Scorpio	251 : 51 : 49	Mars	Saturn	Moon
11	Neptune	Sagittarius	242 : 50 : 55	Jupiter	Ketu	Venus

The occurrence of the ailment can be determined by the significaters of sixth cusp and as such we can see the first time the native complained was on 20th January 2014 when Sun maha dasha and ketu antar and prati antar dasha was in progress.

Case no 41

Female native: born on 29th August 1973 at 0735 hrs. In Mumbai/Worli
Lat. 019:01 N, Long. 072: 49 E

The natal chart shows here with that the lord of ascendant is sun and occupied in own cusp conjoined with Moon and Mercury; here the sign Leo indicates the function of small intestine so also the Moon rules the endocrine function of Pancreas, and Mercury denotes the function of liver. The ascendant with Moon and Mercury are under aspect from Saturn from elevatnh cusp. Further the Sagittarius falls in fifth cusp is afflicted by Rahu and under aspect from Ketu and Saturn. Sign Sagittarius rules the function of large intestine and is afflicted as such disease associated with large intestine is predicted. The planet Jupiter which rules the function of liver and small intestine is occupied in sixth cusp and Capricorn denoting the ailment associated with descending colon and rectum. The planet that rules the elimination of feces from body and as such ano-rectal region is Mars and is occupied in ninth cusp under aspect from Rahu. Uranus is occupied in Virgo indiacting the malfunctioning of small intestine and is conjoined with Venus that rules the finction of pancreas.   Leo that occupies the ascendant is under aspect from Saturn giving rise to the ailments related with gall bladder, which stores the Bile. Sagittarius the sign occupied in fifth cusp is under aspect from Saturn and as Sagittarius denotes the rectum and its function the disease may be related to anorectal region or obstructive type of growth in rectum. Further the lord of eighth cusp is Jupiter which is occupied in sixth cups indicating the serious disease related to colon. The Uranus placed in in Virgo in second cusp aspect the eighth cusp and also afflicts the sign Virgo indicating abnormal growth in intestine. Th Mars that rules the function of discharging feces occupied in Aries aspect fourth cusp which is occupied by Neptune, Neptune being the causative of colon function and structure indicating the tumor growth in colon. Whe the native approached doctor and doctor diagnosed after thourough examination the presence of tumor in colon and advised surgical removal of the same. The native then was required to get hospitalized for surgery and recovered after that. We can see in the chart that star lord of ascendant is Sun occupied in first house is under aspect of Saturn which is sub lord of sixth cusp and twelfth cusp so also the Moon which is Sub lord of ascendant is under aspect of Saturn. The sub lord of eighth house is Jupiter placed in sixth house. The star lord of Sun is Mercury and which is also star lord of eighth cusp and twelfth house as well as is conjoined with Moon which is lord of twelfth cusp. As such the abscessa when confirmed by doctor, the native was required to get hospitalized for surgery. The exact date of occurrence of the disease was not known to native the probable period could be in Mahadasha of star lord of sixth cusp i.e. Mars mahadasha and in Antardasha of sublord of sixth cusp Saturn.The native was operated on 13th June 2016; and was totally recovered and discharged on July 2nd 2016.

Planetary disposition of this natal chart is as given under.

Sr. No	Planet	Zodiac	Degree : Min : Sec	Lord of Zodiac	Star Lord	Sub Lord
01	Sun	Leo	012 : 06 : 17	Sun	Ketu	Mercury
02	Moon	Leo	024 : 31 : 37	Sun	Venus	Mercury
03	Mars	Aries	252 : 30 : 05	Mars	Ketu	Mercury
04	Mercury	Leo	007 : 23 : 31	Sun	Ketu	Rahu
05	Jupiter	Capricorn	160 : 15 : 28	Saturn	Moon	Moon
06	Venus	Virgo	048 : 27 : 36	Mercury	Moon	Mercury
07	Saturn	Gemini	309 : 08 : 37	Mercury	Rahu	Jupiter
08	Rahu	Sagittarius	131 : 02 : 23	Jupiter	Ketu	Saturn
09	Ketu	Gemini	311 : 02 : 23	Mercury	Rahu	Saturn
10	Uranus	Virgo	057 : 05 : 45	Mercury	Mars	Jupiter
11	Neptune	Scorpio	101 : 12 : 55	Mars	Saturn	Moon

Case no 42

Male is native born on 27th August 1986 at 2359 hrs. In Pangri Maharashtra Lat. 018:18N Long. 075:52E

This natal chart shows the ascendant Taurus occupied with Moon and lord of ascendant placed in fifth cusp afflicted with Ketu and under aspect from Rahu denoting the chronic disease related to digestive tract. The Mars which rules the elimination of feces occupied in eighth cusp afflicted with Neptune indicating serious problems associated with colon. The sign Sagittarius that rule the function of intestine occupied in eighth cusp also denotes the diseases related to large intestine; and the lord of Sagittarius Jupiter is occupied in tenth cup in Aquarius. This indicates the ailment associated with digestive system. Moon the causative of secretion of endocrine and exocrine functions is placed in fisrt house and under aspect from Saturn placed and afflicted with Uranus denoting disturbed function of digestive system so also Moon is under aspect from Mars occupied in eighth cusp, which indicates the diseases function of colorectal part of digestive system. The Venus which is causative of function of fluid reabsorption in colon; that leads to formation of hard feces and results into piles or related disorders, is afflicted with Ketu and under aspect from Rahu. The lord of fifth cusp is Mercury is placed in fourth house conjoined with Sun and under aspect of Saturn and Uranus, as Mercury is planet that rules the secretion and that impacts the quality of function of digestive syetem; and there fore the digestive function appears to be disturbed. Further the sign Virgo is occupied in forth cusp is debilitated as under aspect from Saturn and indicates the malfunctioning of sphincters in large intestine that move the idgested food and fecal mass further for fluid reabsorption and elimination of feces causing piles and complications. The Scorpio that rules the anorectal region of large intestine is occupied in seventh cusp afflicted with Saturn and Uranus also causes the malfunctioning of anus.

Further the star lord of ascendant is Venus placed in fifth cusp conjoined with Ketu which is star lord of eighth and twelfth cusp indicating the disease related to digestive system. Further the lstar lord of eighth cusp is rahu which aspect the star lord of ascendane and eighth house. The star lord of Mars is also Venus which is placed in Virgo and under aspect from Rahu. Also the sub lord of ascendant is Jupiter which is also sub lord of sixth house and occupied in Aquarius. The sub lord of twelfth house is Saturn which is also sub lord of eighth cusp and fifth cusp thus all the significators of ascendant, sixth cusp, eighth cusp and twelfth cusp are well connected indicating the occurrence of the disease in dasha period of sixth cusp.

As such for the first time the native reported the ailment to the doctor and was initially advised to consume some medicines after almost two months doctor decided to operate surgically for the piles, thus on 05th February 2014 the native visited doctor regarding the complaint of piles which initially was treated but the doctor advised the surgery as such the native was operated on 10th May 2014. The surgery was successful and the native was discharged on 12th May 2014.

Planetary disposition of this natal chart is tabled as given below.

Sr. No.	Planet	Zodiac	Degree: Min:Sec	Lord of Zodiac	Star Lord	Sub Lord
01	Sun	Leo	100 : 30 : 48	Sun	Ketu	Saturn
02	Moon	Taurus	014 : 58 : 57	Venus	Moon	Jupiter
03	Mars	Sagittarius	229 : 21 : 49	Jupiter	Venus	Rahu
04	Mercury	Leo	091 : 39 : 20	Sun	Ketu	Venus
05	Jupiter	Aquarius	296 : 01 : 11	Saturn	Jupiter	Ketu
06	Venus	Virgo	146 : 33 : 19	Mercury	Mars	Jupiter
07	Saturn	Scorpio	189 : 44 : 15	Mars	Saturn	Venus
08	Rahu	Pisces	329 : 30 : 35	Jupiter	Mercury	Saturn
09	Ketu	Virgo	149 : 30 : 35	Mercury	Mars	Saturn
10	Uranus	Scorpio	204 : 41 : 17	Mars	Mercury	Rahu
11	Neptune	Sagittarius	219 : 27 : 27	Jupiter	Ketu	Saturn

Skeleton and Bones under Horoscope

Human skeleton that serves as frame work of body consists of many individual bones and cartilages. There is also fibrous connective tissue called ligaments and tendons in intimate relationship with the parts of skeleton. Human skeleton consists of two principal sub divisions each with origins distinct from the other and each presenting certain individual features. These are 1) Axial comprising of vertebral column, the spine and much of the skull. 2) The appendicular to which pelvic (Hip) and pectoral (Shoulder) girdles and the bones of the limbs belong. When one considers the relation of these subdivisions of the skeleton to the soft part of human body such as the nervous system, digestive system, the respiratory system, cardiovascular system and voluntary muscles of the muscle system it is clear that the functions of these are different type support, protection, motion. Of these functions support is the most primitive and the oldest, like wise the axial part of the skeleton was the first to evolve. The vertebral column corresponding to the noto cord in lower organism is the main support of the trunk. The central nervous system lies largely within the axial skeleton, the brain being well protected by the cranium and spinal cord by vertebral column by means of the bony neural arches and the intervening ligaments. The distinctive function is protection of heart, lungs and other organs and structures in the chest. The function of these organs involves motion, expansion, contraction, and must have fkexible and elastic protective covering. Such covering is provided by the thorasic basket or rib cage. The connection of the ribs to the breast bone called strnum forms the required covering. The small joints between the ribs and vertebrae permit a gliding motion of the ribs during breathing and other activities. These motions are limited by ligaments attachment between ribs and vertebrae. The third function of skeleton is that of motion. The majority of the skeletal muscles are firmly anchored to the skeleton. Thus the motions of the body and its parts are well protected as well as supported. There are many types of skeletal parts major are as

1) Craneal bones
2) Facial bones
3) Auditory ossicles
4) Hyoid
5) Vertebal column
6) Thorasic cage
7) Pectoral girdles
8) Upper limbs

9) Pelvic girdle
10) Lower limbs

The disorders or diseases of the skeleton are described as any of the diseases of bones or injuries that are major causes of bone abnormality of human skeletal system. Although physical injury causing fracture dominates over diseases; fracture is one of the several common causes of bone diseasesand disease infact is common cause of fracture.

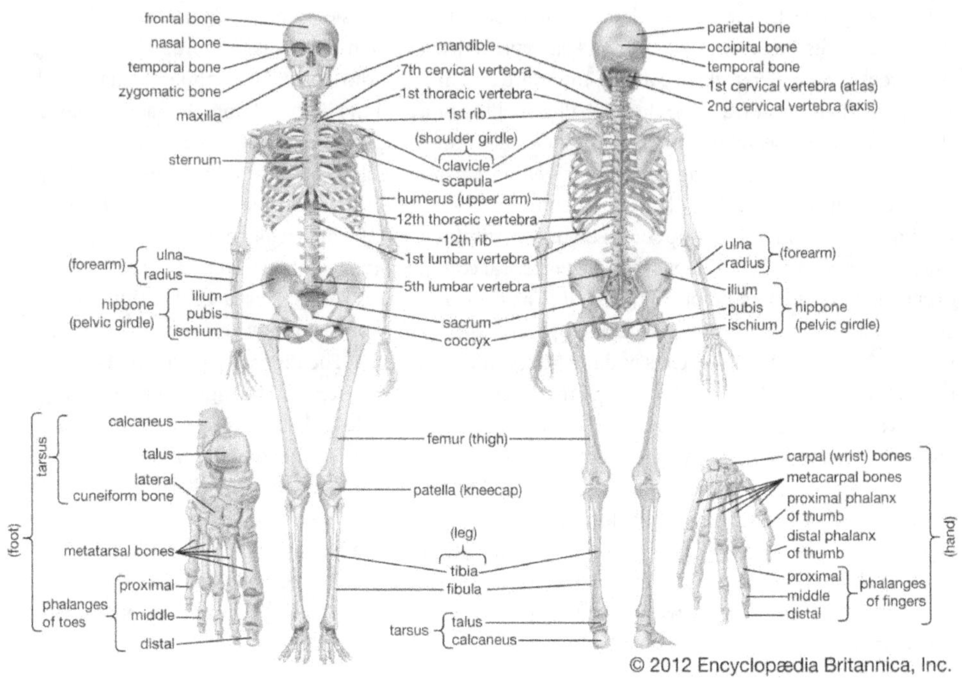

1) Multiple myeloma i.e. malignant proliferation of cells within bone marrow that usually occurs during middle age or later in life and the planet that affect is Saturn either afflicted or under aspect from Mars,or Sun afflicted or under aspect fro Rahuor Uranus. These are more common in male than women and can affect any of the marrow containg bones such as skull etc. The organ involved depends on the cusp that occupies Saturn or Sun.

2) Curvature of spine, any or group of deviations of normal spine curvature including scoliosis, lordosis, kyphosis. The scoliosis is lateral or side ways deviation of spine and is ruled by Mars and Neptune when occupy Capricorn and are under aspect of Saturn or Ketu which include two curves original abnormality and compensatory curve that causes asymmetrical

development of back, chest, or abdominal musculature or cerebral palsy; significant difference in length of legs or malformation or spondylosis, spina bifida. May also occur when Mars and Uranus conjoin in eighth cusp and aspect Sun in second cusp that also leads to fractures, dislocations, hemivertebrae. Also when Neptune and Saturn occupy sixth cusp and are under aspect of Mars causes rickets.

Lordosis is occurred when Mars occupy ascendant in Aquarius and under aspect from Uranus or Ketu that is an increased curvature of lumbar region and may be associated with sondylolisthesis. Inflammation of vertebral disc occurs if Saturn and Sun occupy ninth house and at same time Sagittarius is occupied by malefic planet which also may result from obesity occurs when Jupiter occupy ascendant in Virgo. Kyphosis commonly called round back or humpback is an increased curvature of thorasic vertebral column by the development wedge shaped vertebraeduring adolescence caused by Mars or Jupiter occupy Scorpio and are under aspect from Saturn or Rahu conjoined with Uranus, that may also cause osteoporosis or Tuberculous spondylitis.

3) Aplastic anemia this is adisease in which bone marrow fails to produce an adequate number of cells; there may be lack of all cell types WBC,RBC, Platelates resulting in form of the disease called pancytopenia. This ussualy occurred when the Mars and Moon ar both afflicted with malefic and the Saturn occupied in sixth cusp aspecting Moon.

4) Rickets a disease of infancy and childhood characterized by softening of bones leading to abnormal bone growth and caused by deficiency of vitamin D, when disorder occurs in adults it is known as osteomalacia and is because calcitriol deficiency. The most common planet causes this is Saturn conjoined wit Uranus and under aspect of Mars.

5) Bone cancer; This type of bone cancer is characterized by uncontrolled growth of cells of the bone called bone cancer, different types of bone tissues give rise to different types of bone cancer. Osteosarcoma that develops from the cells that form the bone. Ewing sarcoma of bone develops from immature nerve within the bone, Chondrosarcoma which forms in cartilage tissue principally affect persons above 50 years of age most often causes are hereditary. Even traumatic conditions injuries also contribute. Symptoms are mainly fever, fatigue, and anemia. In all these types principally the Sgittarius sign, Scorpio sign, and Capricorn sign if any of these signs fall in sixth cusp and Saturn, Jupiter, Mars occupied in any cusp if are under aspect of Uranus, Ketu or Rahu causes these types so also if Neptune and Mars ars palced in ascendant and Saturn and Ketu occupy eighth cusp the Bone cancer Is certain to occur.

6) Cervical Spondylosis, this is degenerative disease of neck vertebrae and causing compression of spinal cord or cervical nerve causes cervical spondylitis. Prolonged degeneration of the cervical spine results in narrowing of the spaces between vertebrae, forcing invertebral disc sout of place and thus compressing or stretching the roots of cervical nerves. The vertebrae may themselves be squeezed out of proper alignment. Arthritis developing in reaction to the stress generates new anomalous bone growth called spondylitic bar that impinges on spinal cord interfering with nervous function symptoms include radiating pain, stiffness, of the neck or arms restricted head movment, headaches,spastic paralyses and weakness in arms and legs. Normally it is observed that

malefic in Scorpio, Capricorn, Aquarius or Pisces and if Saturn is afflicted by Rahu the cervical spondylitis is occurred.

7) Rheumatoid arthritis in which progressive inflammatory changes occur through out connective tissue cause irreversible damage to joints. Inflamamtion and thickening of synovial membrane (sacs that hold fluid that lubricates joints) cause irreversible damage to the joint capsule and the articular cartilage as these structures are replaced by scarlike tissue called pannus. This disease is more common in women than men.Mars in saggitarius gives Rheumatoid arthritis, and Saturn and Moon in twelfth cusp cause arthritis. So also Saturn in ascendant and Mars in ninth cusp give the irreversible after inflammatory changes in joints.

8) Craniosynostosis, any of several types of cranial deformities give craniosynostosis; some times accompanied by other abnormalities.that result from premature union of skull vault bones, it is sporadic. Of the various sutures the sagittal (front to back along the topmidline of skull) most frequently fuses prematurely and this causes skull can not grow in width. The vaults become long high and narrow called scaphocephally; if coronal suture (side to side but wideand high) called oxycephally or Aprt syndrome (acrocephalosyndactyle) is rare inherited disorder may be associated with undergrowth of upper jaw. The major astrological correlation here with we find is not in natal chart of patient but in her mother's natal chart if fifth house is occupied by Mars aafflicte by ketu and ninth house be occupied by Saturn may give this disorder while in growth as foetus. Also triangular shaped of head called trigonocephally may be accompanied by brain damage usually occur and surgical proceedings in fisrt few months life can be saved and can minimize the deformities. But mental retardation ussualy occurs. When Saturn occupies fifth cusp and under aspect of Neptune with Mars placed in eleventh cusp may cause this disorder.

9) Graft versus host disease (GVHD) this occurs following bone marrow transplants in which cells in donors marrow attacks tissues of recipient which is meditated by T cells a type of WBCs normally occurring in human body. There are no specific planetary role observed as such but the reaction to recipient cells may be caused due to Uranus occupied with Ketu in eighth house.

10) Fracture In pathology break in bone caused by stress or certain normal and pathological condition may predispose bones to fracture also osteoporosis and other disease that make bones weak causing fracture. When Uranus occupies eighth cusp conjoined with Mars or Uranus occupy sixth cusp with Saturn and aspect Sun in twelfth cusp leads to fracture of bones.

11) Poly myalgia rheumatic is a joint disease that is fairly common in people over age of fifty years. It is characterized by morning stiffness in neck or aching neck and can be detected by erythrocyte sedimentation ratewhich is used in arthritis and often associated with poly myalgia rheumatic. The occurrence of irreversible visual loss. Symptoms include muscle and joint aches, shoulder pain, torso, pelvic girdle pain, Anorexia, weight loss, fatigue, low fever. It is immune response that triggers the production of cytokininwhich cause inflammation. This is probably occurred when Mercury and Mars conjoin in ascendant with Saturn occupies ninth cusp in sign Sagittarius or Capricorn.

12) Peromellia the disease peromellia is congenital absence or malformation of extremities; it is occurred as Thalidomide tragedy in early 1960 caused by errors in formation and development of the limb bud from about fourth to eighth week of intra uterine life. Till date we can not confirmly correlate with exact planetary disposition in mothers natal chart but possibly may be due to afflicted Sun with Rahu and under aspect of Mars and Neptune from eighth cusp with Venus present in fifth cusp.

13) Dislocation Displacement of bones forming joints with consequential disruption of the tissues. Dislocation is caused by stress, forcefull enough to overcome the resistance of ligament, muscle and capsule that hold the joint. This happens because of two things; first being the lack of mental alertness, when it is reduced the accident takes place normally when the Mars occupies eighth place or ascendant and is under aspect of Uranus causes mental disturbance that leads to accidents. Secondly when Saturn occupies sixth cusp and is under aspect from Neptune or Uranus and at the same time Mars is afflicted with Uranus or Ketu this leads to some degenerative changes in body and that leads to porosity of bones which become brittle and easily can be met with accidents causing dislocation. Often the addiction to drugs or alcohol caused when Venus is occupied in second cusp and is under aspect from Saturn or Mars leads to the accident causing dislocation of bones from joints.

14) Fibrous Dysplasia Fibrous dyspla is rare congenital development disorder beginning in childhood and characterized by replacement of solid calcified bone with fibrous tissue often only on one side of the body and primarily in the long bones and pelvic. The disease that appears to result from genetic mutations. When sixth cusp, eighth cusp and twelfth cusp are afflicted or occupied by malefic planets or particularly Rahu, Saturn, Mars then this type of growth occurs most often related to hereditary type and some times part of mutation occurs in intrauterine life and part after birth in childhood or in adolescence.

15) Metatarsalgia This is caused when persistent pains in metatarsal region or ball of the foot and this condition arises when weight of body while standing is forced rest on the centre of the anterior archi.e. on the heads of central metatarsal bones instead of on the inside and out side of the foot. Being postural only corrective posture while standing and some foot excersize can help cure this disorder.

16) Hip fracture This in pathology is a break in the proximal (upper) end of the femure and the condition arises at any age common causes include severe impact falls or car accident and weak bones The Mars in ascendant and any malefic in eighth cusp or Mars and Uranus in eighth cusp along with malefic present is sixth cusp cause the Hip fracture, also the presence of Saturn in Sagittarius in eighth cusp or Scorpio in sixth cusp give rise to these types of accidents and Hip fracture.

17) Tenis Elbow This is an injury characterized by pains at the lateral outer aspect of the elbow. Patient may also complain of tenderness of or palpation of area of concern. Due to overuse of the extensor carpi radials brevis muscles which originates at the lateral epicondyler region of the distal humerous indicates tissues damage. This type of disease normally occurs when Jupiter in conjunction with Ketu and any in sign owned by Venus; is under aspect from other malefic.

18) Marble bone This is a rare disorder which becomes extremely dense hard and brittle. The disease progressesas long as bone growth takes place or continues. The marrow cavities

become filled with compact bone and because increased bone mass crowd the bone marrow and resulting in reduced amount of bone marrow that produces RBC causing severe anemia. There are both congenial and acquired forms of marble bone. Congenital forms are associated with decreased number of osteoclants or decreased osteoclast function leading to frequent fractures. Till date the planetary disposition causing this is not clear but it is noticed that if Moon is afflicted by three malefic in any signs and Saturn and Mars in sixth cusp aspected by Rahu and Sun causes Marble bone disorder.

19) Spondylosis this is non inflammatory degenerative disease of spine resulting in abnormal bone development around the vertebrae and reduced mobility of the interverebral joints. It is primarily a condition of age and occurs much more commonly in men than in women and onset of symptoms are gradual most widely occurring forms ankylosing spondilitis, hypertrophic spondylitis, and the tuberculous spondylitis. This occurs whe malefic occupy Scorpio, Capricorn, Aquarius, and Pisces in any house also Saturn in ascendant and Mars in ninth cusp with Rahu causes spondylitis.

20) Gaut It is metabolic disorder characterized by recurrent acute attacks of severe inflammation in one or more joints. It results from the deposition in and around the joints of Uric Acid salts which are excessive throuout the body in person with disorder. Uric acid is product of Purines compounds that are essential DNA and RNA of many biosynthetic reactions and normally steadily excreted into urine. Gaut accounts for 5% of total cases of arthritis, chondrocalcinosis (pseudo Gaut) is similar to Gaut caused by deposits of calcium pyrophosphate crystals in joint. Thou major cause is unknown excessive alcohol may cause gaut. The sign Sagittarius or Pisces if under aspect from Saturn or Mars leads to Gaut, also Mars in tenth house if afflicted by Saturn causes Gaut.

21) Paget disease of bones is chronic middle aged disease characterized by excessive break down and formation of bone tissue. It is localized unifocal affecting single or many bones. The disease is characterized by excessive bone resorption which is mediated by osteoclatsts and excessive bone formation. The osteoclasts are extra ordinarily active resorbing bone rapidly and at the same time activating a coupling factor that leads to an increase in bone formation by local osteoclasts. This increase may be both excessive and disorganized result in chaotic bone structure with area of excessive bone formation leading to bone weakening and deformities. Ptients are found to have high serum concentration of alkaline phosphatase; an enzyme involved in bone formation. Overgrowth of bones of skull or vertebrae may impinge on spinal cord or nerve causing significant amount of pain. Bone softens and blood to area decrease which may lead to heart problems. This typical disorder occurs when Mars in Capricorn and Saturn and Moon in sixth cusp also when Ascendant is under aspect of Saturn and is occupied by Venus. Also when Saturn and Moon in twelfth are under aspect of Ketu causes this disorder to occur.

22) Osteoarthritis It is disorder characterized by progressive deterioration of the articular cartilage or of entire joint including articular cartilage the synovium (joint lining), the ligament and sub chondralbone may be asymptomatic.

Knee
parasagittal section-lateral to midline of knee

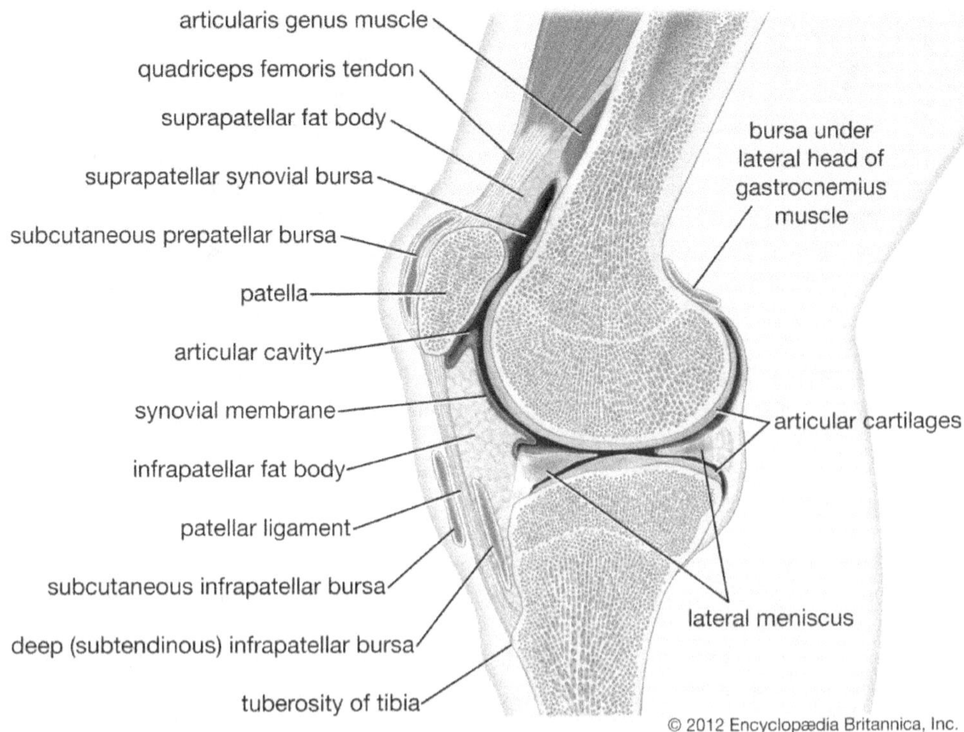

It is most common joint disease and not characterized by excessive joint inflammation and may as such be asymptomatic. As it progresses pain and stiffness in joint in addition to limitations of movement occurs. Coomon sites of discomfort are vertebrae, Knees, Hips that bear much of the weight of the body. The biomechanical forces that place stress on the joints are thought to interact with biochemical and genetic factors contribute to osteoarthritis. In early stage changes in cartilage thickness is affected over passage of time cartilage wears out and subchondrol bone deprived of its protection cover attemts to regenerate the destroyed tissue resulting in increased bonedensity and uneven remodeling of surface of joints. This also causes reduction in synovial fluid which acts as natural joint lubricant and shock absorber. The main Rahu in Sagittarius gives this type of osteoarthritis also conjunction of Mars or Saturn in ninth cusp, tenth cusp, eleventh cusp gives this disorder. Further if Saturn afflicted in tenth, ninth, and eleventh cusp by malefic causes osteoporosis.

23) Bone diseases any diseases any of the diseases or injuries that affect human bones may include hormonal imbalance, malneutrition, and repeated pregnancy. Also congenital dislocations of hipjoint, acetabulum looses the mechanical stimulus for norml growth and development occurs because head of femure does not rest in joint. Poliomelitis, osteopenia,

with vertebral fractures, metabolism related diseases are the result of some bone diseases. Normaaly afflicted ordebilitated Saturn is the main planet responsible for most of the bone diseases.

24) Arthritis; It is inflammation of joints and can be major cause of disabilities occurred in two types osteo arthritis and rheumatoid arthritis. Osteoarthritis is degenerative joint disorder characterized by deterioration of articular cartlage that normally cushion joints. Pain is gradual, onset occurring after prolonged activity and is deep and achying in nature; knee, hip, spine, and fingers joints motion is affected. Muscle weakness predisposed to injuries such as menisculand anterior cuciate ligament tears up, hip can get affected.

25) Stress fractures, any overuse or injury that affect the integrity of bones. Stress fractures result from microdamage and accumulation of micro damage during exercises the body's natural ability to repair the damage occurring can cause pain, weakness and bone that leads to stress fracture. Stress fractures occur mostly in lower extremities and tibia, fibula, metatarsals, navicular bones are involved repeated weight bearing or impact or repetitive loading cycles bones are exposed to micro damage which occur primarily in the form of microscopic cracks, and when given sufficient time it recovers on its own. Healing depends on many factors hormonal nutritional factors etc. The strss fractures are considered as accidents and as such Mars, Saturn in eleventh cusp, if two or more malefic are occupied in ninth, tenth, eleventh cusp gives the stress fractures or create condition that cause stress fractures.

26) Spondylitis it is inflammation of one or more of the vertebrae and takes several forms. The most widely occurring are ankylosing spondylitis, hypertrophy spondylitis, and tuberculous sponylitis. Ankylosing spndylitis is disease of spine characteristically seen in adolescence and young boys. Primarily it gives pain in back and progressively stiffness and limitations of movements are noticed. Then swollen joints, fusion, and deformity of spine are observed. Hypertrophic spondylitis also called as osteoarthritis of spine is degenerative type of spondylitis seen mostly in age group of 50 and above; by destruction of intervertebral disc and growth of spur on vertebrae. The Tuberculous spondylitis is casued by infection by tuberculous bacilli infecting vertebral column. The sign Gemini rules over spine and Pisces pelvic region and any malefic in these sign denotes spondylitis.

27) Osteomyelitis osteomylitis is infection of bone tissue and the condition most commonly caused by staphylococcus aureous which reaches the bone tissue via blood stream or by extension form of local injury. Inflammation follows with destruction of cancellous bones death. Living bone grows around the walls in dead tissue forming involucrum, the content of which gradually reabsorbed as the lesion repaired. Symptoms include bone pain latter swelling and redness may develop around area of infection. The diagnosis confirmed by radionuclide bone scan. Saturn or Rahu in Sagittarius gives infection and Saturn in Leo gives infection of vertebrae and as such if are under aspect of any malefic causes the disease osteomyelitis.

28) Metabolic bone diseases, these are several diseases that cause various abnormalities of bones include osteo porosis, rickets, osteomalacia, osteogenesis, marble bone, fibrous dysplacias.

29) Avascular nacrosis, Death of bone tissue causes by lack of blood to affected area is called as avascular nacrosis. Avascular nacrosis most commonly affect the epiphysis of femure bones, and other commonly affected bones are upper arm, shoulder, Knee, and ankle. Condition often progressive and resulting in joint destruction within few years if untrated. The exact cause is unknown; combination of metabolic factors, mechanical stress, local factors, in affected area that interrupt blood supply may contribute to the cause.

30) Osteoporosis is characterized by the thinning of bone with consequent tendancy to sustain fractures from minor stresses. Osteoporosis is most common metabolic disorder occurred in women after menopause.In affected persons the tiny rigid plates forming the honey combed matrixes within bone gradually become thinner and rod like, and the spaces between them growlarger. Tbone thus become more porous and weaker; these lighter and more fragile bones tend to fracture from minor traumas or stress that ordinarily would have no ill effect. The gradual progression towards osteoporosis result from changes in the balance between the amount of new bone that's formed within body and the amount of bone that is resorbedor broken down to get assimilated. This disease may have arised from decreased bone formation or increased bone resorption. This condition may arise when Saturn occupies the sixth house in either Virgo or Sagittarius and is under aspect from Uranus occupied in twelfth cusp so also when ascendant and ninth house both are afflicted or under aspect from malefic this condition arises.

31) Carpal Tunnel Syndrome This syndrome is condition of numbness, tingling or pain in the wrist caused by repetitive flexing or stressing of fingers or wrist over long period of time. Possibly the most common repititve stress injury in work place isfrequently associated with modern office. It is caused by pressure on median nerve; carpal tunnel is small passage almost completely surrounded by the carpal bones. The patient may experience a temporary loss of control of some of hand muscles and difficulties in picking up or holding objects. They may be awakened at night due to sudden pain in wrist or hand. It is observed that Jupiter in Leo afflicted by Mars or Saturn may cause this syndrome so also when Jupiter and Saturn conjoin in Virgo in fifth cusp leads to this syndrome, the Jupiter in such cases is observed to be weak and debilitated.

32) Restless Leg Syndrome It is a condition characterized by an uncontrollable urge to move the legs; that usually appears during periods of rest, especially while sitting or lying down. Many experience symptoms immediately before onset of slee. Anative with this syndrome experiences various sensations in legs such as pressure, pins, needles, pulling, crawling, or pinching but rarely pains. Occasional involuntarily jerking movements also may occur symptoms may continue to worse with aging if left untreated; cause may include insufficient blood supply, nerve damage, diabetes, anemia, Kidney diseases, infections, such as prostatis and cystis. May occasionally in third trimester. In older people it may precede with onset of Parkinson's disease. The Horoscopic correlation that we can see here in this syndrome are 1) if Saturn, Sun, and Venus be in fifth cusp 2) Mars in tenth cusp conjoined with or under aspect of Saturn 3) IfSun and Mars occupy ascendant and seventh house repectivly this syndrome occurs.

33) Joint diseases; any of diseases or ijury that affect joint are called Joint diseases. Arthritis is most common but there are also many others. Disease of joint may be variously short lived

or exceedingly chronic, agonizingly painfull, or merely nagging and uncomfortable are required to be attened in time in order to avoid the further complications. Two principal categories of joint diseases are important to study. 1) Joint disease in which inflammation is the principal set of sign or symptoms; where in regardless of cause inflammation of joint may cause pains, stiffness, swelling, and redness of skin about joint may occur. Effusion of fluid into the joint cavity is common and examination of fluid is often valuable tool for determining the nature of the disease. Adhesive between the articulating members are frequent resulting fusion with loss of mobility observed. 2) Joint diseases that are without or much less inflammation are also required to be separately examined and treated. Horoscope can show us the relation between arthritis and Saturn, Mercury, and sign Taurus, Virgo, Capricorn and sixth house are most important to study. If Saturn, Mecury or sign Caoricorn, Taurus are afflicted by Rahu or Mars leads to arthritis.

34) Neurofibromatoses. Tis either of two hereditary disorder characterized by distinctive skin lesion that progressively enlarged by benign tumors of nerveous system in type one also known as Raklinghaunsens's syndrome which is much more common and characterized by presence of pale brown spot on skin. Neurofibromas and other tumors may appear in late childhood or early in adult hood, the course of diseases is progressive.Type two is of auditory canal in ear with small spots of café-au-lait spot resulting from genetic mutations. These two diseases are usually occurred when Virgo is placed in sixth cusp and ninth, tenth, eleventh cusps are occupied by malefic or under aspect of malefic planet. Further if two or three malefic planets are placed in Gemini or Pisces then this disorder is observed.

This furthercan well be explained with few natal charts as detailed here with.

Case no 42

A female native born on 07th March 1955 at 1044hrs Nilanga Maharashtra
Lat. 018:22N Long 076:35E

The natal chart shown here with shows Taurus ascendant and the lord of ascendant placed in ninth cusp occupied by Capricorn and Venus the lord of ascendant conjoined with Mercury that denotes the diseases related with connective tissues and the ninth cusp rules the joints. The Saturn that denotes the chronic and obstructive diseases is lord of ninth and tenth house is placed in sixth cusp such indicating the joint diseases that is prolonged and chronic. The Venus is also lord of sixth house shows onset of the disease. Mars that is responsible for blood and bones indicates the disease related to bones and joints; Mars is under aspect of Saturn and placed in twelfth cusp is owner of seventh cusp further confirms the inflammation of knee joints. The lord of fifth house is Mercury which is responsible for the diseases related to ligaments and tissues around joints is occupied in ninth cusp under aspect of Uranus placed in third cusp which is responsible for mysterious disease and as such Mercury indicates the occurrence of inflammation of joins of lower limbs. Moon, planet responsible for the secretion of essential fluids and Blood is occupied in fourth cusp in sign Leo indicating the disease related with blood and synovial fluid that lubricates the joint; Moon is lord of Cancer placed in third house occupied by Uranus that complicates the disease. The bone is also a tissue which is governed by Sun which is occupied in tenth cusp and sign Aquarius denotes the bone disease associated with knee joint. The eighth cusp is occupied by Rahu that aspect Mars in twelfth cusp confirms the knee joint disoreder associated with erosion of joint head, so also the Jupiter which rules the metabolism and growth of new cells is placed in second house with sign Gemini and afflicted with Ketu denotes the rootcause of the disease that lies in disturbed constitution of blood and Bone tissues. As also it is observed that the sign Sagittarius is afflicted with Rahu and under aspect of Sautrn denotes the progressively chronic disease that may need surgical treatments. The sign Virgo is occupied in fifth cusp and in quincunx with Rahu denotes the disease may progreesively damage the other tissues of body.

This also can be confirmed by the significators of ascendant, sixth cusp, eighth cusp, and eleventh cus. The star lord of ascendant is Sun occupied in Aquarius is also star lord of ninth cusp that confrms the disease. The star lord of sixth cusp is mars placed in twelfth house is also star lord of Mercury and Uranus which indicates the intensity of disease; here the Mercury is star lord of twelfth house; the Sub lord of ascendant Mercury causes the severity and hospitalization as it is also sub lord of Mars occupied in twelfth cusp. The sub lord of sixth cusp is Saturn placed in sixth cup aspecting the twelfth cusp and eighth cusp. Saturn is also sub lord of twelfth cusp and sub lord of Sun indicating the progressive deterioration of joints leading to need for surgical procedures. Thus all the significators of ascendant, sixth cusp, eighth cusp and twelfth cusp are well connected indicating the occurrence of the disease, hospitalization and chronic condition of the disease.

The first time the complain regarding painfull knee was reported in the year 1998 June when Mars mahadasha and Saturn antardasha was in progress, native was required to hospitalized on 10th August 1998 when Mars mahadasha   Shani antardasha and Mars prati antardahs was in progress, Where Mars is star lord of sixth cusp and lord of twelfth cusp occupied in twelfth cusp which indicates the severity, Hospitalisation followed by Knee replacement surgery. The native as doctors diagnosed was victim of Osteosrthritis and as such caused deterioration of knee cap requiring surgical procedures.

Planetary disposition of this natal chart is as mentioned bellow.

Sr. No	Planet	Zodiac	Degrees: Min: Sec.	Lord of zodiac	Star Lord	Sub Lord
01	Sun	Aquarius	292: 37 : 38	Saturn	Jupiter	Saturn
02	Moon	Leo	095 : 08 : 58	Sun	Ketu	Mars
03	Mars	Aries	342 : 54 : 14	Mars	Ketu	Mercury
04	Mercury	Capricorn	265 : 31 : 36	Saturn	Mars	Rahu
05	Jupiter	Gemini	056 : 47 : 47	Venus	Jupiter	Venus
06	Venus	Capricorn	249 : 29 : 59	Saturn	Sun	Venus
07	Saturn	Libra	177 : 54 : 34	Venus	Jupiter	Venus
08	Rahu	Sagittarius	218 : 43 : 45	Jupiter	Ketu	Jupiter
09	Ketu	Gemini	038 : 43 : 45	Mercury	Rahu	Jupiter
10	Uranus	Cancer	060 : 38 : 30	Moon	Mars	Jupiter
11	Neptune	Libra	154 : 39 : 04	Venus	Mars	Venus

Case No 43

Male native is born on 02nd October 1965 at 1310 hrs in Karim nagar

With Lat. 018:24N Long 079:06E

The natal chart shows Sagittarius ascendant with lord of ascendant occupied in seventh house.

Seventh House which Rules the diseases of pelvic region, so also the Moon that denotes the diseases related to blood and flesh, the house is also occupied by sign Gemini that denotes disease associated with hands and pectoral girdle. Further the Mars that rules the function of joints and lord of fifth cusp is placed in twelfth cusp afflicted with Ketun in sign Scorpio; whereas the fifth cusp rules the bones and flesh in lower limbs. The sign Virgo that an earthy sign is occupied in tenth house is also occupied by Mercury which is the major planet that rules nervous system, and bone fractures and conjoined with Sun that again a main planet rule the metabolism of formation of bones. The Saturn causative of chronic and prolonged diseases associated with joints and connective tissue of joints is placed in Aquarius in third house that is causative of diseases related to vertebral column. The ninth cusp is afflicted with Uranus in sign Leo that rules the damage of cartilage in joints. The Moon being lord of eighth cusp occupied in ascendant Sagittarius denotes the disease associated with inflammation of joints and swelling. Further we can see in the chart that the requisite signs Taurus, Capricorn, Leo and Scorpio are afflicted and as such we can conclude the disease indicating severe inflammation and swelling of joints. The native visited doctor for diagnosis and treatment and after examination was found suffering from Osteoarthritis showing progressive deterioration of Knee joint. As the doctor advised the treatment for prolonged period and almost irrecoverable nature of disease the native is regularly visiting doctor with some relief from severe pain.

The occurrence of the onset of disease is not exactly known but probably falls somewhere in April 2004 when Mars mahadasha and Jupiter antardasha was in progress, here Mars and Jupiter both are significators of sixth cusp. The native is still under treatment at Narayani Hospital Hyderabad.

Planetary disposition of this natal chart is tabled as bellow.

Sr. No.	Planet	Zodiac	Degrees: Min: Sec	Lord of Zodiac	Star Lord	Sub Lord
01	Sun	Virgo	285 : 31 : 33	Mercury	Moon	Jupiter
02	Moon	Sagittarius	013 : 15 : 12	Jupiter	Ketu	Mercury
03	Mars	Scorpio	335 : 14 : 12	Mars	Saturn	Saturn
04	Mercury	Virgo	289 : 10 : 39	Mercury	Moon	Mercury
05	Jupiter	Gemini	187 : 26 : 18	Mercury	Rahu	Rahu
06	Venus	Libra	328 : 10 : 39	Venus	Jupiter	Venus
07	Saturn	Aquarius	078 : 35 :48	Saturn	Rahu	Moon
08	Rahu	Taurus	164 : 04 : 41	Venus	Moon	Jupiter
09	Ketu	Scorpio	344 : 94 : 41	Mars	Saturn	Rahu
10	Uranus	Leo	263 : 21 : 11	Sun	Venus	Saturn
11	Neptune	Libra	324 : 55 : 05	Venus	Jupiter	Mercury

Case No 44

Male native born on 13th February 1994 at 1710 hrs in Pune Lat. 018:30 N Long. 073:48E

This is classic case of diseases related to deformities formed in spinal coed leading to firther defects in lower limbs. As we see the natal chart first planet that rules the diseases or deformities of Bone Mars is placed in Aquarius that too in Seventh cusp leading to abnormal growth of vertebrae forming curvature of the spinal cord. Mars is afflicted severely with Uranus which indicates mysterious diseases. The ascendant falls in Cancer and the lord of ascednat occupied in ninth house is under aspect of Rahu indicating the disorder related to blood supply of spinal cord. Further the fifth cusp is occupied by Scorpio and afflicted by Rahu denoting the deformities in pelvic bone structure; also the sixth cusp is oocupied by Neptune in Sagittarius that rules the lower part of vertebral column thus indicating the defects associated with spinal cord. The sign Aquarius that rules the lower limbs and motion of feet is occupied by Saturn conjoined with Sun, Venus and Mercury indicating the connective tissue disorder due to afflicted Mercury and bone growth deformities due to afflicted Sun. Further we can note that Mercury being lord of Virgo occupied in third cusp denotes the disease associated with thorasic vertebrae. Mars that rules the growth is occupied in seventh house in sign Capricorn indicates the defective growth of lower limbs and vertebrae in pelvic region. We also can note here is that the lord of fifth cusp Mars is severely afflicted with Rahu in Capricorn. Jupiter the planet that is responsible for growth of bones and function of joints in body is occupied in fourth cusp in sign Libra which indicates the defective growth of vertebral column and exerting pressure on lower limbs to produce further deformity. Saturn aspects the fifth house, that rules the bones in pelvic region indicating the chronic and irreversible diseases of vertebrae. When at the age of 20 years the native was taken to hospital for severe pain in lower back and native was required to bend forward to compenset the pain doctor diagnosed the disease as Scolliosis associated with spinabifida a rare spine disease that allow the abnormal growth of vertebrae leading to deformity.The star lord of ascendant is Saturn is also star lord of fifth and ninth house occupied in eighth cusp. The star lord of sixth cusp is Ketu which is occupied in Turus in eleventh house is aspecting the fifth cusp. The star lord of eighth cusp is Rahu which is also star lord of twelfth cusp Gemini and lord of twelfth cusp is placed in eighth cusp conjoined with Saturn which is star lord of ascendant and lord of eighth cusp. Further the sub lord of ascendant is Mars which is also sub lord of fifth cusp occupied in seventh cusp. The sub lord of sixth cusp is Mercury is lord and sub lord of twelfth cusp and occupied in eighth house conjoined with Saturn. Thus significators of fifth ninth and eleventh cusp are well connected indicating the deformities associated with vertebral column and also significators of ascendant, sixth house, eighth cuap and twelfth house are also well connected showing the occurrence of chronic irreversible disease of bones. The planetary disposition is tabled as bellow.

Sr. No.	Planet	Zodiac	Degrees: min:sec	Lord of Zodiac	Star lord	Sub Lord
01	Sun	Aquarius	210 : 45 : 50	Saturn	Mars	Mercury
02	Moon	Pisces	243 : 37 : 26	Jupiter	Saturn	Saturn
03	Mars	Capricorn	198 : 57 : 43	Saturn	Moon	Mercury
04	Mercury	Aquarius	223 : 23 : 42	Saturn	Rahu	Mercury
05	Jupiter	Libra	110 : 31 : 26	Venus	Jupiter	Jupiter
06	Venus	Aquarius	217 : 20 : 56	Saturn	Rahu	Rahu
077	Saturn	Aquarius	218 : 03 : 49	Saturn	Rahu	Rahu
08	Rahu	Scorpio	125 : 00 : 34	Mars	Saturn	Saturn
09	Ketu	Taurus	305 : 00 : 34	Venus	Sun	Saturn

| 10 | Uranus | Capricorn | 180 : 18 : 34 | Saturn | Sun | Rahu |
| 11 | Neptune | Sagittarius | 178 : 16 : 37 | Jupiter | Sun | Moon |

Case No 45

The female native born on 18th June 2007 at 1315 hrs in Chennai/ Nanganallur

Lat. 013:04N Long. 080:16E

The natal chart is Virgo ascendant and lord of ascendant is placed in tenth that denotes the bone related disease. Further the Jupiter occupied in Scorpio third cups that rules the ears and throat and is under aspect of Mars from Eighth cusp indicating the complicated disease related to ear nose and throat. The Fifth cusp occupied by Neptune and sign Capricorn as such the disease related to bones in ear is indicated; so also the lord of Fifth cusp and sixth cusp Saturn is placed in eleventh cusp conjoined with Venus and Moon in sign Cancer which indicates the disease related to the auditory canal may be maxillofacial bones. Further Mars the planet that is responsible for functioning of bone tissue is occupied in eighth cusp in sign Aries clearly indicating the disease related to ears. The Sixth cusp is occupied by Aquarius and is afflicted with Uranus and Rahu indicating the mysterius disease occurrence is related to intra uterine life, also the Uranus and Rahu are under aspect of Ketu indicates the severity of the disease. The lord of ninth cusp is Venus is occupied in Cancer in eleventh house afflicted with Saturn which gives obstructive and inflammatory diseases.The Sun which rules the growth of Bones in body is placed in Tenth cusp conjoined with Mercury which rules the function of nervous system and is lord of ascendat. The Sun being lord of twelfth house in tenth cusp clarifies the prenatal mutagenic changes in the uterine gives the disease in early childhood. Initially the child was not able to hear the sounds of any frequency and was supposedly assumed to be deaf but later on at the age of twelve years the severe pain in ear and was hospitalized on 25th September 2018, after thorough examination doctors have diagnosed the child with Neurofibromatoses of auditory canal and noted brown spots of Café-au-lait. The neurofibromatoses was result of genetic mutations that started long back in intra uterine life of the child. Unfortunately the details of birth data of the mother were unavailable to find out further probable causes. It is also worth noticing that the significators of the ascendant, sixth cusp, eighth cusp and twelfth cusp are well connected, that led to hospitalization. The star lord of ascendant is Moon which is also star lord of fifth house and ninth house indicating bones and nerves disorder; further the sub lord of ascendant is Mercury occupied conjoined with Sun which is sub lord of ninth cusp. The sub lord of sixth cusp is Moon is also sub lord of Ketu occupied in twelfth cusp, and sub lord of Uranus placed in sixth cusp is Mercury which is lord of ascendant and sub lord Venus. Venus is occupied in eleventh cusp conjoined with Moon, sub lord of sixth cusp. Thus well connected houses ascendant, sixth, fifth, eighth, twelfth indicates abnormal tumor associated with nervous system that gives bone related disease. The native was operated for the surgical procedures but still under treatment and not able to resume normal life.

The planetary disposition of this natal chart is given in this table

Sr. No	Planet	Zodiac	Degrees: Min :Sec	Lord of zodiac	Star Lord	Sub Lord
01	Sun	Gemini	272 : 45 : 41	Mercury	Mars	Venus
02	Moon	Cancer	314 : 01 : 09	Moon	Saturn	Rahu
03	Mars	Aries	211 : 15 : 05	Maars	Ketu	Venus
04	Mercury	Gemini	287 : 26 : 16	Mercury	Rahu	Venus
05	Jupiter	Scorpio	079 : 23 : 59	Mars	Mercury	Venus
06	Venus	Cancer	317 : 47 : 12	Moon	Mercury	Mercury
07	Saturn	Cancer	327 : 06 : 44	Moon	Mercury	Jupiter
08	Rahu	Aquarius	166 : 47 : 27	Saturn	Rahu	Venus
09	Ketu	Leo	346 : 47 : 27	Sun	Venus	Moon
10	Uranus	Aquariius	174 : 43 : 19	Saturn	Jupiter	Mercury
11	Neptune	Capricorn	147 : 55 : 06	Saturn	Mars	Saturn

Case No 46

The male native born on 18th March 1976 at 0430 hrs in Parbhani Maharashtra

Lat. 019:18 N Long. 076: 48 E

The natal chart shows Capricorn falls in sign Capricorn and lord of ascendant Saturn occupies seventh house aspecting ascendant and falls in sign Cancer. The Mars, lord of fourth cusp and eleventh cusp occupied in sixth cusp in sign Gemini, and the lord of sixth cusp Mercury is placed in second house in sign Aquarius conjoined with Venus. The Jupiter lord of twelfth house is placed in fourth house afflicted with Ketu in Aries. Also Moon, lord of fourth house is placed in tenth house afflicted with Rahu and Uranus in sign Libra. This typical combination if studied in toto one thing is clear and that is Uranus being cause of mysterius diseases shows unwarranted or unexpected impact on spinal cord leading to sereous ailment. Further Mars, that is responsible for sudden force applied on vertebral column and also damage to nervous system. Further the Mercury lord of sixth cup is placed in second cusp that rules neck, cervical, vertebrae, and brain stem that is connected to vertebral column and in sign Aquarius indicating the accidental impact on back. Also Saturn is under aspect from Uranus occupied in tenth cusp; the Uranus conjoined with Rahu also indicates the accident that causes serious damage to the nervous system and cervical vertebrae leading to hospitalization. The Sun which is lord of eighth cusp is occupied in third cusp that indicates the impact and damage to Odontoid, the bony peg that forms the joint between upper two vertebrae of neck may get compressed damaging the spinal cord. The accident took place in Mahadasha of Jupiter, antar dasha of Mars and prati antar dasha of Venus was in progress on 10th February 2011. The native was in coma for almost twenty days and got succesfuly recovered and discharged on 20th April 2011 when Mars antar dasha was completed.

Significators of ascendant, sixth cusp, Eighth cusp, Twelfth cusp shows that the accidental damage to the vertebral column was indicated. The star lord of ascendant is Mars is placed in sixth cusp, the star lord of sixth cusp is Jupiter is placed in fourth house afflicted with Ketu; Ketu being star lord of third house occupied by Sun. Sun is lord of eighth cusp and star lord of twelfth cusp. Also the sub lord of ascendant is Jupiter occupied in fourth house, and sub lord of sixth cusp is Venus placed in second cusp conjoined with Mercury which is lord of sixth cusp; the sub lord of twelfth cusp is Sun occupied in Pisces and lord of pisces is Jupiter occupied in fourth house as such well connecting the ascendant, sixth cusp eighth house and twelfth house, indicating the the occurrence of accident and damage due to impact on cervical vertebrae.

The planetary disposition of this natal chart is tabled as given here.

Sr. No	Planet	zodiac	Degree: Min: Sec	Lord of Zodiac	Star Lord	Sub Lord
01	Sun	Pisces	063 : 57 : 14	Jupiter	Saturn	Saturn
02	Moon	Libra	270 : 00 : 58	Venus	Mars	Mercury
03	Mars	Gemini	156 : 12 : 49	Mercury	Mars	Moon
04	Mercury	Aquarius	050 : 30 : 48	Saturn	Jupiter	Jupiter
05	Jupiter	Aries	094 : 33 : 06	Mars	Ketu	Moon
06	Venus	Aquarius	040 : 33 : 12	Saturn	Rahu	Jupiter
07	Saturn	Cancer	182 : 35 : 07	Moon	Jupiter	Rahu
08	Rahu	Libra	291 : 39 : 34	Venus	Jupiter	Jupiter
09	Ketu	Aries	111 : 39 : 34	Mars	Jupiter	Venus
10	Uranus	Libra	283 : 03 : 08	Venus	Rahu	Mercury
11	Neptune	Scorpio	320 : 26 : 34	Mars	Mercury	Venus

Case No 47

Male native born on 13th April 1952 at 1900 hrs in Alibaugh Lat. 018:31N Long. 073:12E

This is classic case of degenerative changes that occur over effect of aging process and the onset and progress of the disease can be well studied. The ascendant in thic case is Libra and occupied by Mars, where Mars is lord of second and seventh cusp. The lord of fifth cusp is Saturn occupied in twelfth cusp aspecting sixth cusp directly and is afflicted with Neptune. Sixth cusp is occupied by Mercury which is lord of ninth cup and twelfth cusp conjoined with Venus, the lord of eighth cusp. Also fifth house is occupied by Rahu in Aquarius. Hrer we can see that the major planet which is cause of degenerative changes in jont and responsible for inflammation of joint, Mars is placed in Libra in ascendant and aspect seventh house occupied by Sun the planet that rules the function of bones conjoined with Jupiter which indicates growth of the disease. Also the lord of ninth house Mercury is placed in sixth house which rules the connective tissue and ligaments is under aspect of Saturn; placed afflicted with Neptune in twelfth house indicating the deterioration of joints and inflammation of joints. Moon, the planet that rules the blood circulation and secretion of synovial fluid that lubricates the joints is placed in Scorpio, second house and under aspect of Saturn indicates the obstructed blood supply to joints and also poor lubrication leading to wearing of articular bone called cartilage in joints. Ketu another malefic planet placed in eleventh house in sign Leoindicates the malfunctioning of bones leading to increased porosity.Thus fifth, ninth and eleventh cusp are occupied by malefic planet giving rise to arthritis associated with inflammation of joints. Also the lord of ascendant and of eighth house Venus placed in sixth house with Mercury the lord of twelfth house indicates the severirty of disease over passage of time. The native when was taken to hospital was diagnosed for Polymyalgia Rheumatica associated with temporal arteritis. The native also complained the morning stiffness of shoulder, and hip joints, loss of appetite and severe fatigue. The disease doctors diagnosed was said to be irreversible in nature and the progress will continue worsening.

The star lord of ascendant is Jupiter is placed in seventh house is also star lord of tenth house and sub lord of eighth cusp, also the star lord of sixth house is Saturn placed in twelfth house is also sub lord of twelfth house and placed intwelfth house afflicted with Neptune. The sub lord of ascendat and lord of eighth house is Venus placed in sixth house and as such all the houses that is ascendant, sixth, eighth, twelfth houses are well connected showing the intensity of the disease and progress.

The occurrence of disease was first noticed when native felt severe pains in shoulder and hip joints with stiffness and fatigue on 30th January 2001 when Venus mahadasha and Antardasha of Saturn was in progress. Unfortunately since then the condition worsened and deteriorated over passage of time. Also the inflammation of knee joints, shoulder joints, and hipjoints continued to increase.

The planetary disposition of the natal chart is tabled as given here with.

Sr. No.	Planet	Zodiac	Degrees: Min: Sec	Lord of Zodiac	Star Lord	Sub Lord
01	Sun	Aries	180 : 21 : 58	Mars	Ketu	Ketu
02	Moon	Scorpio	040 : 29 : 03	Mars	Saturn	Sun
03	Mars	Libra	022 : 59 : 29	Venus	Jupiter	Saturn
04	Mercury	Pisces	166 : 47 : 10	Jupiter	Mercury	Mercury
05	Jupiter	Aries	183 : 07 : 44	Mars	Ketu	Sun
06	Venus	Pisces	161 : 13 : 35	Jupiter	Saturn	Moon
07	Saturn	Virgo	347 : 30 : 08	Mercury	Moon	Saturn
08	Rahu	Aquarius	124 : 46 : 46	Saturn	Mars	Venus
09	Ketu	Leo	304 : 46 : 46	Sun	Ketu	Mars
10	Uranus	Gemini	257 : 01 : 18	Mercury	Rahu	Venus
11	Neptune	Virgo	357 : 03 : 58	Mercury	Mars	Jupiter

Case no. 48

Female native born on 24th December 1951 at 1140 hrs in Pune,

Lat. 018: 30 N Long. 073: 48E

This also is case of age related degenerative changes in body leading to movement relared problems in old age. The Ascendant is Saturn i.e. lord of Aquarius is occupied by Rahu which aspect the seventh house owned by Sun which is placed in eleventh cusp. The Saturn placed in eighth cusp afflicted with Mars and Neptune. The lord of fifth house is Mercury placed in tenth house in csorpio owned by Mars which is placed in eighth cusp afflicted with Saturn and Neptune; this denotes the function of bones and joints is disturbed. Furthe the Jupiter, lord of eleventh house is placed in third cusp i.e. Pisces is under aspect of Saturn, Mars, and Neptune denoting the hyoid bone or thyroid related disorder. The Uranus placed in fifth cusp is i.e. sign Gemini which indicates the function of blood and flesh is directly aspecting the Sun placed in Sagittarius in eleventh cup. Sun rules the bones and jointsis under aspect of Uranus wthe same which is causative of mysterious diseases indicates the disease realted to arthritis and at thyroid. The seventh cusp occupied by Leo, who rules the joints is afflicted by Ketu and also under aspect of Rahu thus indicating the disease related with joints. Further Saturn is the major planet that causes obstructive and inflammatory diseases is placed in Virgo which rules the Purins metabolism that is major amino acid to produce DNA and RNA and gives rise to excess of uric acid in body that gets accumulated in joints to cause inflmation and pain in joints. Also the conjunction of Mars and Saturn in eighth house in Virgo gives the ailment called as Gaut that is because of excess of uric acid in body. The ninth house is occupied by Moon; which is lord of sixth house in Libra indicates the Endocrine secretion or Hormonal disorders in body, the lord of ninth house Venus is placed in conjoined with Moon in ninth house indicates the Endocrine secretion disorder.

The sub lord of ascendant is Saturn occupied in eighth house is sub lord of eighth house afflicted with Mars and Neptune, also the star lord of ascendant is Jupiter placed in second house under aspect of Saturn and Mars is also star lord of ninth house. The sub lord of sixth house is ketu placed in seventh house aspecting the ascendant. Sub lord of twelfth cusp is Mercury placed in tenth house in Scorpio is under aspect of Saturn from eighth house. Thus ascendant, sixth cusp, eighth cusp and twelfth cusp are well connected indicating the disease related to joints and endocrine secretions.

The native complained of vertigo leading to breathlessness was hospitalized when after diagnosis was confirmed to have hyper thyroidism associated with arthritis, the inflammation and swelling of finger joints along with knee and ankles was observed also the hypertension was noticed. The onset of the disease was occurred on 27th Dember 2015 when Mercury mahadasha and Sautrn antar dasha with Mars pratiantardasha was in progress; where Mercury is dasha lord and significator of sixth house. Planetary disposition of this natal chart is given in this table.

Sr. No.	Planet	Zodiac	Degrees: Min: Sec	Lord of Zodiac	Star Lord	Sub Lord
01	Sun	Sagittarius	308 : 25 : 55	Jupitee	Ketu	Jupiter
02	Moon	Libra	250 : 32 : 21	Venus	Rahu	Saturn
03	Mars	Virgo	233 : 25 : 40	Mercury	Mars	Mars
04	Mercury	Scorpio	293 : 36 : 07	Mars	Mercury	Mars
05	Jupiter	Pisces	042 : 02 : 48	Jupiter	Saturn	Moon
06	Venus	Libra	265 : 32 : 52	Venus	Jupiter	Mercury
07	Saturn	Virgo	230 : 54 : 48	Mercury	Moon	Venus
08	Rahu	Aquarius	010 : 40 : 40	Saturn	Rahu	Saturn
09	Ketu	Leo	190 : 40 : 40	Sun	Ketu	Saturn
10	Uranus	Gemini	139 : 12 : 18	Mercury	Rahu	Moon
11	Neptune	Virgo	238 : 15 : 50	Mercury	Mars	Saturn

Case no 49

Male native born on 05th April 1966 at 0715 hrs.in Satara Lat. 017: 42 N Long. 074: 00 E

This chart shows Aries ascendant with lord of house placed in twelfth house conjoined with Sun in Pisces that indicates typical infectious arthritis, or knee infection and inflammation. The second cusp Taurus is occupied by Rahu and being earthy sign denotes disease related to bones and flesh, the lord of Taurus i.e. Venus is occupied in Aquarius in eleventh cusp indicating diseases of legs. Also Venus is afflicted with Saturn indicating disease related to knee joints, beibg conjoined with Mercury lord of sixth cusp Virgo denotes the infection of flesh and bone tissue in knee. Also fifth house is occupied by Uranus placed in sign Leo aspect the Mercury, Saturn, and Venus indicating infectious arthritis of knee joints. Sixth house is occupied by Moon causative of function of blood and fluids in Virgo indicates the cause of infection is through blood stream, as it is under aspect of Mars placed twelfth house. Libra placed in seventh cusp is occupied by Neptune further indicating the disturbed movements of leg joits and severe pains. The eighth cusp is Scorpio occupied by Ketu aspect the twelfth cusp occupied with Mars and Sun indicating the chronic and prolonged nature of disease. The ninth house with sign Sagittarius and lord of this house Jupiter placed in third house in Gemini indicates the continuous growing of the infectious disease of joints. Here the lord of tenth house Capricorn is placed in Aquarius in eleventh house i.e. Saturn which is major planet that gives the chronic and obstructive disease of leg joints, which specifically observed here that native, is suffering from infectious arthritis currently occurred in knee joints with inflammation and pus formation leading to difficulty in even routine movements of knee joints.

The star lord of ascendant is Ketu placed in eighth cusp is also star lord of ninth cusp aspects the twelfth cusp. Also the star lord of sixth cusp is Sun placed in twelfth cusp conjoined with Mars under aspect frpm Ketu. Also star lord of eighth house is Saturn placed in eleventh house conjoined with Mercury which is lord of sixth cusp; further the sub lord of ascendant is Mars which is also sub lord of sixth cusp placed in twelfth cusp conjoined with Sun. The sub lord of eighth cusp is Mercury placed in eleventh house conjoined with Venus which is sub lord of twelfth cusp. Thus all the significators of ascendant, sixth cusp, eighth cusp and twelfth cusp are well connected, and indicates the occurrence, and intensity of the disease. When the infection in knee joints strted giving unbearable pain and very much restricted movements the native approached doctor and was diagnosed as Osteomyelitis i.e. infection of major bone with extensive distruction of the joint. The disease occurred long back before the native complained about the pains on 18th April 2010 when Jupiter mahadasha and Mars antardasha was in progress and Sun pratiantardasha was about to complete, since the Saturn main causative planet of this disease is Saturn it apperars irrecoverable and irreversible with progressive inflammation and infection in other joints. The particularity of the scase is the ignorance of the severity of disease and an unknown fear about the doctor, the native being hailing from microinterior area of village in Satara the disease grpwn to this stage. Also as Moon falls in malefic house indicates the fear factor and constant insecurity complex makes native to bear pain and not to disclose. Another thing that is distinctly observed here is, the economic strata that the native belongs that also kept native away from the appropriate treatment. The planetary disposition of this chart is given bellow.

Sr.	Planet	Zodiac	Degree : Min : Sec	Lord of	Star Lord	Sub Lord

No				Zodiac		
01	Sun	Pisces	351 : 26 : 47	Jupiter	Mercury	Venus
02	Moon	Virgo	165 : 59 : 30	Mercury	Moon	Saturn
03	Mars	Pisces	356 : 59 : 21	Jupiter	Mercury	Jupiter
04	Mercury	Aquarius	329 : 23 : 39	Saturn	Jupiter	Sun
05	Jupiter	Gemini	061 : 30 : 54	Mercury	Mars	Mercury
06	Venus	Aquarius	305 : 04 : 05	Saturn	Mars	Sun
07	Saturn	Aquarius	329 : 32 : 53	Saturn	Jupiter	Moon
08	Rahu	Taurus	034 : 17 : 14	Venus	Sun	Saturn
09	Ketu	Scorpio	214 : 17 : 14	Mars	Saturn	Saturn
10	Uranus	Leo	143 : 04 : 25	Sun	Venus	Saturn
11	Neptune	Libra	208 : 20 : 51	Venus	Jupiter	Venus

Case No 50

Female native born on 11th Jauary 1951 at 1825 hrs.in Pune Lat 018:30N Long 073:48E

In this chart the Cancer ascendant whilst the lord of ascendat placed in eighth house afflicted with Rahu, The lord of eighth cusp Saturn is placed in third house in sign Virgo that rules the lumbar and pelvic bones. The lord of sign Virgo Mercury is placed in sixth cusp conjoined with Sun in sign Sagittarius, under aspect of Uranus placed in twelfth cusp owned by Mercury. As Mercury rules the blood and flesh and sign Sagittarius which denotes the disease related to hip joints. The Mars that rules the function of hip joints and thighs is placed in seventh house with sign Caprocorn conjoined with Venus; Mars in sign Sagittarius denotes the the degenerative changes of hip joints. The lord of sixth house Jupiter is placed in Aquarius under aspect of Ketu and afflicted with Rahu indicates that disease in lumbar region and pelvic region; the further the Jupiter is also lord of ninth house which rules the joints of pelvic region; ninth house is under aspect of Saturn and Neptune placed in third house indicating progressive chronic ailment related to joints of hips and lumbar region of vertebrae. The Uranus occupied in twelfth cup indicates the disease related to legs and long bones, as it denotes the mysterius type of disease.

The fifth hous is occupied by Scorio and is under aspect of Saturn indicates the degenerative type of wearing of bones in pelvic joints. Also the Mars placed in seventh house aspect the ascendant occupied by Cancer that rules the spine and as such denotes the disease related to spine. Further as Mercury occupies in sixth cusp i.e. fourth cusp from Saturn indicates the most disabling form of the disorder of hip joint function. Saturn is known to cause chronic and prolonged typef diseases generally irreversible natue and as it makes a square with Mercury gives rise to the abnormality in hip joints. When the native visited doctor after thorough examination was dignosed for Osteoarthritis associated with subluxation of hip joints.

Further star lord of ascendant is Jupiter occupied in eighth cusp undser aspect of Ketu, which is also star lord of sixth cusp. The star lord of eighth cusp is Mars occupied in seventh house aspecting the ascendant, and is also star lord of twelfth cusp. Sub lord of ascendant is Moon placed in eighth cusp conjoined with Jupiter. The sub lord of twelfth cusp is Mercury occupied in sixth cusp is lord of third house and twelfth cusp indicating well connected ascendant, sixth cusp, eighth cusp, and twelfhth cusp.

The occurrence of disease of hips joints was first noticed when severe pain and difficulty in movements was complained in mahadasha of Ketu, antar dasha of Ketu and prati antar dasha of Mercury was in progress i.e. on 20th February 2008. As the disease is known disorder which is irreversible and progressively getting complicated as on 2018 the native was not able walk normally without support and pains are also increased to unbearable extent.

The planetary disposition of this chart is tabled as given below.

Sr. No.	Planet	Zodiac	Degrees: Min: Sec	Lord of Zodiac	Star Lord	Sub Lord
01	Sun	Sagittarius	177 : 19 : 25	Jupiter	Sun	Sun
02	Moon	Aquarius	226 : 29 : 28	Saturn	Rahu	Venus
03	Mars	Capricorn	208 : 09 : 20	Saturn	Mars	Saturn
04	Mercury	Sagittarius	158 : 50 : 09	Jupiter	Ketu	Jupiter
05	Jupiter	Aquarius	223 : 34 : 10	Saturn	Rahu	Mercury
06	Venus	Capricorn	191 : 24 : 48	Saturn	Moon	Mars
07	Saturn	Virgo	069 : 11 : 14	Mercury	Sun	Venus
08	Rahu	Aquarius	239 : 03 : 09	Saturn	Jupiter	Sun
09	Ketu	Leo	059 : 03 : 09	Sun	Sun	Mars
10	Uranus	Gemini	343 : 44 : 05	Mercury	Rahu	Mercury
11	Neptune	Virgo	086 : 20 : 12	Mercury	Mars	Jupiter

Chapter 23

Skin diseases and planets

Skin disorders vary greately in symptoms and severity and can be temporary or permanentin nature,also may be painless or painful. Some have situational causes and some have genetic causes, also may be minor or may be life threatening. Major skin diseases are discussed herewith for their planetary relation and severity with different types.

1) Acne: Acne is commonly occurring on face in adolescent age or even on shoulders, chest, upper back. Break out on skin composed of black heads or white heads, pimples, or deep paiful cysts, and nodules. Acne may sometimes leave scars behind or darkens the skin, if untreated. Clogged pores of skin cause acne and may be attributed to excess of production of oils called sebum, bacterial infection, hormonal imbalance, dead skin cells, or ingrown hairs. Acne is usually associated with hormonal imbalance experienced during teenage years; it is most common cause of skin condition. Acne may be inflammatory or non inflammatory and it is possible to have multiple types of acne. It is observed that following planetary diposition gives rise to Acne,
If Mercury occupied in eighth cusp with malefic or Scorpio or Capricorn, if Mars be placed in eighth cusp while Moon if placed in fifth cusp and under aspect of Saturn or Rahu. Also if Mars in sign Capricorn be placed in fifth cusp or Mercury afflicted with Uranus may cause acne. Ketu conjoined with Mars be placed in fifth cusp cysts can develop due to clogging of pores and due to bacterial infection acne are likely to leave scar behind.

2) Cold Sores these are red fluid filled blisters that form near the mouth or other areas of face in rare cases may appear on fingers. These may persist for two weeks or more. Commonly virus herpes simplex causes Cold sores. Cold sores are contagious and can spread easily. There is no cure for this disease and there are two types of this virus. Herpes simplex type 1 called HSV1and Herpes simplex type 2 called HSV2which usually called genital herpes. Once the Cold sore is cured; the virus remains hidden and reoccur soon. Normally tingling or burning sensation observed on lips or face before Cold sores occur. These Red blisters are normally painful and tender to touch. Fever, muscle ache, swollen lymph nodes are major symptoms observed. If Mercury or sign Gemini both are afflicted by malefic or placed in malefic house or sign Gemini occupied in sixth cusp and occupied by malefic the cold sores are observed. So also when Sun and Mercury both are under aspect of Saturn, Rahu or Ketu Cold sores are observed.

3) Blisters Blisters are characterized by watery clear fluid filled area on skin may be smaller in size or larger. Normally occur alone or in groups and any where on body. These are also called as vesicles. Common cause is when friction between skin and shoe or any hard surfaces takes place, often annoying and painful or uncomfortable. It heals without any medical treatment. Normally it occurs when skin texture is susceptible to the friction of skin

on hard surface. The major planetary disposition that makes skin vulnerable to friction is, 1) Mars and Mercury conjoined and are under aspect of Saturn or Rahu. 2) Mercury afflicted with Uranus or Saturn 3) if sub lord of ascendant and lord of sixth house is Mercury and is placed in fifth house or in Capricorn the native may suffer from Blisters.

4) Hives; these are itchy raised welts that occur after exposure to allergens. These are flesh colored

   Or red colored spots on skin, known as Urticaria. These normally caused by allergic reaction to medicines or food, or irritant environment. This problem may be alleviated with medicine or food; most rashes go away on its own however chronic cases as well as acompaied by severe reactions may be observed. Here begins to release histamines into blood, these are chemicals that produce in attempt to defend itself against infection and other intruders. Also Hives may be caused as result of stress, tight clothes, and excessive exercise or illness. Dermstographism also is acute form of Hives usually occurs in the form of butter fly marks on skin in rheumatoid arthritisand Lupus, a type of auto immune bone disease or even in thyroids diseases, these get cleared on its own without treatment. Also it is possible to develop Hives as result of excessive exposure to hot or cold temperatures or irritation due to excessive sweating. As there are several potential triggers it is observed that if Sun in ascendant is afflicted with Mars or Saturn or under aspect of Rahu or Neptune Hives occurred. Also if Sun is placed in sixth house afflicted with Ketu or Uranus Further if the ascendant is afflicted with Rahu, Ketu, Uranus, Hives observed to occur. The ninth house if afflicted or under aspect of malefic planet or if Mercury be hemmed in between two malefic Hives occurred.

5) Actinic Keratosis It is about the size of pencil eraser and thick scaly or crusty skin patch normally appears on the skin exposed to Sun for longer time. Usually pink colored but may have brown, tan, or grey color. With

Advancing of age normally rough, scaly spots appearing on hands, arms, or face may be called age spotsand usually developed inareas that have been damaged by years of sun exposure. When skin cells develop Keratinocytes starts to grow abnormally but not cancerous growth, can progress to sqamous cell carcinoma. Primarily it is caused by exposure to sun light or human papilloma virus and major symptoms include hardening of lesion, inflammation, rapid enlargement of the area of lesion, bleeding, redness, ulcerations, and normally cryotherapy used to treat. If sign Libra is occupied by malefic or under aspect of malefic or falls in malefic house Actinic Keratosis is developed also If Mercury in sign of Jupiter or in Libra is under aspect of Saturn, or Mars Actinic Keratosis is developed. Also if lord of ascendant conjoin with Mars in fourth cusp or twelfth cusp or in fourth cusp Mercury placed causes Actinic Keratosis.

6) Rosacea is a chronic skin disease that goes through cycles of fading and relapses. There are four subtypes of Rosacea each has own symptoms. It is small red pus filled bump on the skin present during flare ups and affects only skin on face, nose, cheeks, and forehead; flare ups often occurin cycles experiencing symptoms for weeks or manths at a time then symptoms go away and reappear. Signs of Rosacea are 1) flushing and redness 2) visible broken blood vessels 3) swollen skin,sensitive skin, 5) stinging and burning sensation, 6) dry rough and scaly skin7) oily skin 8) raised patches on skin 9) Thick skin or nose or cheeks 10) large pores 11) blood shots and watery eyes 12) Cysts on eyes 13) diminished vision 14) broken blood vessels on eye lids. If Saturn and Rahu occupy ascendant and sixth cusp or if Mars or Mercury as lord of ascendant or Moon in second or twelfth cusp and under aspect of Rahu Rosacea observed to occur.

7) Carbuncles these are red painful and irritated lump under skin accompanied by body aches, fever, fatigue, because skin crustiness or oozing. These are bacterial infections that form under skin at hair follicles. It is cluster of boils that have multiple pus heads. They are tender and painful; and cause severe infections which could leave scar behind, also called staph skin infection. The mostb obvious first symptom of Carbuncle is red lump under skin and can range from size of small lentil to the medium sized mushroom. The size of lump increases over few days as it quickly becomes filled with pus. It eventually develops a yellow white tip or head that ruptures to drain pus. If the lord of ascendant, Rahu, Moon, Mars, Mercury occupies first, sixth, or eighth cusp Carbuncle develops. Also if Sun, Mars, Mercury, occupy sixth, eighth, or twelfyh cusp Carbuncle will occur.

8) Larex Allergies When a person exposed to Latex irritation occurs, may be in form of Rash within minutes of exposure to latex. Warm itchy red wheels at the site of contact that may take on dry, crusted appearance. Air born latex particles develop cough, runny nose,

sneezing, and itching may occur followed by watery eyes, some times difficulty in breating noticed. There occurs no correlation of planetary disposition or no data is available for this allergy. But in some cases severely afflicted Moon occupied in malefic house is noted that may cause allergy.

9) Eczma White or scaly patches that flake of with affected area becomes red, itchy, greasy, oily, hair loss may occur. Often occurred in babies, childrens and appearing on faces. It is called atopic dermatitis or contact dermatitis or Dishidrotic dermatitis and it affects fingers, palms, soles of feet. It is painful and scaly patches that flake or cracks. Major symptoms include intese itching red or brown spots small red bumps that ooze fluid when scratched, crusty patches of dried yellowish ooze thickened scaly skin. If lord of sixth, eighth, by transit occupies in sixth or Moon and Saturn are in sixth house the disease eczema occurs. Also if Venus and Mars are conjoined inseventh and under aspect of Ketu and Saturn virulent type of Eczema is observed.

10) Psoriasis It is chronic skin disorder and considered as auto immune type; it causes skin to develop scaly patches that are sometimes silvery or red and can be itchy 1) Red patches on skin 2) scaly sometimes sivery skin patches 3) Itchy skin 4) Joint swelling stiffness or pains and apart from this type based symptom are 1) plaque2) guttate 3) inverse 4) pustular 5) erythrodermic . It also can cause symptoms of mental stress, anxiety, and low self confidence or depression. It is non contagiousdisease. The planetry disposition in Psoriasis patient normally we find,

1. If lord of ascendant conjoins with Mercury and under aspect of Saturn and Mars Psoriasis is observed mostly on hands, neck, and upper back.
2. If Jupiter and Saturn occupy sixth cusp and are under aspect of Uranus Psoriasis of lower limb is observed.
3. If lord of ascendant conjoins with Mars or Mercury in sixth cusp or twelfth cusp psoriasis with arthritis is observed.
4. If Venus is afflicted in sixth cusp with Saturn or in eighth with Uranus psoriasis is noticed.
5. If Capricorn falls in sixth cusp and Rahu occupies it psoriasis is observed.
6. If Rahu is placed in third, sixth, eighth, cusp and under aspect of Saturn causes Psoriasis.
7. Also if Moon and Saturn conjoined in Cancer or Scorpio in sixth cusp or eighth cusp psoriasis is observed.

11) Cellulitis cellulitis is common and sometimes paiful bacterial skin disease which is infectious. May first appear Red swollen area that feels hot and tender to touch. The Redness and swelling can be spread quickly. It most often affect the skin of lower limb but can occur anywhere on face and may affect tissues underneath and can spread to lymphnodes or blood stream. Major symptoms of cellulitis include i) Pain and tenderness in affected area ii) Redness or inflammation of skin iii) Skin sore or rash that grows quickly iv) Tight glossy swollen skin v) Feeling of warmth in affected area vi) An abscess with pus vii) Fever. And if become serious gives shaking, chills, feeling ill, fatigue, dizziness, light headedness, sweating may occur. Causes are cuts, bugbites, and surgical wounds. It is usually not contagious. If sublord of eighth cusp is Saturn and in its own starlord or in sixth

cusp or sign Scorpio cellulitis is noticed. Also if Venus under aspect of Mars and afflicted with Ketu cellulitis is likely to cause.

12) Measles or Rubeola Measles is an infectious caused by virus that grows in cells lining the throat and lungsand it is very contagious. It spreads through air, Telltale rash is the hallmark of measles, If goes untreated may lead to complications such as pneumonia, encephalitis. First symptom is cold or flue with fever, cough, running nose, sore throat, followed by red or reddish brown rash forms and spreads down the body. Eventually it covers entire body with blotches of colored bumps, immunocompromised people may not have rashes. If Capricorn which rules the skin is afflicted with Uranus or Ketu and occupied in fifth or sixth cusp gives measles. Also if Rahu is placed in ascendant and aspect the sixth house occupied by Venus in Capricorn indicates Measles. Also when Venus is placed in Scorpio and afflicted with Rahu may give Measles.

13) Basal cells Carcinoma Basal cell Carcinoma is a type of cancer that begins in basal cells,Basal cells line the epidermis. Basal Cells Carcinoma resulta in tumors often look like sores, growth, bumps, scars, or Red patches. It never spreads to other places. It does not metastasizes but still result in disfigurement. If untreated can become life threatening. BCC develops on face, ear, Shoulder, neck, scalp and arms. It is typically painlessand only symptom is growth or change in appearance of the skin. It mostly caused by exposure to radiation, exposure to arsenic, complications from scars, infections Vaccination, tattoos, and burns. Even chronic inflammatory skin conditions. There is strong likely hood of recurrence. 1) If Mercury placed in eighth house, in scorpio or Leo and Uranus in twelfth BCC may be noticed. 2) If Saturn placed in twelfth cusp in sign Leo and afflicted with Mars or under aspect of Neptune from sixth cusp BCC may be occurred.

14) Squamous cell Carcinoma It is type of skin cancer that begins in squamous cells, squamous cells are thin flat cells that make up the epidermis. Squamous cells carcinoma is caused by changes in the DNA of these cells, which cause them to multiply uncontrollably. It often develops scaly, red patches on the skin. This abnormal growth can develop and any where in body but most often found in areas that receive the most exposure to Ultra Violetrays, either from sunlight or from tanning beds or lamps. Condition usually not life threatening but if untreated can become dangerous causing severe complications. In some cases new growth on preexisting scar or mole or birth mark may be noticed. Saturn if conjoined with Mars in sixth or eighth house may give rise to Squamous Cell Carcinoma. Mercury placed in eighth house in scorpio and afflicted with Mars or under aspect of Uranus may cause Squamous Cell Carcinoma.

15) Mellanoma It is one of the least common form of skin cancer but it is deadliest type due to its potential to get spread to other parts of body moles may grow into Mellanoma and biggest clue is asymmetry, Border, Color, Diameter, Evolving,. That mole changes its shape size and color over time. In nail melanoma that causes thinning, or cracking of nail, develop nodular or bleeding becomes wider by cuticle. Conjunction of Jupiter with Ketu in any sign in sixth house may cause Mellanoma to occur. Also if Ketu and Saturn are conjoined in Cancer in eighth cusp Mellanoma is noticed.

16) Contact Dermatitis symptoms of this dermatitis are associated with Allergic contact dermatitis include dry scaly, flaky Skin hives, Skin redness extreme ithing , sunsensitivity,

Cracking, Stiffness in skin, Ulcerations, open sores. Normally caused by allergic contact or irritant cotact or photocontact. Mostly substances like detergent, causes this skin dis order, some times related to JEWELLARY, latex, perfumes, or cosmetics poison oak, or poison Ivy Battery acid bleech, Kerocene, pepper spray, drain cleaners or even hands and legs are constantly exposed to water.

Normally contact dermatitis goes on its own over passage of time. No relevant data or observations found to establish relationship with planetary disposition.

17) Vitiligo in this type of skin disease the cells that are responsible for skin coloration are destroyed, these cells are called melanocytes which no longerproduce skin pigment melanine. And as such that particular area of skin will lose color and turn white. It can develop any where in body; hair may also turn grey. Primary symptom of vitiligo is white patches on skin and can affect any area of body even around eyes. The condition that appears to be hereditary or sometimes auto immune condition may develop Vitiligo, like in scleroderma a disorder of connective tissue or baldness, Type 1 diabetes, pernicias anemia, Addison'sdisease, Rheumatoid arthritis. The most serious side effect that appears in ears and eyes. Rahu and Saturn conjoins in fifth house and are under aspect of Uranus causes Vitiligo to occur. In this case it is irreversible. If Mars is placed in sixth house in fixed sign may give Vitiligo. If Mercury is placed in twelfth house in sign Aquarius and under aspect of Neptune Vitiligo may be noticed. If Saturn is placed in ascendant in sign scorpioor Sagittarius and under aspect of malefic planet or in quincunx with Rahu Vitiligo may be occurred. If Saturn is placed in twelfth house in pisces or Scorpio and under aspect of Mars with Sun anywhere is afflicted with malefic Vitiligo is noticed that is incurable.

18) Leucoderma Quite similar to vtiligo Leucoderma is a skin disease in which white patches on skin tend to lose its natural color and as such regarded as depigmentation of the skin which is marked by localized or complete destruction of melanocyte in the body. The characteristic formation of white spot or patches on the skin. Remain closely bound to each otherun like in vitiligo. In beginning presence of small patches that might get enlarged with the passage of time. It is rare condition there could be several reasons for Leucoderma right from genetic to autoimmune diseases, some of them may include traumatic incidences thermal burns, accidental cuts, eczema, psoriasis and ulcers resulting in form of white patches. Also Leucoderma can be caused by congenital abnormality including tuero sclerosis, partial alberism, and waardenberg syndrome. These symptoms occur much earlier in around adolescent ages, the epithelial tissue also could be result of some immunological conditions like vitiligo, certain chemicals like Butyl phenol also triggers the Leucoderma. Symptoms like grey eyelashes, grey hairs, grey beard, and loss of color of retina of eyes. Other complications include loss of hearing, painful sunburn, changes in vision, and secretion of tears.

The major planet that is responsible for Leucoderma is Saturn with various combinations and permutations with other malefic, including Venus and Mercury.

1) If significator of eighth cusp occupies ascendant and aspect Mercury the Leucoderma is likely to occur.

2) If sublord of eighth house occupies fourth or ninth cusp and under aspect of Uranus or afflicted with Neptune Leucoderma may occur.

3) If sub lord of sixth cusp is either Saturn or in the constellation of Saturn Leucoderma is noticed.

4) If sub lord of sixth cusp is connected to Mercury or in constellation of Mercury Leucoderma will occur.

5) If sub lord of sixth cusp is Mars or in the star of Mars the Leucoderma will be noticed.

6) If the sub lord of sixth cusp signifies the sign Taurus, Leo, Scorpio and Aquarius the Leucoderma is noticed and in this case it leads to complications.

This better can be explained with few examples dicussed herewith.

Case No 51

Natal chart with Aquarius ascendant and lord of ascendant and lord of twelfth house placed in Libra in ninth house, fourth cusp occupied by Rahu in sign Taurus indicating acute skin disorder. Mars the planet that is placed in seventh house conjoined with Moon which is lord of sixth house, Venus lord of ninth and fourth house, and Mercury lord of fifth house and lord of eighth house in sign Leo, indicating origine of disease related to skin on abdominal area. Jupiter lord of eleventh and second house is occupied in tenth cusp afflicted with Ketu and Uranus in sign Scorpio which indicate disease Eczema which was confirmed as Dyshidrotic Dermatitis when diagnosed by doctors. In this chart Mars and Venus are conjoined in Leo further indicating the repeated recurrence of the disease and may prove complicated. Also Saturn aspect eleventh house i.e. sign Sagottarius occupied by Neptune, denotes the sparead may occur in lower limbs. Mercury which is lord of eighth house afflicted with Mars also indicates the disease related to skin and also causing impact on the psychological and behavorial complex that led to depression and frequent irritations due to afflicted Moon. Mars being the lord of third house Aries that rules face and head indicate the occurrence of the disease on facial area.   The star lord of ascendant Jupiter occupied in tenth cusp afflicted with Uranus is also star lord of fifth house owned by Mercury which is also lord of eighth house. Star lord of sixth cusp Mercury which is also lord of eighth cusp is also placed in seventh cusp conjoined with star lord of eighth house and twelfth house, Mars indicating occurrence of complicated Eczema like disease. Sub lord of ascendant is Sun which is also sub lord of eighth cusp is placed in eighth cusp owned by Mercury. Thus all ascendant, sixth cusp, eighth cusp, twelfth cusp are well connected confirming the disease.

Occurrence of the disease was first reported on 20th September 2016 when Moon mahadasha and Rahu antar dasha was in progress and Rahu prati antar dasha was about to finish.

The planetary disposition for this chart is tabled as given here with.

Sr. No.	Planet	Zodiac	Degree : Min : Sec	Lord of Zodiac	Star Lord	Sub Lord
01	Sun	Virgo	226 : 04 : 41	Mercury	Moon	Saturn
02	Moon	Leo	185 : 58 : 02	Sun	Ketu	Mars
03	Mars	Leo	188 : 32 : 36	Sun	Ketu	Jupiter
04	Mercury	Leo	208 : 29 : 57	Sun	Sun	Mars
05	Jupiter	Scorpio	283 : 27 : 19	Mars	Saturn	Rahu
06	Venus	Leo	185 : 00 : 47	Sun	Ketu	Mars
07	Saturn	Libra	250 : 19 : 43	Venus	Rahu	Jupiter

08	Rahu	Taurus	105 : 38 : 46	Venus	Mars	Rahu
09	Ketu	Scorpio	295 : 38 : 46	Mars	Mercury	Rahu
10	Uranus	Scorpio	182 : 29 : 51	Mars	Saturn	Mars
11	Neptune	Sagittarius	303 : 00 : 35	Jupiter	Ketu	Sun

Case No 52

Female - native born on 19th April 1967 at 0350 hrs. In Khopoli Maharashtra Lat. 018:43 N Long 073:20 E This is classic example of native suffering from Leucoderma, since adolescence it was restricted to only upper back and after the age of forty eight spread to all over the body with further complications. The Lord of ascendant is Saturn occupied in second house in sign Pisces conjoined with Mercury which is lord of eighth house ans aspecting eighth cusp indicating severe chronic skin disorder. As Mercury rules the function of flesh and skin is afflicted with Saturn which is lord of twelfth house and aspect eighth cusp sign Virgo which is indicative of skin diseases. Venus, a planet which rules function of tissues is placed in fourth house under aspect of Saturn in Taurus indicates chronic diseases related to dysfunction of skin. Moon that rules the blood and blood cells that gives pigment to skin is placed in sixth cusp in own sign Cancer which is responsible for malfunctioning of flesh and tissue indicates the chronic and prolonged complicated skin disorder. Mars that causes the disfigurement of skin and also responsible for degenerative changes in skin tissue is placed in ninth house afflicted with Ketu giving the disfigurement of skin. Sun that rules the eyes and function of eye related nerves is placed in third cup in sign Aries owned by Mars afflicted with Rahu indicating the disease that may damage eyes. Jupiter which is lord of second house and eleventh house and governs the function of exocrine glands is placed in sixth cusp conjoined with Moon. Thus it is indicative of chronic disfguremnet giving prolonged disease related to skin. Whe we see the star lord of ascendant i.e. Rahu is also sublord of sixth cusp, and star lord of sixth house is Saturn is conjoined with Mercury which is lord of eighth cusp Virgo that indicates the disease Leucoderma as dignosed by doctors which was initially considered as Vitiligois confirmed. Also the Star lord of twelfth cusp i.e. Moon is placed in sixth cusp and sub lord of twelfth cusp; Jupiter is also placed with Moon in sixth cusp. Further the sub lord of ascendant, Venus is placed in Taurus under aspect of Saturn indicating progressive complications and spread of Leucoderma also as Saturn occupied in second house indicates the defects in eyes. As all these significators confirm the disease Leucoderma, and effect over eyes and ears. The occurrence of the disease was reported in early years of adolescence and the first patch was observed on January 1982 considered initially as Vitiligo and when the patches sprad over body till eyes and vision was affected the native went to doctor. At this time it was diagnosed as Leucoderma that has spread to eyes and ears causing damage to retina as it is becoming colorless over passage of time or damage to ears that may hamper the very function hearing.This second confirmation of doctors opinion was occurred in the year 2017 mahadasha of Moon, antardasha of Rahu and Rahu pratiantardasha in month May 2017.

Planetary disposition of this natal chart is tabled as given bellow.

Sr. No.	Planet	Zodiac	Degrees: Min: Sec	Lord of Zodiac	Star Lord	Sub Lord
01	Sun	Aries	064 : 47 : 19	Mars	Ketu	Mars

02	Moon	Cancer	168 : 12 : 13	Moon	Mercury	Mercury
03	Mars	Libra	240 : 05 : 59	Venus	Mars	Mercury
04	Mercury	Pisces	043 : 16 : 35	Jupiter	Saturn	Rahu
05	Jupiter	Cancer	152 : 17 : 00	Moon	Jupiter	Rahu
06	Venus	Taurus	101 : 56 : 11	Venus	Moon	Rahu
07	Saturn	Pisces	042 : 16 : 00	Jupiter	Saturn	Mars
08	Rahu	Aries	074 : 12 : 35	Mars	Venus	Venus
09	Ketu	Libra	254 : 12 : 35	Venus	Rahu	Mercury
10	Uranus	Leo	207 : 33 : 03	Sun	Sun	Moon
11	Neptune	Scorpio	270 : 15 : 15	Mars	Jupiter	Moon

Case No. 53

Female native born on 15th May 2000 at 0445 hrs in Pune Lat. 018: 30 N Long. 073: 52 E

This chart is a typical case we may find as related to Eczema that spread over the fore head. In chart we can see that Aries ascendant occupied with Saturn, Jupiter and Venus. Mars, lord of ascendant is placed in Taurus in second house conjoined with Mercury and Sun indicating the disease related to face and fore head. Fourth cusp occupied by sign Cancer is afflicted with malefic planet Rahu and under aspect of Uranus and Neptune occupied in tenth house denotes the impact of the disease giving disfigurement of face and forehead. The lord of fourth house Cancer, Moon is placed in sixth cusp with sign Virgo indicating skin related disorder. Mars placed in second house conjoined with Mercury and Sun is lord of eighth house aspecting own house occupying sign Scorpio indicates the disfigurement of face associated with skin disorder. Also tenth house in sign Capricorn is afflicted by the planets Nepyune, Uranus, and Ketu denotes the disease is recoverable but may disfigure the face particularly head. When the native first approached doctor for finding out the cause of consistent hairfall and was diagnosed as typical Eczema that causes the disfigurement. Sun that rules the head and face is afflicted with Mars which is lord of eighth cusp also conjoined with Mercury that rules the skin and tissues indicating the skin disorder; Mercury is also lord of sixth house.

Star lord of ascendant is Ketu occupied in tenth house is sub lord of Mercury and under aspect of Rahu which is star lord of sixth cusp. The star lord of eighth house Saturn placed in ascendant conjoined with Venus which is sub lord of eighth cusp and Jupiter which is star lord of twelfth cusp and Jupiter which is sub lord of ascendant. Also the sub lord of twelfth cusp Mars placed with Sun and Mercury. As such ascendant, sixth cusp, eighth cusp, twelfth cusp are well connected so also the causative planets Saturn, Mars and Mercury are well connected. The disease occurred late in adolescence age of 19 years on 20th April 2019 when Rahu mahadasha and Mercury antardasha with Sun praatiantart dasha was in progress. That is mahdasha and pratiantar dasha if Rahu and Sun which are the significators of sixth house.

Planetary disposition is tabled herewith for this natal chart.

Sr.	Planet	Zodiac	Degrees: Min : Sec	Lord of	Star	Sub

No				Zodiac	Lord	Lord
01	Sun	Taurus	030 : 34 : 58	Venus	Sun	Rahu
02	Moon	Virgo	171 : 45 : 11	Mercury	Moon	Venus
03	Mars	Taurus	043 : 56 : 08	Venus	Moon	Jupiter
04	Mercury	Taurus	037 : 35 : 01	Venus	Sun	Ketu
05	Jupiter	Aries	025 : 38 : 02	Mars	Venus	Mercury
06	Venus	Aries	023 : 11 : 12	Mars	Venus	Saturn
07	Saturn	Aries	027 : 06 : 56	Mars	Sun	Sun
08	Rahu	Cancer	094 : 03 : 54	Moon	Saturn	Saturn
09	Ketu	Capricorn	274 : 03 : 54	Saturn	Sun	Saturn
10	Uranus	Capricorn	296 : 55 : 20	Saturn	Mars	Jupiter
11	Neptune	Capricorn	282 : 42 : 15	Saturn	Moon	Rahu

Case No 54

Male native born on 2nd May 1981 at 1245 hrs. in Pune with Lat. 018: 30 N Long. 073: 52 E
The natal chart ascendant is Moon with sign Cancer is occupied and afflicted by Rahu and the sign lord Moon placed in ninth house in Pisces under aspect of Saturn conjoined with lord of ninth house Jupiter. Ffth house with sign Scorpio is occupied and afflicted with Uranus. Saturn which is major planet that gives obstructive or prolonged and chronic diseases and is placed in Virgo that rules the Skin as such afflicting it conjoined with Jupiter that if afflicted by malefic denotes the persistent growth of disease. Saturn aspect Moon placed in ninth house i.e. Taurus owned by Jupiter thus indicating the blood related and skin related disorder that occurs first on upper back side. The Mars that rules the back and shoulder is placed in tenth house Aries conjoined with Venus which rules skin and Sun that rules the bones and blood circulation and Mercury that rules the tissue that forms the skin and as such afflicting the both. Saturn being lord of seventh and eighth house placed in Virgo with Jupiter lord of sixth cusp denotes the disease Psoriasis. Here Mercury that is lord of twelfth and third cusp is afflicted with Mars which is lord of fifth and tenth house indicating the intensity of the disease. Also Moon which is lord of ascendant occupied by Cancer confirms the disease Psoriasis as it is under aspect of Saturn. When we study the significators it reavels that star lord of ascendant is Mercury is occupied in star of Venus which as rule indicates the occurrence of the disease psoriasis; Venus is also star lord of Mercury the main planet that caused the disease. The star lord of sixth house is Venus placed in tenth house conjoined with star lord of ascendant and Venus i.e. star lord of sixth cusp with Sublord of eighth cusp. Further the star lord of eighth cusp is Rahu placed in ascendant indicate occurrence of psoriasis. The star lord of twelfth cusp is Jupiter placed with Saturn and placed inquincunx with Mar indicating disease psoriasis and sign being Virgo denotes the occurrence of psoriasis on leg and upper back of the native. Also as sign Capricorn afflicted with Ketu indicates the affected part is leg, and upper back. The sign Scorpio is afflicted with Uranus in fifhth house denotes the severity of the disease. In this case significators if we see star lord of ascendant i.e. Mercury is placed in tenth house with Mars Venus and Sun indicates the disease psoriasis. The first time occurrence noted was on

20TH February 2015 when it was diagnosed as simple eczemza but after some time when severe itching, pain and warmth feeling at the area of infection doctor diagnosed it as Psoriasis. The Venus and Saturn are significators of sixth cusp andJupiter is lord of sixth cusp. Typically in this case silvery scaly skin was evident but itching and pains were much frequent. The dasha period when diagnosed was Venus Mahadasha with Saturn antardasha and Jupiter prati antar dasha was in progress.

After prolonged treatment of almost one year the itching and pains were reduced and also growth of the area of affection was reduced but total recovery was ssemed to be beyond reach. In this case when initiaaly the symptoms occurred on leg and upper back it was observed that the symptoms on upper back vanished much earlier than those occurred on leg also the ithching and pain on back was little less. Further the swelling on knee was prominent in early stages of the disease and major symptoms in later stage of disease observed were severe depression and irritation that led to frequent quarrels with family members. The self confidence was totally disappeared and in small small thigs the native was seekin help of somebody.

The planetary disposition is tabled as given here with.

Sr. No.	Planet	Zodiac	Degrees: Min: Sec	Lord of zodiac	Star Lord	Sub Lord
01	Sun	Aries	288 : 12 : 11	Mars	Venus	Rahu
02	Moon	Pisces	261 : 25 : 00	Jupiter	Mercury	Venus
03	Mars	Aries	281 : 38 : 37	Mars	Ketu	Mercury
04	Mercury	Aries	293 : 38 : 59	Mars	Venus	Saturn
05	Jupiter	Virgo	067 : 48 : 53	Mercury	Sun	Venus
06	Venus	Aries	294 : 40 : 52	Mars	Venus	Mercury
07	Saturn	Virgo	070 : 19 : 58	Mercury	Moon	Moon
08	Rahu	Cancer	012 : 30 : 03	Moon	Saturn	Mars
09	Ketu	Capricorn	192 : 30 : 03	Saturn	Moon	Rahu
10	Uranus	Scorpio	125 : 12 : 14	Mars	Saturn	Saturn
11	Neptune	Sagittarius	150 : 55 : 36	Jupiter	Ketu	Venus

Case no 55

Native born on 07th April 1976 at 1100 hrs in Pune Lat. 018:30 N Long. 073 : 48 E.

This natal chart shows the classic occurrence of skin ailment growth and disappearance with respect to transit of the planets along with dasha lord period. Gemini ascendant with ascendant occupied by Mars and Moon with the lord of ascendant placed in tenth cusp conjoined with Venus and Sun. Mars that occupies the ascendant is lord of sixth and eleventh house. Saturn which is lord of eighth cusp and ninth cusp is placed in Cancer in second house, Saturn aspect its own eighth cusp Capricorn that rules the skin and fourth house Virgo that rules the tissues. Venus occupied in fifth cusp is afflicted with Rahu conjoined with Uranus that indicate mysterious diseases. Jupiter which is lord of seventh house Sagittarius and tenth house Pisces is placed in Aries in eleventh cusp afflicted with Ketu and under aspect of Uranus indicates the appearance of the disease on face progressively disfiguring it. Sun that rules face and Mercury that rules skin are conjoined in tenth cusp Pisces with Venus which again indicates the occurrence of skin related ail ment on face. Mercury being lord of ascendant and causative of skin tissue diseases conjoined with Sun and Venus. Mars that rules blood and skin is placed in ascendant conjoined with Moon which rules the blood. The Mars is lord of sixth cusp afflicts the Moon and denotes the disorder of skin on face. Interesting is that the sign Pisces and Gemini with sign Libra are afflicted showing the chronic prolonged disorder. The sign Capricorn occupied in eighth cusp is under aspect of its own lord indicating the chronic and inflmatory disease.   The significator study reveals the same observation noted above, as we can see the star lord of Ascendant is Rahu is placed in fifth cusp in star of Sun and star lord of sixth cusp Saturn is occupied in Cancer and in Star of Jupiter aspecting eighth cusp occupied with sign Capricorn indicating severe ailment related to facial skin; Saturn is also star lord of Venus conjoined with Sun which is star lord of eighth cusp and twelfth cusp. Mercury is lord of ascendant and fouth cusp as well as is sub lord of twelfth cusp placed in tenth house. Further Jupiter, sub lord of eighth cusp is under aspect of Rahu which is sublord of ascendant, and under aspect of Saturn which is sub lord of sixth cusp. Thus indicating and confirming the skin disorder observed. The native reported to have complained about the disease to doctors and was diagnosed as Atopic Dermatitis or contact dermatitis that rarely affect the face. Paiful and itchy pathes on face, specifically on surface bellow nose giving intense itching and small red raised bumps that ooze fluid when scratched which initially assumed to be allergic reaction to cosmetics used; later on confirmed Dermatitis. The occurrence of disease was first reported to doctors was on 20th December 2008 when the severity of disease was mild. This shows here with that dasha lord was Saturn which is star lord and sub lord of sixth cusp i.e. in Mahadasha of Saturn and antar dasha of Mars with pratiantar dasha of Saturn was in progress. The planetary disposition of this chart is tabled bellow.

Sr,. No.	Planet	Zodiac	Degrees : Min : Sec	Lord of Zodiac	Star Lord	Sub Lord
01	Sun	Pisces	294 : 00 : 09	Jupiter	Mercury	Mars
02	Moon	Gemini	017 : 15 : 20	Mercury	Rahu	Venus
03	Mas	Gemini	015 : 40 : 49	Mercury	Rahu	Venus
04	Mercury	Pisces	299 : 56 : 10	Jupiter	Mercury	Saturn
05	Jupiter	Aries	309 : 13 : 15	Mars	Ketu	Jupiter
06	Venus	Pisces	275 : 03 : 50	Jupiter	Saturn	Saturn
07	Saturn	Cancer	032 : 35 : 44	Moon	Jupiter	Rahu
08	Rahu	Libra	140 : 35 : 08	Venus	Jupiter	Jupiter
09	Ketu	Aries	320 : 35 : 08	Mars	Venus	Jupiter
10	Uranus	Libra	132 : 20 : 22	Venus	Rahu	Saturn
11	Neptune	Scorpio	170 : 18 : 31	Mars	Mercury	Venus

Case No 56

Male native born on 01st May 1974 at 0244hrs in Mumbai Lat. 018:58 N Long. 072: 49E.

The Aquarius ascendant occupied by Jupiter and lord of ascendant placed in Fifth house Gemini conjoined with Mars clearly indicate repeated acute skin infectious diseases that may not last long. The Venus that governs the skin and growth of skin is placed in Pisces in second house is under aspect of Rahu from tenth house indicates the skin disorder. Mercury that governs the diseases related to skin and connective tissue is placed in third house conjoined with Sun that rules the head and face is under aspect of Uranus which is known for mysterious diseases denotes the infectious diseases related to connective tissue. Further fourth house is occupied by Ketu in sign Taurus indicates the arm and armpit area of skin is infected. Mars, main planet that rules the skin disorder in afflicted with Saturn in Gemini occupied in fifth cusp also indicates the acute and painful skin disorder. Moon which rules the blood and fluid of the body is placed in seventh cusp Leo under aspect of Saturn indicate the disease related to blood stream infection. Here Moon is also lord of sixth house indicating occurrence of disease. The sign Virgo that rules the abdomen and pelvic area is placed in eighth house. The tenth cusp is occupied by Uranus in sign Libra confirms the skin disease that is acute but of repeatedly occurring as the Uranus always indicates mysterious diseases first ignored then becoming difficult to treat. Also tenth cusp is Scorpio afflicted with Rahu and Neptune which indicates the infection of bacterial type damaging the skin. Further the sign Sagittarius placed in eleventh house is under aspect of Saturn and Mars also denotes the disease related to skin. If significators are studied we find that star lord of ascendant Rahu is placed in tenth house aspecting second house occupied by Venus with sign Pisces. Venus is sublord of sixth cusp and twelfth cusp. Further the star lord of sixth cusp is Saturn occupied in fifth house with Mars is sub lord of ascendant. Also star lord of eighth cusp is is Moon placed in seventh house aspecting ascendant. The star lord of twelfth cusp is Sun placed in Aries in second house conjoined with Mercury whilst Mercury is sub lord of eighth cusp. Sub lord of twelfth cusp is Venus placed in second house occupied by sign Pisces aspect the eighth cusp. Thus ascendant, Sixth cusp, eighth cusp, and twelfth cusp are well connected indicating the disease. Occurrence of disease first noticed was on 25th May 2008 when native suffered from itchy raised welts on thighs and legs getting vanished on its own but reappearing soon, which developed small pusfilled blisters giving itching and pain even wearing clothes was painful. Whe the native reported to the doctor for diagnosis; after examination doctor diagnosed it as Urticaria also called Hives. It was established by doctor to be result of some medicines native was consuming to treat digestive problems. The exact substance yet unknown, it is believed to be some herbal medicine administered by unqualified medical professional. After stoping the use of that substance the Hives were also disappeared without medicine. It is note wothy here that healthy persons also can aquire diseases just by ignoring the hazards with unknown herbs and consuming it. The occurrence was in Mahadasha of Moon and antar dasha of Saturn while pati antar dasha of Venus was in progress. Planetary disposition of this natal chart is tabled bellow.

Sr. No.	Planet	Zodiac	Degrees : Min : Sec	Lord of zodiac	Star Lord	Sub Lord
01	Sun	Taurus	030 : 34 : 58	Venus	Sun	Rahu
02	Moon	Virgo	171 : 45 : 11	Mercury	Moon	Venus
03	Mars	Taurus	043 : 56 : 08	Venus	Moon	Jupiter
04	Mercury	Taurus	037 : 35 : 01	Venus	Sun	Ketu
05	Jupiter	Aries	023 : 38 : 02	Mars	Venus	Mercury
06	Venus	Aries	023 : 11 : 12	Mars	Venus	Saturn
07	Saturn	Aries	027 : 06 : 56	Mars	Sun	Sun
08	Rahu	Cancer	094 : 03 : 54	Moon	Saturn	Saturn
09	Ketu	Capricorn	274 : 03 : 54	Saturn	Sun	Saturn

| 10 | Uranus | Capricorn | 296 : 55 : 20 | Saturn | Mars | Jupiter |
| 11 | Neptune | Capricorn | 282 : 42 : 15 | Saturn | Moon | Rahu |

Case no 57

Male native born on 15th July 1972 at 1635 hrs. Pune Lat. 018:30N Long. 073:52E.

This natal chart is Scorpio ascendant with lord of ascendant occupied in ninth cusp with sign Cancer indicative of skin disorder, Mars which is lord of ascendant and lord of sixth cusp placed in ninth cusp Cancer conjoined with Mercury which is lord of eighth cusp and Ketu as such severely afflicted. The lord of second cusp Sagittarius is occupied by Jupiter also lord of fifth house. Rahu major planet that aspect the ninth house and Mars, Mercury indicating the skin disease also as it afflicts the Cusp with sign Capricorn which denotes the skin disease on legs indicates the chronic and prolonged type of skin disorder. The lord of Capricorn Saturn which is also lord of fourth cusp Aquarius is occupied in seventh cusp; Saturn being causative of inflammatory and obstructive type of diseases aspect ascendant and afflicts the sign Taurus indicates occurnce of Psoriasis type of chronic disease. Also Venus that rules the skin is also lord of twelfth cusp and afflicted with Saturn indicates the severe inflammation of skin on legs. Eighth cusp with sign Gemini is occupied by Sun that rules the Head and face is lord of tenth house which is occupied by Moon, Main planet that rules the blood circulation denotes the disease related to skin and blood. The eleventh cusp with sign Virgo that rules the legs and hips is afflicted with Planet Uranus that is known to cause mysterious diseases indicates the delay in diagnosis of the disease and proliferation of disease all over body as result.

The star lord of ascendat is Mercury which is lord of eighth cusp is placed conjoined with sub lord of eighth cusp. Further the star lord of sixth cusp is Sun which is lord of tenth house placed in eighth cusp. Also the star lord of eighth cusp Jupiter which is also star lord of twelfth cusp is placed in second cusp aspecting eighth cusp. Sub lord of ascendant is Moon which is also sublord of sixth cusp is placed in tenth house owned by Sun occupied in eighth cusp. Sub lord of eighth cusp is Saturn placed in seventh house aspecting ascendant conjoined with Venus which is sub lord of twelfth cusp. Thus all the ascendant, sixth cusp, eighth cusp, twelfth cusp are well connected indicating the occurrence of Psoriasis.

The occurrence of disease first noticed on 25th March 2011 when the skin disease deteriorated severely the native visited doctor, and then was diagnosed as Psoriasis. At this time the skin had developed silvery scaly patches which were itchy and painful; also the native had complained about severe depression leading to nervous disorder. The occurrence first noted was on 25th March 2011 when Rahu mahadasha, Moon antardasha was in progress with Jupiter prati antardasha.

The planetary disposition of this natal chart is tabled as given bellow.

Sr. No.	Planet	Zodiac	Degrees:Min:Sec	Lord of Zodiac	Star Lord	Sub Lord

01	Sun	Gemini	239 : 33 : 55	Mercury	Jupiter	Moon
02	Moon	Leo	297 : 18 : 34	Sun	Sun	Sun
03	Mars	Cancer	257 : 09 : 04	Moon	Mercury	Mercury
04	Mercury	Cancer	265 : 23 : 38	Moon	Mercury	Rahu
05	Jupiter	Sagittarius	037 : 27 : 20	Jupiter	Ketu	Rahu
06	Venus	Taurus	205 : 28 : 03	Venus	Mars	Rahu
07	Saturn	Taurus	202 : 04 : 50	Venus	Moon	Venus
08	Rahu	Capricorn	062 : 44 : 49	Saturn	Sun	Jupiter
09	Ketu	Cancer	242 : 44 : 49	Moon	Jupiter	Rahu
10	Uranus	Virgo	320 : 57 : 44	Mercury	Moon	Venus
11	Neptune	Scorpio	009 : 14 : 05	Mars	Saturn	Venus

Case no 58

Female native, born on 17th September 1993 at 1307 hrs. in Sangli Maharashtra

Lat. 016: 55 N Long. 074: 37 : E

This istypical case in which we can study onset of Acne proliferation and scars left behind after recovery. It is not worthy here that the ascendant with sign Sagittarius is occupied with malefic that is Uranus and Neptune and lord of the house placed in tenth cusp occupied by Virgo which rules the skin; Jupiter, lord of ascendant is conjoined with Sun, lord of ninth houseand Moon, which is lord of eighth house with Mars which is lord of twelfth house and Mercury, lord of seventh and tenth hose. Also twelfth house is occupied by Rahu in sign Scorpio aspecting cusp sixth house with sign Taurus. This indicates the appearance of Acne repeatedly recurring nature. Further leaving behind the scar it is disfiguring the face. Mercury that rules theskin with Moon that rules the tissues and blood are afflicted with Mars denotes the acute small wounds appearing on face. Here the important to note that is sign Virgo also rules the hormones and as it is afflicted with Mars and under aspect of Ketu denotes malfunctioning; indicating imbalanced hormonal function which also might have caused the acne on face.

The star lord of ascendant is Ketu placed in sixth cusp in Taurus, Star lord if sixth cusp Sun is occupied in tenth cusp which is under aspect of Ketu and conjoined with sub lord of ascendant. Sub lord of sixth cusp is Venus placed in nineth cusp and twelfth cusp; also star lord of twelfth cusp is Saturn which is also sub lord of eighth cusp indicating occurrence of disease. In fact when the native approached doctor for advice on the recurring occurrence of acne it was diagnosed as acne getting spread over face and even chest and upper part of back. It initially composed of black heads with deep painful cysts and nodules leaving scars after getting cure. Doctor diagnosed first as result of bacterial infection but later on found to have related to hormonal imbalance.

Planetary disposition of this natal chart is tabled as given bellow.

Sr. No.	Planet	Zodiac	Degrees:Min:Sec	Lord of Zodiac	Star Lord	Sub Lord

01	Sun	Virgo	270 : 39 : 20	Mercury	Sun	Rahu
02	Moon	Virgo	287 : 36 : 22	Mercury	Moon	Saturn
03	Mars	Virgo	299 : 40 : 53	Mercury	Mars	Saturn
04	Mercury	Virgo	285 : 51 : 32	Mercury	Moon	Saturn
05	Jupiter	Virgo	294 : 37 : 56	Mercury	Mars	Rahu
06	Venus	Leo	241 : 01 : 28	Sun	Ketu	Venus
07	Saturn	Aquarious	061 : 11 : 08	Saturn	Mars	Mercury
08	Rahu	Scorpio	342 : 54 : 51	Mars	Saturn	Rahu
09	Ketu	Taurus	162 : 54 : 51	Venus	Moon	Rahu
10	Uranus	Sagittarius	024 : 29 : 52	Jupiter	Venus	Mercury
11	Neptune	Sagittarius	024 : 38 : 51	Jupiter	Venus	Mercury

Case No 59

Female native born on 14th November 1956 at 1120 hrs in Pune Lat 018:30 Long 073:48E
This is Capricorn ascendant natal chart lord of ascendant and second house Aquarious
Saturn occupied in Scorpio afflicted with Rahu, which denotes the skin disorder related to
legs. Mars occupied in second house Aquarious indicating the blood stream infection; Mars
is lord of fourth cusp and eleventh cusp occupied by Saturn afflicted with Rahu indicates
further the disease that is chronic and prolonged with severe inflammation. Moon that rules
the blood stream and secretion of body fluids placed in Pisces in third house. Uranus that is
responsible for mysterious and inflammatory diseases placed in seventh cusp in Cancer
owned by Moon aspecting the ascendant indicates inflammation of skin on legs. Fifth cusp
occupied by Ketu aspect directly Saturn occupied in eleventh cusp indicates the severe
inflammation and painful skin disorder. The Jupiter that rules the growth of tissues
underneath skin is occupied in ninth cusp with sign Virgo conjoined with Venus that rules
the skin disfigurement indicates the disease related to legs. Mercury, lord of sixth cusp; that
rules the skin and nerve supply to skin is placed in tenth house in sign Libra afflicted with
Neptune and conjoined with Sun that rules the skin indicates and is lord of eighth cusp the
skin disorder that may get worsened. Furthe the sign Capricorn in ascendant is under
aspect of Saturn indicating disease related to skin of legs.   The star lord
of ascendant is Sun, which is lord of eighth cusp is placed in tenth cusp afflicted with
Neptune. The star lord of sixth cusp is Mars occupied in second house aspecting the eighth
cusp. The star lord of eighth cusp is Ketu which is also star lord of twelfth cusp aspect the
eleventh cusp occupied by Rahu that is sub lord of rwelfth cusp also the sub lord of
ascendant is Jupiter placed in ninth house conjoined with Venus. Further sub lord of sixth

cusp, Moon is placed in third cusp aspecting sub lord of ascendant Jupiter; Sub lord of eighth cusp Rahu is also sub lord of twelfth cusp placed in Scorpio occupied by Saturn. Thus ascendant, sixth cusp, eighth cusp, and twelfth cusp are well connected indicating the occurrence of the disease. The first time, disease noticed was on 02nd June 2018 when Moon mahadasha Moon Antardasha and Mecury prati antar dasha was in progress. Moon being the sub lord of sixth cusp and Mercury is the lord of the sixth house. The disease that doctor diagnosed as Cellulitis with cause was unknown.

Planetary disposition of this natal chart is tabled as given here with.

Sr. No.	Planet	Zodiac	Degrees:Min:Sec.	Lord of zodiac	Star Lord	Sub Lord
01	Sun	Libra	298 : 35 : 18	Venus	Jupiter	Venus
02	Moon	Pisces	068 : 57 : 42	Jupiter	Saturn	Venus
03	Mars	Aquarius	057 : 00 : 14	Saturn	Jupiter	Venus
04	Mercury	Libra	299 : 22 : 38	Venus	Jupiter	Sun
05	Jupiter	Virgo	242 : 53 : 11	Mercury	Sun	Jupiter
06	Venus	Virgo	262 : 56 : 01	Mercury	Moon	Sun
07	Saturn	Scorpio	310 : 30 : 36	Mars	Saturn	Sun
08	Rahu	Scirpio	305 : 58 : 48	Mars	Saturn	Mercury
09	Ketu	Taurus	125 : 58 : 48	Venus	Sun	Mercury
10	Uranus	Cancer	193 : 43 : 48	Moon	Saturn	Rahu
11	Neptune	Libra	277 : 41 : 39	Venus	Rahu	Rahu

Chapter no 23

Herniated growth under horoscope

A hernia occur when an internalorgan or other body part protrudes through the wall of of muscles or tissues that normally contains it, most hernias occur within abdominal cavity between chest and hips. The most common forms of the hernias are mentioned bellow.

1. Inguinal hernia. In men the inguinal hernia is passage way for spermatic or blood vessels leading to testicles.

   In women the inguinal canal contains the round ligament that gives support for women. In an inguinal hernia fatty tissue or part of the intestine pokes into the groin at top of inner things is most common type of hernia and affects more often men than women. This is abdominal tissue dis order occurred when

   a) Sign Cancer falls in fifth house with degrees 07:20:00 to 08:06:40and is occupied by Saturn.

   b) Sign Cancer falls in fifth cusp with degrees 24:06:40 to 26:06:40 and occupies Mars.

   c) Sign Virgo falls in fifth house with degrees 01:13:20 to 03:13:20 and is occupied by Rahu or Ketu.

d) Sign Cancer falls in sixth cusp with degrees 26:06:47 to 27:53:20 and under aspect of Saturn.

e) Sign Virgo falls in sixth cusp with degrees 15:40:00 to 17:46:00 and fifth house is occupied by Mars.

2. Femoral hernia; Fatty tissue or part of intestine protrudes into the groin at the top of inner thigh is called Femoral Hernia.Femoral hernias are much less common than inguinal hernias and occur when

    i. Sign Virgo falls in fifth house with degrees 019:40:00 to 20:26:40 and sixth cusp is occupied by Uranus.

    ii. Sign Virgo in fifth cusp with degrees 23:20:00 to 24:06:40 and occupied by Mars.

    iii. Sign Virgo in fifth house falls with degrees 24:06:40 to 26:06:40 and occupied by Saturn.

3. Umbilical Hernia, Fatty tissue or part of intestine pushes through the abdomen near navel

    i) Libra falls in fifth house with degrees 04:53:20 to 05:33:20 and is occupied by Mars or Ketu.

    ii) Scorpioin fifth cusp falls with degrees 12:53:20 to 14:53:20 and sixth cusp is occupied by Saturn.

4. Hiatal Hernia - Part of stomach pushesup into chest cavity through an opening indiaphragm.

    i) When signs Scorpio falls in sixth cusp with degrees 26:06:40 to 27:53:20 and occupies Jupiter.

    ii) Sign Leo falls in fifth cusp with degrees 07:33:20 to 09:20:00 and Saturn is placed in sixth cusp.

    iii) Sign Virgo falls in sixth cusp with degrees 07:00:00 to 07:46:00 and Jupiter be occupied conjoined with Saturn.

Other types of hernias rarely occurred are

1. Incisional Herniain which tissue protrudes through the site of an abdominal scar from a remote abdominal or pelvic surgery.

2. Epigastric Hernias in which fatty tissue protrude through the abdominal areas between navel and lower part of sternum.

3. Spigelin Hernia in this type intestine pushes through the abdomen at the side of abdominal muscles bellow navel.

4. Diphragmatic Hernia Organs in abdomen move into the chest through an opening in diaphragm.

Inguinal and femoral hernias are due to weakened muscles that may have been present since births or associated with aging and repeated strains on the abdominal area and groin areas. Such strain may come from physical exersion, obesity, pregnancy, frequent coughing or straining on toilet due to constipation. Adults may get umbilical hernia by straining abdominal area, being over weight, or after giving birth. The cause of Hiatal hernias is not fully understood but weakening of diaphragm with age or pressure on abdomencould play a role.

The major symptoms of Hernia in abdomen or groin can produce a noticeable lump or bulge that can be pushed back in or that can disappear when lying down. Laughing, crying, coughing, or physical activity may make the lump reappear after it has been pushed in.

1. Swlling or bulge in groin or scrotum.
2. Increased pain at the site of the bulge.
3. Pain while lifting.
4. Increase in the bulge size over passage of time
5. Dull aching sensation.
6. A sence of feeling full or signs of bowel obstructions.

    In case of hiatal hernias there is no bulge on the outside of the body. Instead symptoms may include heart burn, indigestion, and difficulty in swallowing. Sometimes frequent regurgitation and chest pain are noticed.

Case No 60

A female native born on 14th August 1975 at 2000hrsin Khandala Pune

Lat. 018:30N Long. 074:01E

This natal chart shows Aquarius ascendant with lord of ascendant placed in sixth cusp with Sun which is lord of seventh cusp. Lord of second house Jupiter is placed in Aries in third cusp under aspect for Uranus indicating abnormal growth of tissues or obesity. Mars which is lord of third and tenth cusp placed in fourth cusp afflicted with Ketu in sign Taurus. Lord of sixth cusp Moon is placed in tenth house afflicted with Rahu and Neptune and under aspect from Mars and Ketu in Scorpio. Lord of fifth cusp Mecury is placed in seventh cusp conjoined with Vwnus which is lord of fourth and ninth cusp. Eighth house is occupied by sign Virgo lord of this house is placed in seventh house. It is important to note here is that the fifth cusp Gemini is hemmed in between two malefic Mars and Saturn indicating abnormal growth in abdomen. Further Jupiter which governs the growth of tissues and flech in body is under aspect of Uranus indicating the the abnormal growth of tissues in stomach. The sign Virgo occupied in eighth cusp with degrees 23:13:19 is also under aspect of Ketu and sixth house occupied by Saturn indicates the Herniated groth that caused due to obesity and strain arising out of physical exersion. Also it is noticed that the sign Leo is occupied by Mercury lord of eighth cusp which denotes the disorders of abdomen. The native complained about the pain and discomfort several times and was diagnosed as inguinal hernia that gives bulging in lower abdomen and causing pain intermittently which subsides when in rest. As Saturn is lord of twelfth house the native was hospitalized and surgical procedures were performed thrice but even after the surgical procedures the Hernia reoccurs. This chronic and obstructive type of disorder is caused due to Saturn placed in sixth house with lord of Leo i.e. seventh house Sun. Sign Cancer in seventh house also causes such types of abnormal growth in abdomen when afflicted with Saturn. The star lord of ascendant is Rahu occupied in tenth cusp with Moon which is lord of sixth cusp; where sixth cusp is occupied by Saturn which is star lord of sixth house. Moon is also star lord of twelfth cusp and eighth cusp. Sub lord of ascendant is Venus placed in seventh house conjoined with Mercury which is lord of eighth cusp. Also the sub lord of sixth cusp Rahu is occupied in tenth house conjoined with Moon which is star lord of twelfth cusp. Further the sub lord of eighth cusp Sun is placed in sixth house conjoined with Saturn which is star lord of sixth cusp. Sub lord of twelfth cusp is Jupiter placed in third house is under aspect of Saturn which is star lord of sixth cusp and conjoined with Sun, sub lord of eighth cusp. Thus ascendant, sixth house, eighth house, and twelfth house are well connected with each other indicating occurrence, and progression of the disorder. Important point to note here is that the sign Gemini also when falls in fifth cusp which if hemmed in between two malefic or is under aspect of malefic or the lord of this house Mercury is debilitated or afflicted shows the Herniated growth in body. And the symptoms mentioned earlier i.e. bulging, pain while lifting or movements, dull aching sensation are observed. It is also important to note that when Saturn occupies sixth house some or the other ailment is certain to exists in body that depends on other planets. The occurrence of this herniated growth was first reported in the year 2013 on 15th October when Ketu mahadsha and Rahu mahadasha was in progress and Rahu antardasha was started. First operated on 20th January 2014 when Saturn pratiantardasha was in progress.

Planetary disposition for this chart is tabeld as given bellow.

Sr. No.	Planet	Zodiac	Degrees:Min:Sec	Lord of zodiac	Star Lord	Sub Lord
01	Sun	Cancer	177 : 39 : 59	Moon	Mercury	Jupiter
02	Moon	Scorpio	273 : 58 : 55	Mars	Saturn	Saturn
03	Mars	Taurus	096 : 19 : 04	Venus	Sun	Mercury
04	Mercury	Leo	190 : 40 : 43	Sun	Ketu	Saturn
05	Jupiter	Aries	061 : 11 : 00	Mars	Ketu	Venus
06	Venus	Leo	196 : 48 : 59	Sun	Venus	Moon
07	Saturn	Cancer	152 : 07 : 36	Moon	Jupiter	Rahu
08	Rahu	Scorpio	273 : 07 : 25	Mars	Jupiter	Rahu
09	Ketu	Taurus	097 : 07 : 25	Venus	Sun	Saturn
10	Uranus	Libra	245 : 28 : 22	Venus	Mars	Sun
11	Neptune	Scorpio	285 : 30 : 34	Mars	Saturn	Jupiter

Blood Vessels and Role of Planets

The Blood vessel disorders generally referes to the narrowing, hardening, or enlargement of arties and veins. It is often due to the build up of fatty deposit in the lumen of blood vessels, or infections of the vessel walls. It may develop into more critical health problems like myocardial infarction, stroke or heart failure which are some of major reasons of death. There are many causes contributing to blood vessel disorders including high blood cholesterol and calcium levels, blood clot formation and inflammation of arteries. It is found that age sedentary lifestyle, diets rich in lipids, smoking, diabetes and family history of cardiovascular diseases are common risk factors. A mild degree of blood vessel disorder may be symptomatic. Types of blood vessel disorders are as follow.

1. Atherosclerosis- Atherosclerosis is a developmental diseasein the large arteriesdefined by accummlation of lipids, macrophages and fibrous materials in the intima; when the endothelial cell of blood vessel is damaged. It looses the ability to regulate itself. It results in inflammation as the macrophages interrupt the vessel wall. Macrophages take up lipoproteins to form foam cell walland release growth factor cytokines to attract more macrophages and smooth muscle scales. Aplaque is formed and proliferate to a larger size,

gradually accluding the blood flow. It causes different complications that affect whole body. Atherosclerosis causes peripheral arterial diseases and main sign that rules the arteries and Veins is sign Sagittarius and sign Aquarius, planets Saturn and Mars, Mercury, Jupiter, and Ketu.

i)   If sixth cusp is occupied by Sagittarius and the sub lord of sixth cusp is placed in twelfth cusp the atherosclerosis is occurred.

ii) If fourth cusp is occupied by Capricorn and Sun be placed in fourth and if under aspect of Saturn or Ketu the native is certain to suffer from Atherosclerosis.

iii) If sixth house is occupied by Capricorn and Jupiter be placed in ascendant, and is under aspect of sub lord of sixth cusp the native is likely to suffer from Atherosclerosis.

2. Aneurysm This is a localized enlargement of arteries, and characterized by ballon like bulge. It results from abnormal weakening of blood vessel wall. Common types of aneurysm include abdominal aortic aneurysm and intra cranial aneurysm. Most of aneurysms exceptintra cranial aneurysms are mainly caused by atherosclerosis.

   If fourth cusp is occupied by Sagittarius and sub lord of sixth house be placed in Capricorn conjoined with Sun the native is likely to suffer from abdominal aneurysm.

3. Reynauds disease it is rare peripheral vascular syndrome that narrows blood vessel generally in hands and feet due to cold or stress ful emotions. It is recognized by the reduction of blood flow and toes with periodic spasm and results in drastic color change to white or blue. The disease may further develop into ischemic pain and necrosis of fingers and toes. The pathology of raynauds disease starts with the activation of sympathetic nervous system triggered by or feeling of stress.

   When Moon occupies sixth cusp and in sign Sagittarius and Sun be placed in eighth house under aspect of Saturn the native is likely to suffer from Raynaud's disease.

4. Venous thromboembolism it is common peripheral disease. It is defined by occlusion of venous blood vessels by blood clots. There are two major types of Venous thromboembolisms,

   i.   Deep vein thromboembolism which is often found in the calf accompanied with swelling of limbs along the deep vein.

   ii. Pulmonary embolism this causes chronic pulmonary hypertension.

Venous Rhrombo Embolism is the third deadliest cardiovascular disease in the world. Haemostasis is the rapid development of blood clots for the pupose of reducing blood loss. On the contrary venous clots are formed much slower in terms of several days or even weeks. Abnormality of coagulation during haemostasis, changes in blood flowand endothelial failure may trigger.

i)   If Venus occupies twelfth cusp as sub lord of sixth cusp and Sun is occupied in eighth cusp the native is likely to suffer from Venous Thrombo Embolism.

ii) If Jupiter placed in eighth cusp as sub lord of sixth house and Sun be in placed in fourth cusp, also ascendant is occupied in fixed sign the native is likely to suffer from Venous Thrombo Embolism.

iii)   If ascendant occupies eighth cusp and under aspect of Saturn and also sub lord of
sixth house conjoins with Sun native is likely to suffer from Venus Thrombo
Embolism.

5.   Erythromelagia. It is clinical disorder causing redness, burning sensation and intense pain
in limbs. It is more common in lower limbs than upper limbs. Erythromelalagia initiated
from dysfunction of peripheral nerves which thickens the blood vessel walls, resulting in
hypraemic flow in limbs.

If Saturn be placed in sixth house with Jupiter and sub lord of sixth house is
occupied in twelfth house the native is likely to suffer from Erythromelalgia.

6.   Stroke Stroke is serious condition of the of blood vessel disorder caused by stop of bllod
supply to the brain cells with ceased oxygen sypply from blood will die in a million per
second. Not only it is one of the major causes of death around the world, it is also the cause
of permanent disability. Two major types of strokes include ischemic stroke which is caused
by atherposcleosis in the brain and haemorrhagic stroke which is the bleeding in brain due
to weakened blood vessel wall inside the brain.

i.   If Sun be placed in fourth cusp in sign Taurus, and sub lord of sixth cusp is placed in
eighth house conjoined with Mars; the native is likely to suffer from stroke.

ii.   If Sun occupies in fourth cusp in sign Scorpio and conjoins with sub lord of sixth
cusp and conjoins with sub lord of sixth cusp and is under aspect of Saturnthe native
is likely to suffer from stroke.

iii.   If Sun occupies sixth cusp with sign Virgo and sub lord of sixth cusp is placed in
eighth cusp native is likely to suffer from stroke.

Case No 51
To explain this particular blood vessel disorders we may study few example as given
bellow.
Native born on 15th August 1970 at 1605 hrs. in Mumbai Lat. 018:57N Long.
072:49E

This natal chart shows Sagittarius ascendant with lord of ascendant occupied in eleventh house in
sign Libra under aspect of Saturn placed in Aries in fifth cusp Moon lord of eighth cusp is placed in
second house in sign Capricorn under aspect of Mars from eigth cusp. Further lord of twelfth cusp
Mars is occupied in eighth cusp conjoined with Sun which is lord of ninth house. Lord of sixth cusp
Venus is placed in tenth cusp occupied by Virgo afflicted with Uranus. Also Mercury lord of seventh
cusp and tenth cusp is placed in ninth cusp sign Leo afflicted with Ketu. Twelfth cusp is occupied by
Neptune which aspect sixth cusp. Here Sun occupied eighth cusp which is lord of ninth cusp and
afflicted with Mars which is lord of twelfth cusp indicates diseases related with blood vessels, and
Moon lord of eighth cusp which rules the Blood circulation is also under aspect from Mars, lord of
twelfth cusp, denotes the disease related to blood vessels and also dysfunction of wall of vessel in
lower limb.   Also star lord of ascendant Ketu is placed in ninth house Leo
afflicting Mercury which is sub lord of twelfth cusp and sub lord of sixth cusp. Star lord of eighth

cusp is Saturn occupied in fifth cusp. Sub lord of ascendant is Mercury which is also sub lord of sixth cusp and twelfth cusp is under aspect of Rahu and afflicted with Ketu. This indicates that native is likely to suffer from blood vessel wall dysfunction. The occurrence of disease was reported on 23rd February 1999 when Mahadasha of Rahu, antar dasha of Mercury and prati antar dasha of Moon, when doctor diagnosed the disease as Venous Thrombo- Embolism; with serious damage to leg causing severe pains, inflammation and swelling.

The planetary disposition of this natal chart is tabled as given bellow.

Sr. No.	Planet	Zodiac	Degrees : Min : Sec	Lord of zodiac	Star Lord	Sub Lord
01	Sun	Cancer	238 : 44 : 02	Moon	Mercury	Saturn
02	Moon	Capricorn	034 : 43 : 19	Saturn	Sun	Saturn
03	Mars	Cancer	234 : 35 : 57	Moon	Mercury	Rahu
04	Mercury	Leo	266 : 05 : 14	Sun	Venus	Ketu
05	Jupiter	Libra	306 : 30 : 29	Venus	Mars	Moon
06	Venus	Virgo	284 : 02 : 30	Mercury	Moon	Jupiter
07	Saturn	Aries	148 : 48 : 53	Mars	Sun	Mars
08	Rahu	Aquarius	069 : 50 : 41	Saturn	Rahu	Jupiter
09	Ketu	Leo	249 : 50 : 41	Sun	Ketu	Saturn
10	Uranus	Virgo	282 : 54 : 32	Mercury	Moon	Rahu
11	Neptune	Scorpio	334 : 40 : 45	Mars	Saturn	Saturn

Chapter no 24

COVID 19 and relation with planetary disposition

Current pandemic corona infection has created havoc all over the worl claiming over 300 000 lives with after almost three months with no assured remdy in hand. Let us here first study the word Pandemic often used to denote the spread of the disease. Not all infectious diseases terms are created equal, though often they are mistakenly used interchangeably. The distinction between the words Pandemic, Epidemic and Endemic is regularly blurred; evenby medical experts. This is because the definition of each term is fluid and changes as disease become more or less prevalent over time. While conversational use of these words might not require precise definitions knowing the difference is important to help you better understand public health news and appropriate public health responses.

Let us understand the basic definitions;

An Epidemic is disease that affects a large number of people within the community population or region. A Pandemic is an epidemic that spread over multiple countries or continents.

Endemic is something that belongs to particular population or country.

And as such we can see term Pndemic important letteris P as P denotes passport to get spread over countries or continents when endemic becomes Pandemic. Epidemic which is actively spreading new cases of disease substantially exceed what is expected; more broadly it's used to describe any problem thas out of control, such as the opiod epidemic. An epidemic is often localized to to region but the number of those infected in that region is significantly higher than normal for wxample whe COVID 19 was limited to Wuhan, China it was an epidemic; the geographical spread turned it into Pandemic on the other side Maleria is endemic to the part of Africa also Ice is endemic to Antartica. Having understood the COVID 19 disaster one thing is very clear and that is Human immune system which is at stake due to CORONA virus; this is the major reason we find so many lives that COVID19 claimed. The another thing we have to understand is that instead of finding planetary relationship with what is happening in world we can easily correlate it with individual and those individuals who are prone to the disease may only be targeted to make their immunity work and fight with COVID19. For every one to understand self is easier than to understand Universe and future. Further these Pandemics are as assumed are not the result of Universal Movements like transit of major planet or effect of any meteoroids but it was human error and to find out the human error we will have to understand planetary disposition. Practically for all purposes few endocrine secretions and the fluids secreted in human body are the causative of emotions, and immunity. And as such if we under stand the basic planetary disposition as to who is susceptible to this Pandemic and extend treatment to him only, shall reduce the load over the medical machinery we use now to fight with the disease. This well can be explained if we understand what immunity is and what factors it works well or works weak.

The one characteristic feature of the specific immune system is that it normally distinguishes between self and non self and only reacts against non self.

Immune system is bodys defense system against infactions and other harmful invaders. Without which human would constaly get sick from bacteria, viruses etc. Immune system is made up of specisl cells, tissues, and organs that work togetherto protect us. The Lymph or lymphatic system is a major part of immune system; it's a network of lymphnodes, and vessels. Lymphatic vessels are thin tubes that branch like blood vessels through out the body and carry clear fluid called lymph. Lymph contains tissue fluid, waste product, and immune system cells. Lymph nodes are small bean shaped lumps of immune systemcells that are connected by lymphatic vessels. They contain white blood cells that trap viruses, bacterias and other invaders including cancer cells. White blood cells are the cells of immune system and are made in one of human lymph organs, the bone marrow, other lymph organs include the spleen and thymus. When our immune system does not work the way it should; called as immune system disorder and we may

i)   Be born with weak immune system called primary immune deficiency disorder.

ii) Get a disease that weakens our immune system, called as acquired immune deficiency disorder

iii) Have an immune system too active; thus may happen with an allergic reactions.

iv) Have an immune system that turns against body tissues of own body called as auto immune disease.

1. Severe combined immunodeficiency disorder.

It is an example of an immunodeficiency disorder that is present at birth; childrens are in constant danger from bacterial or viral or fungal infections. This disorder sometimes called as Bubble boy disease. In 1970s a boy had to live in sterile environment inside the plastic bubble. Childrens with Severe Combined Immunodeficiency Didorder are found to have missing important white blood cells. This is inreference with planetary dispositions we study we may find that

i) Jupiter is placed in eighth cusp with sub lord Moon and under aspect of Ketu or Uranus the native is likely to suffer from SCID.

ii) If Mercury conjoined with Mars in sixth cusp and sub lord of sixth cusp be placed in eighth cusp, also Mercury is under aspect of Saturn or Uranus SCID may occur.

iii) If Jupiter occupies in sixth cusp with sign Cancer, Scorpio, or Virgo and sub lord of sixth cusp be occupied in eighth house native is likely to suffer from SCID.

iv) If Jupiter occupies Cancer in sixth cusp with sub lord of eihghth cusp conjoined the native if likely to suffer from SCID.

v) If Saturn occupies Scorpio in sixth cusp and sub lord of eighth cusp conjoins with Saturn native is certain to suffer from SCID.

2. Temporary acquired immune deficiency disorder.

Human immune system can be weakened by certain medicines or substances, for example this can happen to people on chemotherapy treatment for Cancer. It can also happen to people following organ transplant who takes medicines to prevent organ rejection. Also frequent infections like flue virus, mononeucleosis, measeles, can weaken the immune system for brief time. Immune system can even be weakened by excessive smoking, acohol, poor nutrition.   Following are some planetary dispositions

i) If Moon be placed in sixth cusp in sign Gemini, and Rahu or Ketu be occupied in eighth cusp native may have temporary acquired immune deficiency disorder.

ii) If Moon be placed in in sixth house in Virgo or Pisces and under aspect of Saturn or Mars native may suffer from this disorder.

iii) If Mars conjoined with Saturn or Ketu in sign Aries or Leo native may hae to suffer from temporary immunodeficiency disorder.

3. Acquired Immunodeficiency Syndrome

Acquired immune deficiency syndrome or AIDS, also called as Human Immunodeficiency Virus, is an acquired viral infection and destroys the important white blood cells threreby weaken the immune system. People with AIDS or HIV become seriously ill with infections that are called opportunistic infections because they take advantage of weak immune system.

i. If Moon and Mars conjoined in eighth cusp and sub lord of sixth cusp is also sub lord of eighth cusp the native is likely to get affected by HIV.

ii.   If Moon falls in Leo or Scorpio in eighth cusp native may suffer from HIV.

iii.   If Saturn, Moon, and Venus conjoined in sign Virgo or Scorpio sixth cusp with sub lord of sixth cusp occupies eighth cusp native is likely to suffer from HIV.

If you are born with certain genes; your immune system may react to substances in the environment that are normally harmless then these substances are called as allergens. Having an allergic reaction the most comman example of an overactive immune system are dust, mold, poolens, and foods, some conditions caused by and overactive system are, Asthma in which response in lungs can cause coughing, wheezing, and trouble breathing. Asthma can be triggered by common allergens like dust or pollen or by tobacco smoke. Eczema is also caused by allergens an itchy rash known as atopic dermatitis. Allergic rhinitis, causes eezing, runny nose, sniffingof nasal passages from indoor allergens like dust, and pets or outdoor allergens like pollen or molds.

In 2003 an Pndemic of severe acute respiratory syndrome affecting 26 countries and resulted in more than 8000 casees since then a small number of cases occurred as result of laboratory accidents or possibly through animal origine. It appears to have occurred mainly during second week of illness which corresponds to the peak of virus excretion in respiratory secretions and stools; and when cases with severe disease start deteriorating clinically. It was eventually contained contained by means of syndromic surveillance, prompt isolation of patients, and strict enforcement of quarrentine of all contacts and in some areas to down enforcement of community quarrentine. By interrupting all human to human transmission was effectively eradicated.   By contrast in February 2020 within matter of two months since beginning of outbreak of COVID 19 more than 1,997,666 confirmed cases and 126,597 deaths world over this difference even after taking same measures in terms of infectious period, transmissibility, clinical severirty and extent of community spread. The main transmission route is thought to be espiratory droplets although viral shedding via feaces has also been reported for both Viruses.

The angiotensin converting enzyme 2 (ACE2) found in lower respiratory tract of human being has been identified as receptor used for cell entry for both SARS-CoV and COVID19. Risk factor for severe disease outcomes are old age and combordities. The progression for patients with severe disease follows a similar pattern in both viruses with progression to acute respiratory distress syndrome. However the similarities end here, the pandemic trajectory looks different. Therefore if current planetary disposition is observed it is seen that as of February 28th 2020; Sun, Mercury both the planets that rules breathe, pulmonary function are afflicted with Neptune. So also the planet that rules the function of immunity system Venus is also afflicted with Uranus a planet that rules the mysterious diseases. This shows that who so ever having Sun occupied in eighth house with ketu, Rahu, or Uranus in natal chart irrespective of zodiac sign that falls in eighth cusp are having threat to threir lives. Furthermore Saturn if occupied in sixth sign in sign Scorpio. Libra or Sagittarius also have threat to their livesas currently Saturn is occupied in Capricornand Uranus in Aries. So also it can be seen that in natal chart of any person if Sun is occupied in eighth house with any malefic or in sign Capricorn or Scorpio. If Moon be placed in twelfth cusp in sign Aries and under aspect of Saturn also at the same time Sun is placed in eighth house with Mars or Uranus the native will suffer from COVID 19 infection. The threat to life will be certain if Mars is placed in fourth cusp and is infected by COVID19. Few further planetary dispositions amy also have threat to lif if the native is infected.

1. If lord of ascendant is in movable sign and lord of eighth cusp is in dual sign the death due to pandemic occurs if infected.
2. If lord of ascendant is in fixed sign and lord of eighth cusp isalso in fixed sign the death due to infection by COVID19 may occur.
3. If lord of ascendant is in dual sign and lord of eighth cusp is in fixed sign there is threat to life of native if suffer from COVID 19 infection.
4. If sun and Venus conjoined in Aries in eighth cusp and under aspect of Saturn threat due to life due to COVID 19 may be there.
5. If Sun is occupied in sign Aries, Leo, Sagittarius, or Pisces there will be hospitalization due to COVID 19 may be required but threat to life will not be there.
6. If Sunis placed in Cancer in eighth house or if Sun is placed in fourth cusp in sign Cancer or Gemini or Virgo the native may be required to be hospitalized for serious infection due to COVID19.
7. If Sun is placed in Gemini, Virgo, or Aquarius in sixth cusp native mabe required to be hospitalized due to COVID19 but threat to life will not be there.
8. If Sun is placed in fourth cusp and in sign Scorpio or Taurus native gets infected by COVID19 and there is threat to life.
9. If Saturn is occupied in sixth cusp and in sign Cancer, Scorpioor Pisces and in quincunx with Sun, Mars the native is certain to get infected from COVID 19 but danger to life will not be there.
10. If Saturn is placed in sign Taurus, Leo, or Scorpio and under aspect from Uranus or Ketu then native is likely to suffer from infection due to COVID19. Threat to life is likely but not certain.

To understand the function of human immunity system one must understand the protein immunoglobulines and there types related to teir functions. Immunoglobulines are glycoprotein molecules that are produced by plasma cells in response to an immunogen and which function as antibodies from the finding that they migrate with globular proteins, when antibody containing serum is placed in an electrical field. General functions of immunoglobulines are

1. Antigen binding – Immunoglobulines bind with specifically to one or few closely related antigens. Each immunoglobulin actually binds to specific antigens determinant. Antigen binding by antibodies is the primary function of antibodies and can result in protection of host. The valency of antibody referes to the number of antigenic determinents that an individual antibody can bind. The valency of all antibody molecules is at least two and sometimes more.
2. Effector functions- Frequently the binding of an antibody to an antigen has no direct biological effect. Rather the significant biological effects are consequences of secondary effector functions of antibodies. The immunoglobulins mediate veriety of their effector functions; usually the ability to carry out a particular effector function requires that the antibody binds to its antigen. Not every immunoglobulin will mediate all effector functions and such effector function includes i) Fixation of complement which result in the lysis of cell and release of biologically active molecules.
ii) Binding to various cell types, the phagocytic cells,

lymphocytes, platelates, mast cells and basophils have receptors that bind immunoglobulins. This binding can activate the cells to perform some functions. Some immunoglobulins bind to receptors on placental tropoblasts which result in transfer of immunoglobulin across the placenta; as a result the transferred maternal antibodies provide immunity to the foetus and newborn child. Although different immunoglobulins can differ structurally they all are built from the same basic unit.

a) Heavy and light chain structure, all immunoglobulins have four chain structures as their basic unit they are composed of two identical light chain and two have identical heavy chains.

b) Disulfide bonds. There are two types of Disufide bonds first being interchain disulfide bonds, the heavy chain and light chain are held together by interchain disulfide bonds and by non covalent interactions. Another type is called intrachain disulfide bonds, which binds within each of polypeptide   chain; there are also intrachain disulfide bonds.   Immunoglobulin classes, subclasses, types and subtypes can be derived into five different classes in amino acid sequences in the constant region of heavy chain. All immunoglobulins within given class will have very similar heavy chain constant region. The differences can be detected by sequence studies or more commonly by serological means.

1) IgG this is Gammaheavy chains molecule.
2) IgM this is Mu. Heavy chains molecule
3) IgA alpha heavy chain molecules
4) IgD delta heavy chain molecules
5) IgE epsilon heavy chain molecules.

These are further divided into subclasses based on small differences in amino acid sequence in constant region of heavy chain. These differences are most commonly detected by serological means. Immunoglobulines considered as population of molecules are normally very heterogenous because they are composed of different classes and subclasses each of which has different types and subtypes of light chain and different immunoglobulin molecules can have different antigen binding properties because of different VH and VL region. IgG is the most versatile immunoglobulin because it is capable of carrying out all of the functions of immunoglobulin molecules. Binding to cell are Macrophages, monocytes, some lymphocytes. IgG is good opsonin i.e. enhances phagocytosis. IgM normally exists in pentamer but also can exists as monomer functions as receptor for B cells; however for Tdependant antigen a second signal provided by looper T cell   is required before B cells are activated. IgA is major class of immunoglobulins in secretions, tears, colostrums, mucous; IgA is important in local immunity and bind to some same cells, lymphocytes. IgD is found in lower level and role in serum is uncertain, it does not bind complement.

IgE is least common serum Ig since it binds tightly to basophils and most cells even before interacting with antigen. IgE levels are helpful indignosing parasitic infections, eosinophilia have receptor for IgE.

IgG increases in

1) In chronic granulomatosus infection

2) Infections oof all types
3) Hyper immunization.
4) Liver disease
5) Malnutrition
6) Dysproteinemia
7) Diseases associated with hypersensitivity granuloma, dermatological disorder.
8) Ig myeloma
9) Rheumatoid Arthritis.

Decreases in

i) Lymphoid aplasia
ii) Selective IgA deficiency
iii) Ig A myeloma
iv) Chronic lymphoblastic leukemia

IgM increases in

i) Trypanosomiasis
ii) Actinomycosis
iii) Malaria
iv) Infectious mononucleosis.
v) Lupus Eryhtromatosus.
vi) Rheumatoid arthritis.

Decreases in

i) Lymphoproliferative disorder
ii) Lymphoid aplasia
iii) IgG and IgA myeloma
iv) Chronic Lymphoblastic Lukemia.

IgA increases in

i) Cirrhosis of Liver
ii) Certain stages of collagen and other auto immune disorders.
iii) Chronic infections.
iv) IgA myeloma

Decreases in

i. Hereditary telangiectasia.
ii. Immunologic deficiency.
iii. Lymphoid aplasia.
iv. IgG myeloma
v. Acute and chronic lymphoblatic leukemia.

IgD increases in chronic infections.

IgE increases in

i)   Atopic skin disease like eczema.
ii)   Hay fever.
iii)   Asthma.
iv)   Anaphylactic shock
v)   IgE myeloma

After considering the above facts it will be crystal clear that in case of infection by COVID19 the immunoglobulin Ig G levels will be increased and before that if immunity is perfect the IgM levels will be high denoting the infection had occurred and gone. Here if we take note it will be observed that we need not panic for every patient that comes with symptoms like COVID19 and just looking at the natal chart we can take decision to consider for tests or not after giving gestation period for the disease to penetrate the body. It can be seen here that the COVID19 infection can be confirmed by conducting tests IgG and IgM, as IgG shall get us the indication of immunity level of the patient and IgM shall indicate whether the infection already exists or occurred and accordingly we can take dicision to quarrentine the patient or to hospitalize the patient and exactly same can be observed just by lookink at the birth chart of the patient.

Thus sub lord of sixth cusp, if is significator of eighth and twelfth cusp then patient will be required to be admitted to hospital but if sub lord is not the dasha lord during the period then patient will not be required to be hospitalized. Further if sub lord of sixth cusp is in movable sign recurring disease may occur and dasha period of the same planet is in progress the patient may be required to be hospitalized and threat may occur to life, if it is in fixed sign then irrecoverable disease may occur, and if in dual sign then the patient may be required to be hospitalized for short period and may recover soon.

It may sound funny but the fact is each person has to face the predestined situation and sickness during the period of sub lord of sixth house or of the concerned cusp. In case of immunity level of patient is observed we may find that same patient shows very good immunity at a time and may become pray to disease at other time indicating the immunity has gone down, which represents the period as it changes with the planetary disposition changes and as such ruling planets are required to be studied to understand whether patient will respond to the medication well or may be required to be hospitalized. It is there fore if we learn to llok at the natal chart we may decide instantly the course we may be required to follow. It is very true that in Pandemic and Epidemic time every body including doctor is passing through phase of psychological tension and as such naturally follow the more practiced path to try to save the life of victim; and the more practiced part being medical treatment we render it to patient which may or may not find response and exactly may or may not has an answer in Astrology. It is always beneficial for doctors or medical experts to acquire knowledge of Astrology in order to decide quickly at the time of emergency as planetary disposition if under stood will definitely make you aware of the hidden part of the situation. In case patient approached to you is not serious and you are confident to administer the treatment for his illness many times it is seen that the response level of patient decides the effect of medicines or treatment rendered to him which may sometimes yield very encouraging results and sometimes discouraging due to the different response level of the patient. It may also be noted that mere having expertise in particular field may or may not yield same results at all the time but atleast one can have the hint of what May going to happen. As in case of one COVID Patient history of whom I am furnishing details here with it may clarify that it was certain that course of events taking place indicating the worst but at the same time having understood, the effort might have been put differently to save the patient.

Case no 53

A female patient born on 27th November 1980 at 1530 hrs in Pune Lat. 018:30 Long. 073:52E

History; a female patient on 3rd March travel to Mumbai in cab for attending marriage of relative, no one of whom participated were having history of foreign travel or any signs of illness. On fourth March the female returns back to Pune in same cab; here even taxi driver also had no airport pick up or foreigner traveler in month of February and asymptomatic. On sixth March the female travels to some village for meeting and comes back the same day. Even on 7th March female had no symptoms of any illness. All of sudden female shows on 8th March sore throat, dry cough and no relief with inhalation or gargles, still at home all the day. On 9th she visited her family doctor for the symptoms and was advised the symptomatic treatment. On 10th March the gough increased and as such the female stays at home for rest. On 11th March the female felt marginally better and as such on 12th March traveled to another city for work, and also visited in laws house. On 13th March again visited the family doctor who again advised symptomatic treatment but no relief. On 15th March she was required to be hospitalized for breathlessness and was unable to complete her sentence. Doctor conducted tests and Xrays found some Pneumonia symptoms and accordingly was advised some antibiotics and rest in hospital. The following day she was shifted to ICU and was put on some antiviral drugs. Her swab samples were sent for H1N1 to virology institute and the report was negative on 18th March. On 19th March gradual clinical worsening occurred and was required ventilator and elective intubation. On 20th March only the reports made available indicting she had tested positive for COVID 19. Last breath was on 20th March. In this case it was certain that the worsening of sickness is going to happen but had it been thought of astrological view the doctor would have considered the patient serious evn well before she was admitted to hospital not I cansay doctors would have saved her but still better course of treatment with early diagnosis could have helped the doctors to save their trouble at eleventh hour.

This case in astrological point of view if we study we may find few indications as to how stars and planets intervene our life. This natal chart shows the Aries ascendant and lord of ascendant occupied in ninth house in Sagittarius. Sixth house is occupied by Jupiter afflicted with Saturn and lord of sixth house Mercury that falls in sign Virgo and conjoined with Venus. Lord of fifth cusp Sun occupied in eighth cusp afflicted with

Uranus and Neptune, indicates the obstructive and acute diseases related to chest may occur. Lord of eighth house Mars is placed in ninth cusp Sagittarius aspecting Moon, indicating hospitalization for pulmonary diseases may be there, so also the psychology of the native is appears to be always depressed and immunity also may be less. The Moon also is under aspect of Mars which indicates reduced immunity function and native may fall sick frequently. Venus lord of second house Taurus is placed in Own house Libra in seventh cusp under hemmed in between Saturn and Uranus that rules the mysterious diseases. This shows that native may fall sick due to blood related diseases frequently. The lord of fifth house Sun is placed in eighth cusp afflicted with Neptune indicating severe infectios several times in life and native may also suffer from breathing troubles. Star lord of ascendant Ketu is placed in tenth cusp aspects directly Moon placed in fourth cusp. This denotes the reduced immunity with repeated recurrence of respiratory diseases. Star lord of sixth cusp is Venus placed in seventh house hemmed in between Saturn and Uranus, aspecting directly ascendat. And is also sub lord of ascendant, indicating frequent reduction in immunity level. Sub lord and Star lord of eighth cusp Saturn is occupied in sixth cusp conjoined with Jupiter which is star lord of twelfth cusp and aspect twelfth house. Further sub lord of ascendant Venus placed in seventh cusp conjoined with sub lord of twelfth cusp Mercury which is also sub lord of sixth cusp and this denotes the reduced level of confidence leading to reduced immunity.

After few days of treatment native was totally recovered and resumed the normal life and business. It was also noticed that when ever the native finds she is psychologically depressed was suffered from respiratory diseases like cough and cold. Further if we look at the chart it is noticed that Lord of ascendant Mars aspect the Moon and is occupied in star of Ketu indicating the strength required to resist diseases or odds in life is much less and the native either psychologically gets depressed and develops cranky mood or succumbs to cold and cough. On several occasions she was told to get Cognitive behavioral therapy and also was given Rational Emotive Therapy. When returning back from Mumbai on 4th March native reported in depressed and disgusted mood that she did not receive desired treatment from her relatives and was not given important which actually triggered the syndrome but then some how was given solace by her husband and mother. On 8th March when symptoms of cold and cough occurred she took rest inspite of visiting doctor and it was only 9th evening when she suffered severe sore throat and headache visited her family physician who was aware of her nature and accordingly got treated but in vein. When on 16th she developed severe trouble with fever, headache and breathlessness was required to hospitalized

It is noticed here is that initially the swab testing reports were negative showing nosign of any seriousness but still not responding to the treatment. And here it is note wothy to point that when on 16th native was required to get hospitalized when Venus mahadasha was in progress and Mercury antardasha with Rahu prati antardasha was passing. Where Venus is star lord and Mercury is sub lord of sixth cusp this indicates hospitalization and may be athreat to life. Thus considering all these facts it will be clear that if few minutes are spent on the reading of natal chart can get us clue about the further progress of ailment that gives us way to decide the mode of treatment.

Sr. No.	Planet	Zodiac	Degrees: Min: Sec	Lord of Zodiac	Star Lord	Sub Lord
01	Sun	Scorpio	221 : 44 : 07	Mars	Saturn	Moon
02	Moon	Cancer	108 : 44 : 43	Moon	Mercury	Ketu
03	Mars	Sagittarius	250 : 28 : 20	Jupiter	Ketu	Saturn
04	Mercury	Libra	204 : 02 : 19	Venus	Jupiter	Mercury
05	Jupiter	Virgo	161 : 54 : 16	Mercury	Moon	Rahu
06	Venus	Libra	190 : 32 : 43	Venus	Rahu	Saturn
07	Saturn	Virgo	163 : 51 : 34	Mercury	Moon	Rahu
08	Rahu	Cancer	110 : 43 : 39	Moon	Mercury	Venus
09	Ketu	Capricorn	290 : 43 : 39	Saturn	Moon	Venus
10	Uranus	Scorpio	212 : 51 : 12	Mars	Jupiter	Rahu
11	Neptune	Scorpio	238 : 10 : 27	Mars	Mercury	Saturn

To understand the role of natal chart and KP sublords we can study one more example given herewith.

Case no 54

Native born on 24th February 1952 at 1134 hrs in Pune Lat. 018:38N Long. 073:48E

This natal chart showing Taurus ascendant with lord of ascendant placed in ninth cusp with Moon which is lord of third house and Venus also is lord of sixth cusp is under aspect of Mars placed in sixth cusp. Also lord of ninth cusp occupied by Venus conjoined with Moon is Saturn placed in fifth cusp afflicted with Neptune. Saturn being planet known to cause obstructive and inflammatory diseases is also lord of tenth house which is occupied by Sun conjoined with Mercury, lord of fifth house and afflicted with Rahu; Sun also is under aspect of Ketu indicates reduced level of immunity leading to frequent infections. Also Mars the lord of twelfth and seventh house is placed in sixth house which denotes the respiratory diseases. Further lord of eighth cusp is Jupiter placed in eleventh cusp Pisces and is under aspect of Saturn and Neptune indicating the pulmonary disorders. Interesting to note here is that though the sixth cusp, afflicted Moon, and Pisces occupied by Jupiter shows the severe infection but does not show any sign of threat to life. Nd this due to the fact that the very link that connects the ascendant, Sixth cusp, Eighth cusp and twelfth cusp is missing some where that indicates though the disease will occur but no threat to life. In addition if we see the history of the native it is found that on 15th March the native had visited Mumbai for some family function which was attended by about four hundred peoples and when returned on 17th March was not showing any sign till 25th March; all of sudden on 25th March the native shows some symptoms like sore throat, fever and headache was taken to doctor. After few days passed the symptoms become further severe and as such were required to get admitted to hospital. On 27th March when swab test was sent to Institute of Virology the native was still serious till 29th and again sudden there was bit improvement in health. On 2nd April when reports were available as COVID19 positive and confirmed infected there was further improvement in the health of the native observed and ventilater was removed. The native then was dischrged declared recovered from COVID 19. It is very important here to note that even though the age of person is more vulnerable to the disease and complications were expected, despite of all odds the native responded to the treatment positively and got recovered. If we try to understand the the route cause we see that the Moon placed in ninth house with Venus which is lord of ascendant shows elevated levels of endorphins and serotonins that increases the immunity level and native's response to treatment was positive.

Also we can see further that the star lord of ascendant is Sun placed in tenth cusp conjoined with Mercury which is star lord of twelfth house. And this was the reason the native was required to get hospitalized. Star lord of sixth cusp is Mars placed in sixth cusp aspects the twelfth cusp. The sub lord of ascendant is Saturn placed in fifth cusp is also sub lord of sixth cusp placed in sign Virgo owned by Mercury and Mercury is placed in tenth cusp with Rahu and Sun. it can be clear thath here the connectivity breaks and threat to life gets eliminated. Saturn is also sub lord of sixth and twelfth cusp that led to hospitalization. The occurrence of the disease was on 17th March was in progression of maha dasha of Mercury and antardasha of Mars and in prati antardasha of Venus, where Mars is sub lord of sixth cusp Mecury is star lord of twelfth cusp.

Planetary disposition for this natal chart is tabled as given below.

Sr. No.	Planet	Zodiac	Degree : Min: Sec	Lord of Zodiac	Star Lord	Sub Lord
01	Sun	Aquarius	281 : 23 : 26	Saturn	Rahu	Saturn
02	Moon	Capricorn	265 : 38 : 59	Saturn	Mars	Rahu
03	Mars	Libra	170 : 28 : 04	Venus	Jupiter	Jupiter
04	Mercury	Aquarius	283 : 11 : 57	Saturn	Rahu	Mercury
05	Jupiter	Pisces	321 : 44 : 07	Jupiter	Mercury	Sun
06	Venus	Capricorn	250 : 33 : 48	Saturn	Moon	Moon
07	Saturn	Virgo	140 : 58 : 58	Mercury	Moon	Venus
08	Rahu	Aquarius	277 : 23 : 32	Saturn	Rahu	Rahu
09	Ketu	Leo	097 : 23 : 32	Sun	Ketu	Rahu

| 10 | Uranus | Gemini | 046 : 57 : 47 | Mercury | Rahu | Venus |
| 11 | Neptune | Virgo | 148 : 14 : 59 | Mercury | Mars | Saturn |

In all these cases if we study the status of Moon and its relations with sixth cusp and ascendant which makes it more vulnerable to psychological diseases and consequently the immunity disorders. And thus it is very important to know the basic cause of immunity disorders and ultimately all types of infections; which indicate further that, it is not worthy to understand the planetary aspects on Universal causes like pandemics and epidemics which take mass of population into account and as such normally seen in that perspective instead an individual can be centred and if studied may reveal more secrets of Pandemics and Epidemics. In any pandemic or epidemic situation other measures which reduce the contacts are necessary but important measures that is required is the combating fear factor and negativity that if spread may reduce the very immunity necessary to fight with the infection. As such in pandemic situation or critical conditions; the medical treatments and psychological treatments are equally important to be administered. Firstly it is of utmost importance to understand the patient's psychological condition because it decides ultimately the level of body response to the medicines and treatment. This can briefly be understood by not only looking at the birth chart but also the condition of Moon placed in the chart because it denotes the Serotonin level, Endorphine level and frequency of mood swing as it will give you the exact psychological status of pwtient and you can plan the course of treatment to be administerd. In these cases Serotonin and Endorphin levels always determine the very IgG and IgM levels and accordingly decision can be taken on how to handle the patient. It was assumed earlier that the GP's in old days to be family friends rather than the doctors that helped patients to talk openly with doctor and doctors can decide the mode of treatment. In mid1950's Dr. Albert Ellis, reknowned clinical psychologist trained in psychoanalysis, bcame disillusioned with slow progress of his patients. He observed that they are tended to get better when they changed their ways of thinking about themselves, their problems, and the world. Dr. Ellis reasoned that any therapy would progress faster if the focus was directly on the patient's beliefs. There are umpteen numbers of examples we find when the serotonin and endorphin levels in body increased the recovery rate also had increased not only but the pain bearing capacity also increased. In pandemics like Spanish flu or Covid19 it is noticed by number of physicians that first symptos they observed was atypical headache associated with fear, impaired mental ability, and all these symptoms result in the reduced immunity level. In many cases doctors have noticed and recorded in patients history that fever was present which vanishes without any antipyretic drugs but just when doctors looks at the patient and through a smile with confidence and connection with the feelings of patients. Thus in case we just look at the natal chart and assess the position of Moon we can differentiate our way to treat the patient and get better results. People to large degree consciously or unconsciously construct emotional difficulties such as self blame, self pity, clinical anger, and hurt, guilty, shame, depression, and anxiety, behavior tendencies like procrastination, compulviveness, and avoidance. Dysfunctional ways and pattern of thinking, feeling, and behavingare contributing too much disturbances and lead to impairment of immunity function.

Chapter no 25

A short course on clinical Astrology

Clinical astrology is a science which helps us to find out planetary influences which cause various diseases afflictions and accidents. It gives clear picture of planets and and its relations with diseases; what disease will be caused under different planetary conditions, occurrence of such diseases, and whether or not the disease will prove fatal.To hava sund cpondition and robust health the first house called ascendant and lord of ascendant shoylbe strong, under aspect of benefic planets as well as lord of ascendant should be strong. The sixth cusp and lord of sixth cusp are also important to study. Astrology and medicine are intimately linked in as much as the science of healing forms an important part of remedial astrology. Sun is natural significator of human living beingand gives health and energy. It should be strong and free from maleficinfluence to give good health. Moon, the planet that rules nervous system functions and moods; should also be from affliction.   Further sixth, eighth, and twelfth cusp is afflicted to as malefic houses; that give results as far as health and accidents are considered. Sixth house is called as house of diseases gives resultantly ill health in the planets dasha period. Iany chart look to the planets in sixth house from ascendant and sixth cusp from Moon, lord of sixth cusp and sign occupied in sixth cusp. These all combined together will produce a clue about the disease and the part of the body affected by the disease, for example Venus occupies sixth cusp is bad to cause diseases related to reproductive system or organs; especially if it is afflicted by Saturn or Mars or any nod. Moon is watery planet and if conjoined with or aspected by fiery planet like Mars it may cause instability of thought and make native violent, furious, abusive, and treacherous. Besides these there are there are three houses in chart called malefic three sixth, eighth and twelfth. The body of Time personified has been divided into ttwelve parts i.e. twelve zodiacs.

Sr. NO.	Zodiac	Part of body of time personified
01	Aries	Head
02	Taurus	Face
03	Gemini	Neck
04	Cancer	Cervical, Collarbone, Thorasic region.
05	Leo	Heart, Lungs, Upper abdomen, Vertebrae.
06	Virgo	Lower abdomen, Liver, lower vertebrae.
07	Libra	Kidney, Pelvic joints, Lumbar region.
08	Scorpio	Reproductive organs, Colon.
09	Sagittarius	Thighs, Femure.
10	Capricorn	Knee joints.
11	Aquarius	Shanks, Ankles.
12	Pisces	Feet

Also Aries, Leo, Sagittarius rule Vitality, and Vigour.

Taurus, Virgo, Capricorn rule Bones, and Flesh

Gemini, Libra, Aquarius rule pulmonary function

Cancer, Scorpio, Pisces rule Blood, and fluids of body. Zodiacs further divided into twelve houses called cusps.

Sr. No.	Cusp or House no.	Body Parts of time personified
01	Ascendant or first cusp	Head, brain, Face, Nose, nature of person.
02	Second cusp	Face, eyes, nose, Tongue, Teeth, Neck, collar Bones, Throat.
03	Third cusp	Breathing, ears, growth of body
04	Fourth cusp	Heart, Lungs, Chest, Blood, Body fluids.
05	Fifth cusp	Upper abdomen, nervous system, Kidney, Vertebrae.
06	Sixth cusp	Lower abdomen, Reproductive organ, Lumbar region.
07	Seventh cusp	Reproductve organs, Diaphragm, Pelvic joints.
08	Eighth cusp	Colon, Rectum, External features of reproductive system.
09	Ninth cusp	Thighs, Femure bone, flesh.
10	Tenth cusp	Knees, joints, Flesh, Feet.

| 11 | Elevanth cusp | Pulmonary function, Blood circulation, Nervous system. |
| 12 | Twelfth cusp | Eyes, Blood, body fluids. |

The cusps from second to sixth govern right side of the body and cusps from seventh to twelfth govern left side of the body in reverse order. Some planetary combinations are summerised as given under.

1) Heart diseases and role of planets.

   Heart disease can be manifested by several factors and one of thease several factors are hypertension, paralysis, angina, depression and vascular diseases. It involves planets like Sun, Moon, Mars, and signs Cancer, Fourth cusp, and fifth cusp. Affliction to Sun, Leo and the fifth cusp cause heart ailments. Affliction of Sun, Moon, Mars, and any relation of these planets and signs with malefic or are in malefic house and lord of sixth cusp or Virgo sign gives heart ailments. Also conjunction of Sun, Saturn, and Jupiter in fourth affects the heart function, Saturn, affects, the valves of the heart or arteries or it enhances the deposition of fatty layers in arteries. Neptune affects the heart through drugs, smoking. Uranus causes ailments of nerves of heart and lungs, Urenus and Jupiter if conjoined brings about dialation of heart and Mars damages the pertonium of heart with strain.

2) Eye diseases are caused because of following planetary conbinations.
   i. Second cusp and Sun rule the right eye, and twelfth cusp and Moon rules the left eye.
   ii. If Sun and Moon occupy malefic house and also there is malefic influence on second cusp and twelfth cusp even loss of eye sight is indicated.
   iii. Venus governs natural lenses of eyes and if it afflicted or is occupied in sixth cusp vision may be impaired.

3) Brain diseases and role of planetary combinations.
   i. Sun is significator of brain and nervous function and if severly afflicted may cause ailments of brain.
   ii. Mercury is responsible for nerves and functions of nervous system and as such if afflicted by maefic or be placed in sixth or eighth cusp nervous system disorders may cause. Diseases like head aches, neuralgia, neurasthenia, palpitation, delirium may occur.
   iii. Mars is known to produce aggressive nature and angry hot constitution that leads to nervous break down or severe depression; it also causes blood flow disruption to brain and leading to major injuries to nervous system.
   iv. Moon is significator of psychological functions of nervous system and as such if afflicted or occupied in malefic house and under aspect of malefic planets may cause mental ability impairment, degenerative changes, structural defects, and infections such as meningitis.
   v. Saturn is known to produce obstructive and inflammatory diseases of nervous system, and as such may cause persistent or sudden onset of headaches, loss of feeling and tingling, loss of muscle strength, memory loss, lack of coordination.
   vi. Aries rules cranium and if falls in sixth cusp and occupied by malefic plaet like Rahu or Ketu it may casuse tremors and seizers, back pain which radiates to the feet and toes or other parts of body.

vii.   First cusp or ascendant rules the brain and nature of native and if afflicted and under aspect of malefic planets like Uranus or Ketu may lead to muscle wasting, slurred speech, new language impairment i.e. expression or comprehension.

viii.   If Moon and Mercury conjoin in fifth cusp or lord of fifth cusp is Mrecury or Moon and is afflicted severly or falls in sixth cusp and under aspect of Saturn may cause muscle rigidity, memory loss, weakness, loss of sight.

ix.   Epilepsy or mental inefficiency is caused when Moon, Mercury, fifth house, and lord of fifth house and lord of ascendant or Leo sign are considered and are under aspect of malefic or afflicted severely then functional disorders, dizziness, neuralgia, parkinson's disease or alzhemeimer disease may occur.

4) Dental problems and planetary combinations.

i.   Tooth loss are occurred when Mars in ascendant in watery sign and is under aspect of Saturn.

ii.   Conjunction of Sun with Saturn in watery sign in ascendant may cause gradual tooth decay and finally loss.

iii.   If Sun in ascendant and or in sixth house and under aspect of Saturn loss of tooth occurs.

iv.   If Saturn in seventh cusp in signs other than Capricorn and Aquarius especially in Sagittarius, Taurus, Aries and Saturn is afflicted with Ketu uneven teeth or uncouth teeth may be observed.

v.   If Pisces in ascendant with Jupiter occupied it broad and protruding teeth may occur.

vi.   Jupiter in first house and Saturn in sixth cusp may also cause the early decay of tooth leading to removal.

5) Autism; planetary combinations and autism.

i.   Second house if occupied by malefic and also Jupiter is placed in sixth cusp defect in speech may be noticed.

ii.   If Mercury and sign Taurus both are afflicted simultaneaously and second house is occupied by Uranus loss of hearing and dumbness may be produced.

iii.   If Ketu in sign Gemini occupies second house and is under aspect of Saturn may cause stammering, delayed voice pronouncation and hearing loss may be reported.

iv.   Afflicted Rahu with Mars or Saturn in Taurus or second house may cause delay in speaking.

v.   If Mercury occupies sixth cusp or eignth cusp in Aries and Jupiter in twelfth cusp afflicted severely may cause irreversible Autism.

vi.   Jupiter in sixth or eighth cusp in sign Taurus or Aquarius and is under aspect of malefic may cause deafness.

vii.   Saturn in second or twelfth cusp in sign Pisces or Gemini is under aspect of Ketu or Uranus may cause defects in cochlea and loss of hearing may occur.

viii.   Third cusp, eleventh cusp, and ninth cusp or planets Sun, Moon ,Mars or Saturn are afflicted may lead to deafness.

ix.   Fifth, twelfth cusp and Jupiter and Mars are afflicted simultaneously deafness may be noticed.

6) Paralysis and cerebral haemorrhage, planets responsible
   i.   Mercury if afflicted in malefic house by Npetune or Mars may cause paralysis.
   ii.   Influence of Saturn and Rahu on ascendant simultaneously and lord of eighth cusp
          occupies sixth cusp cerebral haemorrhage may be caused even death may occur.
   iii.   Mercury if occupies sixth cusp and is under aspect of Saturn or Ketu nervous
          disorder bue to to haemorrhage in cranial artery may occur.
   iv.   Saturn if placed in sixth cusp conjoins with Mercury or Sun and is under aspect of
          Ketu may cause paralysis.
   v.   Saturn if occupies ascendant in Pisces and afflicted with Rahu and simultaneously if
          Uranus occupies eighth house paralysis folloed by death may occur.
   vi.   If ascendant, Sun, Moon and Saturn are under aspect of Mars or Ketu or Neptune,
          facial palsy may occur.
   vii.   If ascendant is under aspect of Saturn and Rahu simultaneouly and sixth cusp is
          occupied by Ketu paralysis may occur.
7) Liver diseases and planetary combinations.
   i.   Bilious planet like Mars or Sun if afflicted in in fifth house or in Virgo with Saturn or
          Uranus liver cirrhosis may occur.
   ii.   Leo or Virgo in sixth cusp occupied by malefic like Rahu or Ketu liver diseases may
          occur.
   iii.   If Jupiter in sixth house is afflicted with Ketu and under aspect of Saturn or Mars
          diseases related to pancreas or liver may occur or gall bladder stone may develop.
   iv.   If fifth cusp is afflicted by Scorpio or Aquarius and sixth cusp is occupied by Jupiter
          under aspect of ketu may give diseases related to liver in this case liver transplant
          also may be required
   v.   Leo if occupied by Rau and Jupiter placed in sixth cusp and simultaneously if Moon,
          Mars are afflicted with malefic liver dysfunction may be observed.
   vi.   If Rahu conjoined with Mars in fifth cusp and sixth house is occupied by Jupiter in
          sign Capricorn liver dysfunction may occur.
8)   Apendicitis disorder and planetary combinations.
   i.   If Virgo is occupied by Saaturn or Ketu and sixth cusp is occupied by Jupiter and
          Uranus Appendix infection and surgical removal may be required.
   ii.   If Sun occupies sixth cusp afflicted with Rahu and lord of sixth cusp is placed in
          eighth cusp appendix infection may take place.
   iii.   If Venus conjoined with Sun or Mars in sixth cusp and under aspect of malefic
          appendix may get infected and even rupture may occur, that threats the life.
   iv.   If sixth cusp is occupied by Jupiter conjoined with Venus and under aspect of Saturn
          from twelfth cusp appendix may develop severe infection and surgery may be
          required.
   v.   If in sixth house sign Taurus falls and is occupied by Ketu PPendix may get infected.
9) Hypertension or Hypotension and planetary combination.

Blood pressure is measured in terms of millimeter of mercury and apparatus used is called
sphagmomanometer, and average normal systolic blood pressure at age of 20 years is 120 mm
of Hg. and diastolic of 80 mm of Hg. However there is wide range of narmal blood pressure for

different people and the same person may have different circumstances for example excitement blood pressure shoots up and genrally increases with age and body weight; low blood pressure called hypotension is normal for many people and with others it may result from malnutrition or extended bed restand weakness. High blood pressure affects first the heart and blood vessels; and indirectly other organs. Hardening of arteries is perhaps the chief danger of continuos hypertension. A heart attack is usually a case of coronary thrombosis, the usual symptoms of high Blood pressure are shortness of breath after slight exertion, digestion, or vertigo, eye trouble, pain of tightness in chest, persistent headache, fatigue, swelling of ankles or abdomen. Astrologically the Sun, Mars rule over the heart.

i. Moon if becomes isolated and Mars is afflicted may cause problems related to blood pressure.
ii. A weak moon and at the same time if Mars is under aspect of Saturn may cause hypertension.
iii. A debilitated Mars in fourth house and If Moon occupies sixth house afflicted with Saturn Hypotension may cause due to malnutrition.
iv. Is Sun afflicted in ascendant with Saturn and Mars aaspect it Hypertension may be observed.
v. Mars in quadrant of Jupiter or quincunx with Jupiter may cause Hypertension due to constricted blood vessels.
vi. If Jupiter and Venus conjoin in Leo in fourth cusp and are under aspect of malefic may cause hypertension due to progressive increase in fatty layer deposit on wall of arteries.
vii. Sun afflicted with Saturn and in quadriquadrant or sextant of Mars gives Vasculatis which is denoted by inflammation of blood vessels leading to hypertension.
viii. Mars squaring or in conjunct with Jupiter and under aspect of Saturm may cause blood pressure.

10) Hydrocele

Hydrocele is caused due to dysfunctional fluid absorption in scrotum and is caused when Mars is placed in eighth house afflicted with Rahu in Scorpio.

11) Herniated growth in body and planets.

i. Herniated growth in abdomen is caused when sign Libra occupies seventh cusp and is occupied by Ketu.
ii. Lords of ascendant, sixth cusp, eighth cusp and twelfth cusp are well connected and Virgo falls in ascendant herniated growth may occur.
iii. If eighth cusp is occupied by malefic and lord of eighth cusp is afflicted with Rahu any where in chart may cause herniated growth
iv. If lord of ascendant, fifth cusp, eighth cusp and twelfth cusp are related with each other herniated growth may occur.
v. Rahu if placed in Leo and Sun conjoins lord of second house with Saturn occupies third cusp herniated growth may take place.
vi. If Mars is afflicted with Ketu in sixth or eighth cusp herniated growth may occur.
vii. If Mars conjuncts with Saturn and Rahu in sixth cusp herniated growth may occur.
viii. If Jupiter is afflicted with Rahu in eighth cusp herniated growth may occur.

ix. If lord od ascendant occupies eighth cusp and is afflicted with Rahu and simultaneously under aspect of Mars herniated growth may occur.

12) Prostate gland disorders and planetary combinations.

i. If lord of ascendant in sixth cusp and Moon is in watery sign under aspect of malefic prostatitis may occur.

ii. If malefic in sixth, seventh, or eighth cusp and lord of sevent cusp occupies sixth cusp prostate gland cancer may be noticed.

iii. If Saturn in seventh cusp and under aspect of Mars and lord of sixth cusp is placed in eighth cusp prostate gland cancer may be noticed.

iv. If Venus occupies fiery sign or airy sign in sixth or eighth cusp prostatitis may occur.

v. If Mars is placed in seventh cusp and is under aspect of Ketu or Rahu prostate gland disorders are noticed.

vi. If Venus as lord of eighth cusp occupies sixth cusp in watery sign prostatitis may be noticed.

vii. If Saturn conjoins with Ketu in in eighth cusp and under aspect of Mars prostatitis may be noticed.

13) Splenomegaly i.e. enlargement of spleen and planets.

i. If Saturn occupies seventh cusp and Moon is hemmed in between two malefics splenomegaly is noticed.

ii. If Moon is hemmed in between two malefic and Sun occupies Capricorn in sixth splenomegaly is observed.

iii. If Moon and Ketu occupy ascendant owned by Saturn and in Saturn be placed in sixth cusp splenomegaly is noticed.

iv. If Aquarius, Ascendant and Moon are under aspect of malefic simultaneously splenomegaly is observed.

v. If Mars occupies ascendant and lord of sixth house is hemmed in between malefic splenomegaly is noticed.

vi. If Sun placed in ascendant and under aspect of Mars as lord of sixth cusp splenomegaly is observed.

vii. If Sun, Moon and Mars together placed in sixth cusp splenomegaly may be noticed.

viii. If Saturn is conjoined with Moon in sixth or eighth cusp as lord ascendant splenomegaly may be noticed.

14) Female reproductive system and planetary combinations.

i. If sixth cusp and Virgo occupied by malefic hormonal disorder may be noticed.

ii. If seventh house and Libra are afflicted with malefic hormonal disorder may be noticed.

iii. If eighth cusp and Scorpio are occupied by malefic hormonal disorder may be noticed.

iv. Mars in fiery sign occupied in eighth cusp with moon placed in sixth cusp growth of polyps or cysts is noticed in ovaries.

v. If Saturn placed in fifth house and Mars occupies eighth cusp Amenorrhea is observed.

| | vi. | If Venus afflicted any where in chart and fifth cusp is occupied by Mercury conjoined with Ketu Polycystic ovarian disorder is noticed. |

vi.   If Venus afflicted any where in chart and fifth cusp is occupied by Mercury conjoined with Ketu Polycystic ovarian disorder is noticed.

vii.   If Mars occupies fifth cusp and under aspect of Saturn and Venus placed in eighth cusp dysfunctional bleeding is observed.

viii.   If Moon is placed in sixth cusp and Saturn occupies sixth cusp painful menstruation is noticed.

ix.   If Moon is afflicted with Mars in fifth cusp and under aspect of malefic polycystic ovarian syndrome is noticed.

x.   Moon and Mars or Moon and Saturn or Moon and Rahu or Moon and Ketu occupies fifth cusp hormonal imbalance associated with Pelvic Inflmmation Disease is observed it may lead to infertility.

xi.   If Libra or Seventh cusp or Lord of seventh cusp is afflicted and Mars occupies sixth, eighth or twelfth cusp and under aspect of Saturn endometriosis is observed.

xii.   If Fifth cusp is occupied by Mercury afflicted with Saturn and Mars placed in eighth cusp Polycystic ovarian disorder may be observed or in this case infertility occurs but cause goes unnoticed.

15)   Pregnancy and delivery of child, a corelation with planetary combinations.

i.   Ketu in fifth cusp may cause painful delivery sometimes ceaserian may be required.

ii.   Jupiter afflicted with Ketu in fifth cusp causes miscarriages and abortions.

iii.   Jupiter in sixth or eighth cusp afflicted with malefic may cause repeated abortions.

iv.   Malefics in sixth, eighth and twelfth cusp with Moon occupies fifth cusp indicates miscarriages and infertility.

v.   Malefic in fifth, seventh and ninth cusp and Moon occupy eighth cusp gives caeserian birth to child.

vi.   Moon in fifth in sign Virgo, Leo, or Scorpio and under aspect of Mars may cause infertility due to unknown reason.

vii.   Exchange of lord of fifth and eighth cusp may cause pelvic inflammation disorder making it severe to cause infertility.

viii.   Mars, Saturn, and Rahu placed in fifth cusp may cause intrauterine tumor which may lead to infertility.

ix.   If Sun is placed in fifth cusp and under aspect of Mars with Moon occupy sixth cusp may cause premature birth with spastic child.

x.   If Sun and Rahu or Sun and Ketu occupy fifth house infertility due to dysfunctional ovaries is noticed.

xi.   If malefic present in fifth cusp or aspect it without connection of any benefic; fallopian tubes blockages are observed.

16) Stomach and planetary combinations.

i.   If sign Virgo occupies sixth cusp with Jupiter stomach ailments are noticed.

ii.   If Leo occupy fifth cusp and under aspect of Saturn abdominal diseases are observed.

iii.   If Ketu placed in fifth cusp and Jupiter occupies sixth cusp frequent abdominal diseases are noticed.

iv.   If Sun occupies eighth cusp and Jupiter is placed in sixth irritable bowel syndrome is observed.

v.   If Mars conjoined with Mercury in sixth cusp may cause ulcers and colic pains.

vi.   If Rahu occupies sixth cusp conjoined with Jupiter gives mal functioning of large intestine and colon.

vii.   If Venus is afflicted with any malefic in sixth cusp repeated indigestion and nauseatic feeling may be noticed.

viii.   If Venus conjoined with Moon in watery sign in fifth cusp dropsy or excessive fluid retention in body or oedema may be noticed.

ix.   If lord of ascendant and Sun occupies eighth cusp piles or colorectal diseases are noticed.

x.   Sun, Saturn, and Ketu if occupy sixth cusp in sign Virgo frequent abdominal pains with malfunctioning od digestive system is observed.

17) Skin disorders and planetary combinations

i.   Mercury occupied in second house and under aspect of Moon gives Eczema or Dermatitis.

ii.   Saturn in sign Libra occupied in third cusp if conjoins Mars skin diseases are observed.

iii.   Sun, Moon, and Mars conjointly placed in sixth cusp may cause Eczema.

iv.   If Moon and Mars occupied in sixth cusp are under aspect of Saturn causes fungal infections. Also known to cause Cellulitis.

v.   If Saturn occupies ascendant and and is under aspect of Mars Psoriasis may be noticed.

vi.   If Moon placed in second house with watery sign and under aspect of malefic is noticed to give acne that leaves scarmarks on facial skin.

vii.   If if Sun conjoins with Saturn in ascendant and is under aspect of Ketu gives measles and scars on skin.

viii.   If malefic presents in sixth cusp conjoined with Mercury and also under aspect of Rahu likely to cause Carbuncles that gives pain.

ix.   If Rahu is placed in sixth cusp conjoined with Mercury and under aspect of Saturn is likely to cause psoriasis.

x.   If Moon occupies sixth cusp conjoined with Mercury and under aspect of Mars may cause Vitiligo or Leucoderma.

xi.   If Moon in Virgo in sixth house hemmed in between two malefic causes pigmentation on skin and sometimes allergic reactions on skin.

xii.   If Moon occupies Sagittarius in eighth cusp conjoined with Mercury and under aspect of Mars gives Eczema.

xiii.   If Moon conjoined with Saturn in Pisces, Cancer, Capricorn or Taurus and under aspect of Rahu may cause serious skin diseases.

xiv.   If Jupiter conjoins with Saturn with weak Moon in tenth cusp and Mars in ascendant gives chronic Eczema.

xv.   If Moon occupies Sagittarius in sixth cusp and under aspect of Saturn or Mars gives dry skin that frequently gives infectuins.

xvi. If fifth or ninth house is occupied by Mars and Saturn with sign Taurus and Capricorn respectively may cause fungal infections.

18) Fracture of bones and planetary combination.
   i. Sun conjoins with Moon, Saturn, or Mars in eighth cusp, Fifth cusp, and ninth cusp bones are likely to get fractured due to reduced bone marrow density.
   ii. If Rahu, Mercury, Saturn may cause decay in tooth causing tooth problems.
   iii. If Moon occupies sixth cusp conjoined with sixth cusp and under aspect of Uranus causes accidends and bone fracture.
   iv. Moon placed in ascendant Saturn in fourth cusp and Mars occupies tenth cusp bone fracture may occur.
   v. Saun in ascendant Saturn in fifth and Moon occupies eighth with Mars in ninth cusp may cause fracture of bones due to disease called Marble bone disease.
   vi. If Mars occupies Capricorn or Aquarius bone fracture may be occurred.
   vii. If Moon placed in second house, mars placed in fourth cusp, and Sun in tenth cusp may cause bone fracture due to calcium deficiency syndrome.
   viii. If Sun occupies fourt house Saturn occupies eighth cusp and Moon placed in tenth cusp bone fracture may occur.
   ix. If Saturn placed in second house Moon placed in fourth cusp and Mars placed in tenth cusp bone fracture may occur.
   x. If Sun and Saturn occupies third cusp and Mars conjoined with Uranus may cause bone fracture.

19) Diabetes and planetary combination.
   i. If Saturn and Rahu aspects Jupiter in any cusp function of Pancreas and leads to Diabetes.
   ii. If Jupiter and Sun conjoines in any sign on Rahu-Ketu axis function of Pancreas is suffered leading to diabetes.
   iii. If Venus occupies sixth cusp and Jupiter placed in Twelfth cusp diabetes is noticed.
   iv. If lord of fifth cusp conjoined with lord of sixth or lord of eighth cusp or lord of twelfth cusp diabetes is noticed.
   v. If retrograde Jupiter is afflicted in sixth or eighth cusp with Mars disbetes is occurred.
   vi. If Jupiter in the star of Saturn and Venus occupies eighth cusp diabetes is noticed.
   vii. If Saturn occupies sign Cancer and Veus placed in eighth cusp diabetes is observed.
   viii. If Moon is afflicted by Saturn and Venus occupied in sixth cusp Diabetes is observed.
   ix. If Jupiter occupies star of Rahu and is afflicted by Rahu diabetes is noticed.
   x. If Jupiter is debilitated and occupies sixth or eighth cusp or twelfth cusp and is afflicted by Saturn, Rahu or Mars diabetes is noticed.
   xi. If a malefic occupies ascendant and Venus occupies eighth cusp and also Jupiter is afflicted diabetes is noticed.
   xii. If malefic occupies Ascendant and Moon and Jupiter both are afflicted then diabetes is noticed.
   xiii. If malefic is occupied in eighth conjoined with Venus and Jupter is afflicted any where diabetes may occur.

xiv.   If malefic occupies eighth cusp and simultaneously Jupiter and Moon both are afflicted diabetes is observed.

xv.   If Venus with malefic occupies ascendant or eighth cusp diabetes may be occurred.

xvi.   If Venus occupies eighth cusp and afflicted diabetes may be observed.

xvii.   If Moon in Cancer or Scorpio afflicted by malefic diabetes is noticed.

xviii. If Venus occupies eighth cusp and under aspect of malefic diabetes is occurred.

xix.   If Mercury occupy Sagittarius or Pisces and conjoined with Sun diabetes may be observed.

xx.   If seventh house is occupied by watery sign occupied by Saturn and sixth cusp is occupied by Sun, Mars, or Rahu diabetes is observed.

xxi.   If Mars, Saturn, Rahu, or Ketu in watery sign insixth, eighth cusp, or twelfth cusp then diabetes is observed.

xxii.   If lord of sixth cusp, eighth cusp, in watery sign or malefic in sixth, eighth, twelfth cusp in watery sign may cause diabetes.

Dedicated in Loving memory of my Beloved Wife Sau. Vidya

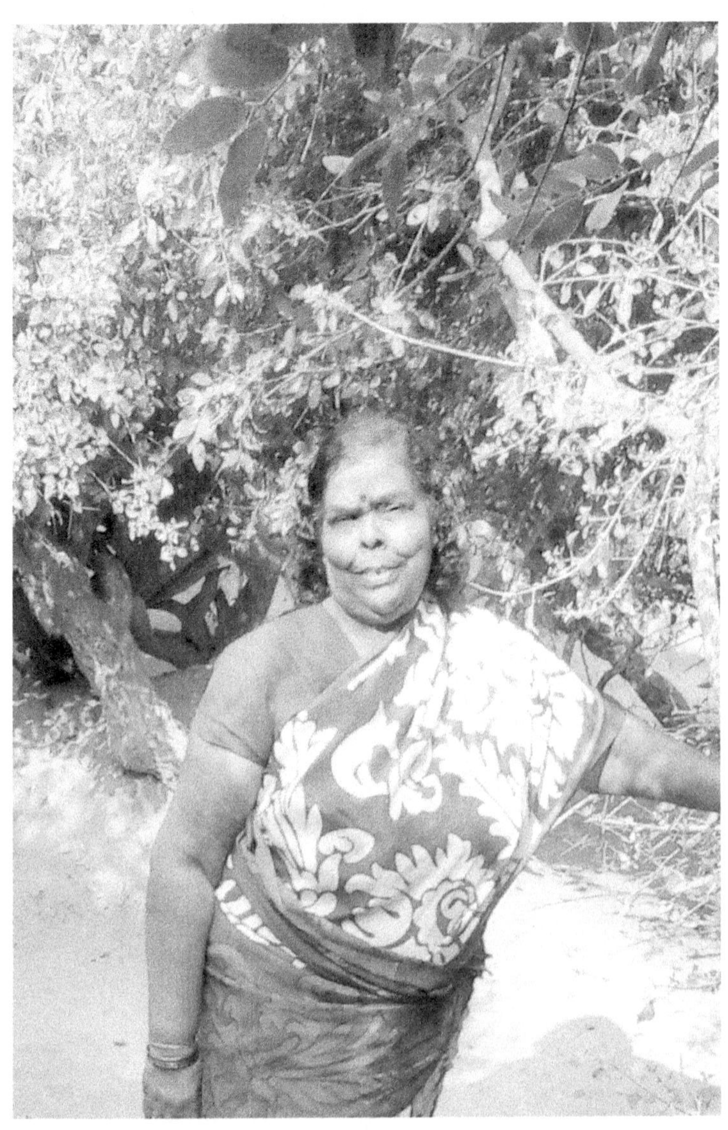